Blood-Derived Products for Tissue Repair/Regeneration

Blood-Derived Products for Tissue Repair/Regeneration

Special Issue Editors

Isabel Andia
Nicola Maffulli

MDPI • Basel • Beijing • Wuhan • Barcelona • Belgrade

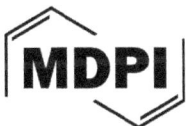

MDPI

Special Issue Editors
Isabel Andia
Instituto de Investigaciones
Sanitarias Biocruces bizkaia
Spain

Nicola Maffulli
University of Salerno
Italy

Editorial Office
MDPI
St. Alban-Anlage 66
4052 Basel, Switzerland

This is a reprint of articles from the Special Issue published online in the open access journal *International Journal of Molecular Sciences* (ISSN 1422-0067) in 2019 (available at: https://www.mdpi.com/journal/ijms/special_issues/PRPBiol).

For citation purposes, cite each article independently as indicated on the article page online and as indicated below:

LastName, A.A.; LastName, B.B.; LastName, C.C. Article Title. *Journal Name* **Year**, *Article Number, Page Range.*

ISBN 978-3-03921-860-8 (Pbk)
ISBN 978-3-03921-861-5 (PDF)

Cover image courtesy of Isabel Andia.

Contents

About the Special Issue Editors

Isabel Andia is the Principal Investigator and Head of the Regenerative Therapies Laboratory at Biocruces bizkaia Health Research Institute, Bizkaia, Spain. After years of research in neurochemistry, she was introduced to the biology of platelet-rich plasma (PRP) by Dr. A. T. Nurden in Bordeaux, France. Her current research interests include translational medicine and biomedical innovation using biological technologies such as platelet-rich plasma (PRP) to enhance the body's ability to regenerate. Staying active while aging is the hope of every "baby boomer", a hope too often compromised by sports injuries. To maintain the healthiest possible lifestyle, Isabel Andia is committed to regenerative therapies research. She firmly believes that progress in this field may lead to innovative solutions for a number of health problems, in particular osteoarticular pathology, overuse tendon disorders, and difficult-to-heal wounds.

Nicola Maffulli, the most highly cited author in Orthopaedics, Professor Maffulli is a Consultant Orthopaedic and Sports Injury Surgeons. He has published close to 1,200 peer reviewed articles in scientific journals and 12 books, and has described more than 40 new surgical techniques in the fields of knee, foot and ankle, fracture, and sports surgery. Many have now become the standard of practice in these fields. A keen free-style wrestler in his younger days, his dream of going to the Olympics was granted in London: he organised the medical services for the wrestling tournament at the London 2012 Olympics.

International Journal of
Molecular Sciences

MDPI

Editorial

Blood-Derived Products for Tissue Repair/Regeneration

Isabel Andia [1,*] and Nicola Maffulli [2,3]

1   Regenerative Therapies, Biocruces Bizkaia Health Research Institute, Cruces University Hospital,
    48903 Barakaldo, Spain
2   Department of Musculoskeletal Disorders, University of Salerno School of Medicine and Dentistry,
    84084 Salerno, Italy; n.maffulli@qmul.ac.uk
3   Barts and the London School of Medicine and Dentistry, Queen Mary University of London,
    London E1 2AD, UK
*   Correspondence: isabel.andiaortiz@osakidetza.eus; Tel.: +34-946007964

Received: 9 September 2019; Accepted: 12 September 2019; Published: 17 September 2019

check for
updates

Medical interest in "blood-derived products for tissue repair/regeneration" has old roots, starting with chronic wounds in the 1980s, and boosted by sports medicine at the beginning of the millennium, when elite athletes treated with platelet rich plasma (PRP) resumed competition earlier than expected. Linking blood-derived products and healing mechanisms is a past milestone that has uncovered distinctive therapeutic approaches for disparate medical conditions. As exemplified in this issue, the transversal nature of blood derived therapies encompasses research that falls in a variety of medical fields: Eye surface in ophthalmology [1], regeneration of bone defects and periodontal tissues in dentistry [2–4], osteoarticular pathology, e.g., meniscal repair [5], knee osteoarthritis [6] or radiocarpal osteoarthritis [7]. It also reflects that research in this field encompasses in vitro [4,8–10] and in vivo [1,2] experimentation, clinical veterinary [11] and clinical studies [3,5–7] representing all the stages of translational research.

We fully acknowledge the explosive growth of research interest in this area, but never have the stakes been higher. After nearly three decades of research, two key questions remain unanswered: What can blood-derived products offer to help understand the intricacies of healing mechanisms? What can we do to foster PRP research and take the benefits it can offer to the varied unmet medical needs? Answering both questions means that we can identify the crucial elements that boost the healing mechanism, and that we can refine formulations to fit with tissue needs in each clinical application.

A holistic approach to deciphering the participation of PRPs in healing mechanisms starts from understanding that the PRP actions are more than those attributed simply to the fact that they contain a vast array of powerful growth factors (GFs). The presence of various GFs in platelets' alpha granules and their involvement in boosting tissue healing grounded the hypothesis of the clinical use of PRPs, but we should also consider that there is controversy about whether platelet number (concentration factor relative to peripheral blood) and growth factor concentration is paramount in PRP formulations. While traditional approaches of tissue healing research focused on separate GFs, for example recombinant human platelet-derived growth factor (rhPDGF-BB), recombinant human fibroblastic growth factor (rhFGF) or recombinant human epidermal growth factor (rhEGF), have shown some clinical benefits in difficult-to-heal wounds, they provide a limited understanding of healing mechanisms. As postulated by system biology, "networks are more than the sum of the parts", and this premise helps understanding the difficulties in finding quality parameters able to control efficacies of the different blood derivatives.

In this issue, two reports have focused on the molecular composition of blood-derived products [9,10]. As proposed by Kardos et al. [9], exhaustive scrutiny of the molecular content can provide a guide for developing better formulations tailored to specific tissue/organs' needs.

However, because of the intrinsic complexity of the process of healing, molecular description is not sufficient, and functional in vitro assays can help to differentiate which formulation is more appropriate for a given pathology and/or perhaps different formulations in the different healing stages. Therefore, a priori, there is not a sole effective formulation and different blood derived products may be indicated for the specific tissue needs. Grounded on this idea, Jeyakumar et al. [8] drew parallels between PRP formulation/preparation protocols and healing mechanisms. They evidenced some advantage of hyper-acute autologous serum in enhancing chondrocyte proliferation, while PRP was more useful to stimulate extracellular matrix synthesis and enhance the anabolic/catabolic protein balance in the context of engineered cartilage constructs.

Research could foster new ways of thinking, and can assist in elucidating which blood derivative works better in specific tissues in specific conditions. The molecules released from blood derivatives may transiently form part of the immediate cell microenvironment (local milieu), thereby activating cell function in different tissues/organs. However, different cell phenotypes behave differently in functional terms when exposed to blood derivatives. Moreover, Chellini et al. [12], in a narrative review about skeletal muscle healing, reported that not a single cell phenotype but the collaborative interactions and crosstalk between different cell phenotypes can be modified by PRP. Moreover, platelet poor plasma, PPP, is capturing the attention of researchers in the field of muscle regeneration as it drives cells into the myogenic differentiation pathway and lacks pro-fibrotic factors such as TGF-β1.

Blood derivatives are also interesting as adjuvants, as part of either combination therapies or combination products. Seen in this light, Pomini et al. [2] developed a method to enhance bone formation using platelet-rich fibrin combined with bioOss®(a popular bone filler) and associated to photobiomodulation therapy, in dentistry. Likewise, current research [1] also evaluates the possibility of combining PRP releasate with hyaluronan to treat corneal epithelial defects. In the clinical context, the combination of adipose tissue (more specifically microfat) with PRP is explored as an innovative therapy to treat wrist OA (osteoarthritis) [7].

PRP research must lift its gaze to bigger accomplishments. This will require an improved understanding of repair, which in turn would support treatment strategies, patient selection and the development of precise application procedures. We hope that the identification of biomarkers will help to stratify patients, bringing about more efficient and accurate therapies, better understanding of healing mechanisms and more rational use of PRP therapies and foster the development of new combinational treatments.

Conflicts of Interest: The authors declare no conflict of interest.

References

1. Suárez-Barrio, C.; Etxebarria, J.; Hernáez-Moya, R.; Del Val-Alonso, M.; Rodriguez-Astigarraga, M.; Urkaregi, A.; Freire, V.; Morales, M.C.; Durán, J.A.; Vicario, M.; et al. Hyaluronic Acid Combined with Serum Rich in Growth Factors in Corneal Epithelial Defects. *Int. J. Mol. Sci.* **2019**, *20*, 1655. [CrossRef] [PubMed]
2. Pomini, K.T.; Buchaim, D.V.; Andreo, J.C.; Rosso, M.P.D.O.; Della Coletta, B.B.; German, Í.J.S.; Biguetti, A.C.C.; Shinohara, A.L.; Rosa Júnior, G.M.; Cosin Shindo, J.V.T.; et al. Fibrin Sealant Derived from Human Plasma as a Scaffold for Bone Grafts Associated with Photobiomodulation Therapy. *Int. J. Mol. Sci.* **2019**, *20*, 1761. [CrossRef] [PubMed]
3. Panda, S.; Karanxha, L.; Goker, F.; Satpathy, A.; Taschieri, S.; Francetti, L.; Das, A.C.; Kumar, M.; Panda, S.; Fabbro, M.D. Autologous Platelet Concentrates in Treatment of Furcation Defects-A Systematic Review and Meta-Analysis. *Int. J. Mol. Sci.* **2019**, *20*, 1347. [CrossRef] [PubMed]
4. Kawase, T.; Nagata, M.; Okuda, K.; Ushiki, T.; Fujimoto, Y.; Watanabe, M.; Ito, A.; Nakata, K. Platelet-Rich Fibrin Extract: A Promising Fetal Bovine Serum Alternative in Explant Cultures of Human Periosteal Sheets for Regenerative Therapy. *Int. J. Mol. Sci.* **2019**, *20*, 1053. [CrossRef] [PubMed]
5. Kaminski, R.; Maksymowicz-Wleklik, M.; Kulinski, K.; Kozar-Kaminska, K.; Dabrowska-Thing, A.; Pomianowski, S. Short-Term Outcomes of Percutaneous Trephination with a Platelet Rich Plasma

Intrameniscal Injection for the Repair of Degenerative Meniscal Lesions. A Prospective, Randomized, Double-Blind, Parallel-Group, Placebo-Controlled Study. *Int. J. Mol. Sci.* **2019**, *20*, 856. [CrossRef] [PubMed]

6.   Guillibert, C.; Charpin, C.; Raffray, M.; Benmenni, A.; Dehaut, F.X.; El Ghobeira, G.; Giorgi, R.; Magalon, J.; Arniaud, D. Single Injection of High Volume of Autologous Pure PRP Provides a Significant Improvement in Knee Osteoarthritis: A Prospective Routine Care Study. *Int. J. Mol. Sci.* **2019**, *20*, 1327. [CrossRef] [PubMed]

7.   Mayoly, A.; Iniesta, A.; Curvale, C.; Kachouh, N.; Jaloux, C.; Eraud, J.; Vogtensperger, M.; Veran, J.; Grimaud, F.; Jouve, E.; et al. Development of Autologous Platelet-Rich Plasma Mixed-Microfat as an Advanced Therapy Medicinal Product for Intra-Articular Injection of Radio-Carpal Osteoarthritis: From Validation Data to Preliminary Clinical Results. *Int. J. Mol. Sci.* **2019**, *20*, 1111. [CrossRef] [PubMed]

8.   Jeyakumar, V.; Niculescu-Morzsa, E.; Bauer, C.; Lacza, Z.; Nehrer, S. Redifferentiation of Articular Chondrocytes by Hyperacute Serum and Platelet Rich Plasma in Collagen Type I Hydrogels. *Int. J. Mol. Sci.* **2019**, *20*, 316. [CrossRef] [PubMed]

9.   Kardos, D.; Simon, M.; Vácz, G.; Hinsenkamp, A.; Holczer, T.; Cseh, D.; Sárközi, A.; Szenthe, K.; Bánáti, F.; Szathmary, S.; et al. The Composition of Hyperacute Serum and Platelet-Rich Plasma Is Markedly Different despite the Similar Production Method. *Int. J. Mol. Sci.* **2019**, *20*, 721. [CrossRef] [PubMed]

10. Marck, R.E.; Gardien, K.L.M.; Vlig, M.; Breederveld, R.S.; Middelkoop, E. Growth Factor Quantification of Platelet-Rich Plasma in Burn Patients Compared to Matched Healthy Volunteers. *Int. J. Mol. Sci.* **2019**, *20*, 288. [CrossRef] [PubMed]

11. López, S.; Vilar, J.M.; Sopena, J.J.; Damià, E.; Chicharro, D.; Carrillo, J.M.; Cuervo, B.; Rubio, A.M. Assessment of the Efficacy of Platelet-Rich Plasma in the Treatment of Traumatic Canine Fractures. *Int. J. Mol. Sci.* **2019**, *20*, 1075. [CrossRef] [PubMed]

12. Chellini, F.; Tani, A.; Zecchi-Orlandini, S.; Sassoli, C. Influence of Platelet-Rich and Platelet-Poor Plasma on Endogenous Mechanisms of Skeletal Muscle Repair/Regeneration. *Int. J. Mol. Sci.* **2019**, *20*, 683. [CrossRef] [PubMed]

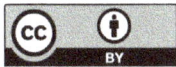

International Journal of
Molecular Sciences

MDPI

Article

Hyaluronic Acid Combined with Serum Rich in Growth Factors in Corneal Epithelial Defects

Carlota Suárez-Barrio [1,†], Jaime Etxebarria [1,2,†], Raquel Hernáez-Moya [1], Marina del Val-Alonso [1], Maddalen Rodriguez-Astigarraga [1], Arantza Urkaregi [3], Vanesa Freire [1,4], María-Celia Morales [1], Juan Antonio Durán [4,5], Marta Vicario [6], Irene Molina [6], Rocío Herrero-Vanrell [6] and Noelia Andollo [1,*]

[1] Department of Cell Biology and Histology, School of Medicine and Nursing, University of the Basque Country, BioCruces Health Research Institute, Begiker, 48940 Leioa, Spain; carlotasb.8@gmail.com (C.S.-B.); JAIME.ECHEVARRIAECENARRO@osakidetza.eus (J.E.); raquel.hernaez@ehu.eus (R.H.-M.); marina_mdv@hotmail.com (M.d.V.-A.); m.rodriguezastigarraga@gmail.com (M.R.-A.); vanesafreire@hotmail.com (V.F.); celiamoralesgonzalez@gmail.com (M.-C.M.)
[2] Department of Ophthalmology, University Hospital of Cruces, BioCruces Health Research Institute, Begiker, 48903 Barakaldo, Spain
[3] Department of Applied Mathematics and Statistics and Operational Research, BioCruces Health Research Institute, 48940 Leioa, Spain; arantza.urkaregi@ehu.eus
[4] R & D Department, Instituto Clínico-Quirúrgico de Oftalmología, 48006 Bilbao, Spain; duran@icqo.org
[5] Department of Dermatology, Otorhinolaryngology and Ophthalmology, School of Medicine and Nursing, University of the Basque Country, BioCruces Health Research Institute, Begiker, 48940 Leioa, Spain
[6] Pharmaceutical Innovation in Ophthalmology (InnOftal) UCM Research Group 920415. Department of Pharmaceutics and Food Technology, Faculty of Pharmacy, Complutense University, 28040 Madrid, Spain; mvicario@farm.ucm.es (M.V.); iremm@farm.ucm.es (I.M.); rociohv@farm.ucm.es (R.H.-V.)
* Correspondence: noelia.andollo@ehu.eus; Tel.: +34-94-601-3295
† These authors contributed equally to this work.

Received: 18 February 2019; Accepted: 30 March 2019; Published: 3 April 2019

check for updates

Abstract: The aim of this study is to assess if an adhesive biopolymer, sodium hyaluronate (NaHA), has synergistic effects with s-PRGF (a serum derived from plasma rich in growth factors and a blood derivative that has already shown efficacy in corneal epithelial wound healing), to reduce time of healing or posology. In vitro proliferation and migration studies, both in human corneal epithelial (HCE) cells and in rabbit primary corneal epithelial (RPCE) cultures, were carried out. In addition, we performed studies of corneal wound healing in vivo in rabbits treated with s-PRGF, NaHA, or the combination of both. We performed immunohistochemistry techniques (CK3, CK15, Ki67, ß4 integrin, ZO-1, α-SMA) in rabbit corneas 7 and 30 days after a surgically induced epithelial defect. In vitro results show that the combination of NaHA and s-PRGF offers the worst proliferation rates in both HCE and RPCE cells. Addition of NaHA to s-PRGF diminishes the re-epithelializing capability of s-PRGF. In vivo, all treatments, given twice a day, showed equivalent efficacy in corneal epithelial healing. We conclude that the combined use of s-PRGF and HaNA as an adhesive biopolymer does not improve the efficacy of s-PRGF alone in the wound healing of corneal epithelial defects.

Keywords: corneal epithelial defect; cornea regeneration; serum eye drops; plasma rich plasma (PRP); serum derived from plasma rich in growth factors (s-PRGF); hyaluronic acid (NaHA); wound healing

1. Introduction

Integrity of the corneal epithelium is a critical requirement for correct vision function [1]. The maintenance of the epithelium is based on a balance among limbal stem function, tear quantity and quality, the eyelid anatomy and function, and corneal sensitivity [2]. In cases of corneal injury, healing mechanisms are activated involving cell proliferation, migration and reattachment of the epithelium to its extracellular matrix, and cell differentiation. Factors needed for corneal wound healing are provided by the tear film, aqueous humor, and limbal blood vessels. Furthermore, cornea epithelium by itself is a rich source of cytokines that contribute to modulate the wound healing process [3].

Sometimes, corneal wounds persist over time and are resistant to conventional treatment, such as artificial tears or topical antibiotics [4], lateral tarsorrhaphy [5], bandage contact lenses [6], punctual plugs [7], and amniotic membrane transplantation [8]. Different topical growth factors have been also tested in these persistent epithelial defects [9–13]. As wound healing demands a balanced combination of different mediators, blood derivatives have been used to treat corneal epithelial defects, including autologous serum [14] and platelet rich plasma [15]. One of these, s-PRGF (a serum derived from plasma rich in growth factors) has already been used successfully as a treatment for eye disorders [4,16,17] and its effectiveness has been proved in wound healing [4,18]. s-PRGF has been proved to stimulate proliferation and migration of epithelial cells [18]. It has a moderate platelet concentration and its leukocyte content has been removed [19,20].

On the other hand, eye barriers and the continuous turnover of tears can alter the absorption of drugs instilled in the eye, so, although eye drops are an easy-to-use treatment, they must be instilled frequently and/or at high concentrations to achieve therapeutic levels in the tissues. The high frequency of instillation can induce a non-compliance of treatment by patients. The development of vehicles capable of adhering to the conjunctival and/or corneal tissue is an interesting alternative for increasing the bioavailability of ophthalmological medications. With this aim, hydrogels and polymer micelles [21], biodegradable nanocapsules or HA coated nanospheres, and niosomes have been reported as agents for the release of drugs on the ocular surface [22–24]. The role of liposomes has also been investigated, although their potential is limited due to their short half-life on the ocular surface and relatively low stability [23]. HA-coated liposomes have also been used to facilitate the entry of drugs into human corneal epithelial (HCE) cells [25]. In all these cases, HA-coated nanovehicles allow greater concentrations of the transported drug to enter into the cornea.

Other authors have tried other vehicles with well-known mucoadhesive properties, with the intention of increasing the contact time of various drugs in the corneal tissue. Thus, the concomitant use of 0.5% carboxymethylcellulose, 0.2% HA, or 0.3–0.5% hydroxypropylcellulose associated with topical 0.5% timolol has been studied. In this case, combination with HA did not show improved efficacy with respect to timolol alone [26]. However, some authors have concluded that an increase of drug viscosity reduces its systemic absorption, so it could enhance the exposition of treatment to the ocular surface [27].

Topical surfactant molecules (perfluorohexiloctane), as well as ophthalmic inserts of methylpropylcellulose (Lacrisert®), have been developed with the intention of increasing the residence time of the tear on the ocular surface and therein improving the quality [28,29]. Another strategy to prolong the contact of drugs with the ocular surface is the use of contact lenses that slowly release the drug over several weeks [30].

Specifically, to extend the contact time of the platelet lysates with the damaged ocular surface, Sandri and colleagues studied their combination with molecules with mucoadhesive properties, such as polyacrylic acid and chitosan [31]. Similarly, the combination of HA with autologous serum has also been studied, suggesting that HA would facilitate the gradual release of growth factors and increase its duration and effect on the ocular surface, so fewer instillations would be needed [32].

HA is a bioadhesive molecule produced by the cells of the corneal matrix and is one of its main components. It is a polyanionic glycosaminoglycan composed of disaccharide subunits of N-acetyl glucosamine and D-glucuronic acid [33]. Depending on the number of disaccharides bound, hyaluronic acids of different molecular weights will be formed. Among its characteristics, it is noteworthy that it is biocompatible, biodegradable and non-toxic, and non-irritating [34,35]. It also possesses a high capacity for binding to water and has a viscous and pseudoplastic fluid behavior with the ability to act as a mucoadhesive polymer, which makes it possible to increase the residence time in the eye, in addition to reducing friction during blinking and extraocular movements when it is being used as a natural lubricant of the ocular surface that reduces epithelial damage [36]. A negative charge would facilitate adhesion to the ocular surface, giving theoretically more corneal bioavailability to the molecules associated with hyaluronic acid [37].

High molecular weight HA has immunosuppressive and anti-inflammatory properties by reducing the migration of inflammatory cells [38] and by specifically inhibiting certain metalloproteases that degrade the extracellular matrix [39]. It also has anti-angiogenic properties [40] and analgesic effects [41]. However, small fragments of HA can have a proinflammatory and pro-angiogenic effect [42]. In our work, we used intermediate molecular weight HA, as we wanted to assess its mucoadhesive capacity for s-PRGF and not its anti-inflammatory synergy.

All commercial ophthalmic hyaluronic acids used as artificial tears contain concentrations between 0.1% and 0.4% hyaluronic acid. In order to mimic real clinical situations, the concentration used in our work was 0.1% for in vitro assays and 0.2% for in vivo experiments.

Therefore, the beneficial effect of HA both in vitro and in vivo, as well as Platelet Rich Plasma (PRP), seems to be evident, both in the field of traumatology [43] and in corneal epithelial wound healing [18,44].

Given this "state of the art", the aim of this study is to test if combining both treatments, s-PRGF and HA, is synergistic in terms of in vitro migration and proliferation of corneal epithelial cells and in vivo reduction of the time (or reduced posology) of corneal wound healing.

2. Results

2.1. In Vitro Proliferation Assays in Rabbit Primary Corneal Epithelial Cells and Human Corneal Epithlial Cultures

We studied cell proliferation at 0, 24, 48, and 72 h in rabbit epithelial cells (RPCE) and HCE cultures under the following treatments: 45% s-PRGF; 45% s-PRGF + 0.1% sodium hyaluronate (NaHA) (combined treatment); 0.1% NaHA; 10% FBS as a positive/reference control; and 1% BSA as a negative control.

Results showed that in RPCE cultures all treatments produced a time-dependent proliferation pattern, with no significant differences within treatments at 72 h (Figure 1A). Viability in RPCE cultures exposed to different treatments was very similar in all cases. We observed that viability in the first 24–48 h (Figure 1B,C) was higher with FBS, the standard or reference culture medium. However, differences decreased over time, especially under s-PRGF and control (BSA) treatments. Thus, after 24 h of treatment, we observed highly significant differences between FBS and NaHA, alone or combined with s-PRGF, and between FBS and the control treatment (Figure 1B). However, there were not significant differences between FBS and s-PRGF at 24 h ($p = 0.42$). In addition, we found significant differences in cell viability between cells cultured with s-PRGF in comparison to those cultured with both NaHA treatments.

Thus, proliferation of RPCE cultures at 24 h was similar for FBS and s-PRGF treated cultures and higher than cultures under the other treatments. At 48 h, we found significant differences within treatments compared to FBS, with these being less than those at 24 h and completely disappearing at 72 h (Figure 1B–D).

In summary, NaHA, whether combined or not with s-PRGF, did not enhance either proliferation capability or viability in RPCE cultures.

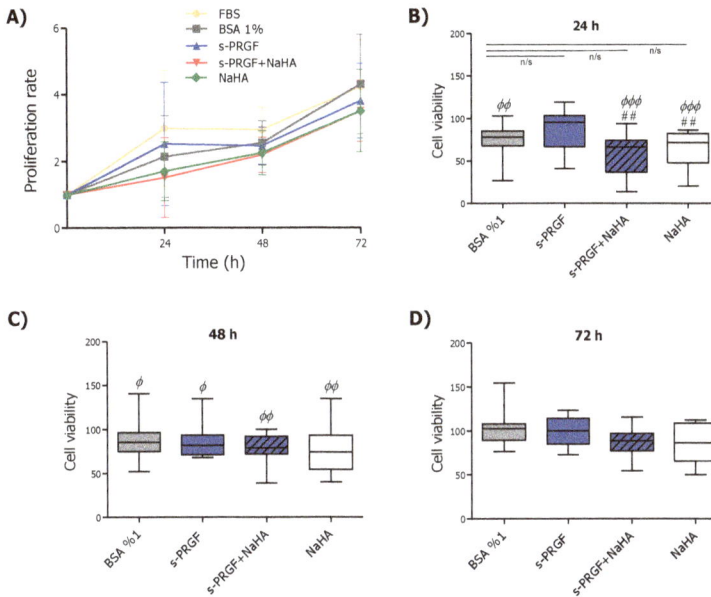

Figure 1. Effect of serum derived from plasma rich in growth factors (s-PRGF), alone or combined with sodium hyaluronate (NaHA), (**A**) on the proliferation and (**B–D**) viability of rabbit primary corneal epithelial (RPCE) cultures. Cultures were exposed for 24, 48, and 72 h to 10% FBS; 45% s-PRGF; 45% s-PRGF and 0.1% NaHA (combined treatment); 0.1% NaHA; and 1% BSA as a negative control. Proliferation results are expressed as proliferation rate ± standard deviation of viable cells with respect to viable cells at t = 0. Viability results are expressed as percentages versus that with FBS (100% viability). Statistically significant differences with respect to FBS (Φ) or to s-PRGF (#) (## $p < 0.01$; ^{Φ} $p < 0.05$; ^{ΦΦ} $p < 0.01$; ^{ΦΦΦ} $p < 0.001$; n/s, not significant. Kruskal-Wallis test, Dunn test with Bonferroni correction to Multiple Comparisons).

Results concerning HCE cultures showed a time-dependent proliferation pattern, except for the 1% BSA control treatment, while s-PRGF, with or without NaHA, produced a decrease in proliferation at 24 h which was not statistically significant (Figure 2A). All treatments, especially 10% FBS, showed a higher proliferation rate that the control treatment. In addition, we saw a positive tendency for higher proliferation when cells were cultured with NaHA compared to s-PRGF or the combined treatment.

Regarding viability, we do not see significant differences between FBS and NaHA during the first 48 h (Figure 2B,C). In addition, besides the FBS treatment, only the non-combined treatments showed significant (s-PRGF) or very significant (NaHA) differences compared to the control treatment at 48 and 72 h (Figure 2C,D).

In conclusion, s-PRGF and NaHA treatments showed better proliferative patterns in HCE cells, whereas the combination of both did not improve it.

HCE cultures

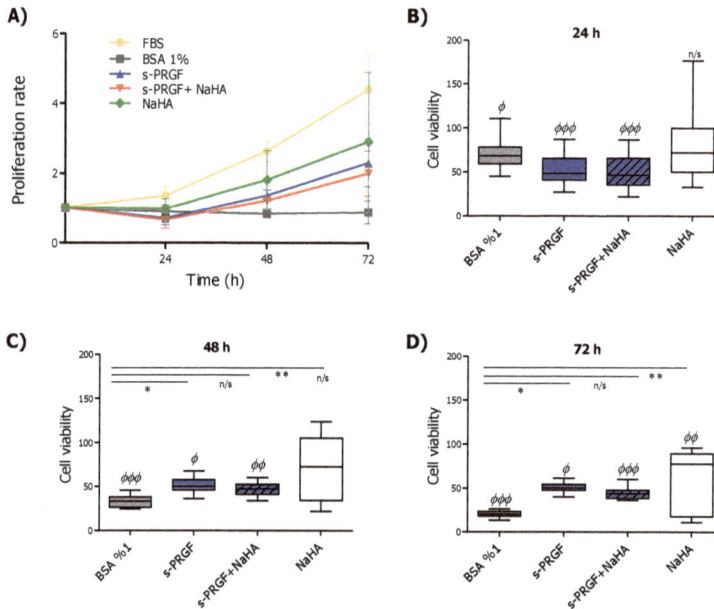

Figure 2. Effect of s-PRGF, alone or combined with NaHA, on the (**A**) proliferation and (**B–D**) viability of human corneal epithelial (HCE) cells. Cultures were exposed for 24, 48, and 72 h to 10% FBS; 45% s-PRGF; 45% s-PRGF and 0.1% NaHA (combined treatment); 0.1% NaHA; and 1% BSA as a negative control. Proliferation results are expressed as proliferation rate ± standard deviation of viable cells with respect to viable cells at t = 0. Viability results are expressed as percentages versus that with FBS (100% viability). Statistically significant differences with respect to BSA (*) or to FBS (Φ) (* $p < 0.05$; ** $p < 0.01$; ^{Φ} $p < 0.05$; ^{ΦΦ} $p < 0.01$; ^{ΦΦΦ} $p < 0.001$; n/s, not significant. Kruskal–Wallis test, Dunn test with Bonferroni correction to Multiple Comparisons).

2.2. In Vitro Scratch Wound-Healing Assays in RPCE and HCE Cultures

In order to evaluate the capability of the different treatments to promote migration and re-epithelialization on RCPE and HCE cultures, we scraped off rounded areas on cell monolayers and treated them with the following treatments: 45% s-PRGF; 45% s-PRGF + 0,1% NaHA (combined treatment); 0,1% NaHA; 10% FBS as a positive/reference control; and 1% BSA as a negative control. We measured the re-epithelialization process at 0, 12, 24, 36, 48, 60, and 72 h.

We did not find significant differences within treatments at any time when studying wound healing evolution in RPCE cultures (Figure 3A). However, when we analyzed the percentage of wells in which the defect in the monolayer had completely resolved, we found evident differences in cultures treated with NaHA (alone or combined) with respect to other treatments (Figure 3B–D). Additionally, a smaller number of completely resolved defects in cultures treated with the combined treatment was observed, with this result being statistically significant from 48 h.

RPCE cultures

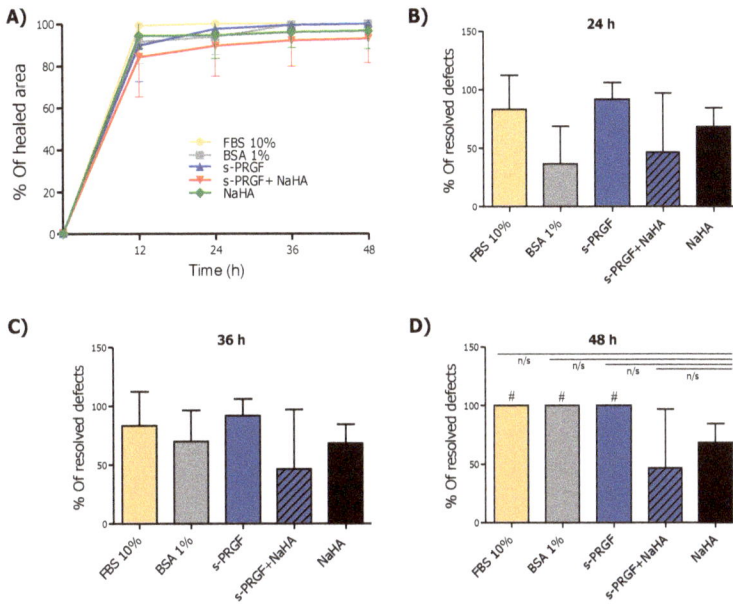

Figure 3. Effect of s-PRGF, alone or combined with NaHA, on the re-epithelialization of rabbit primary corneal epithelial (RPCE) cultures. Cultures were exposed for 72 h to 10% FBS; 45% s-PRGF; 45% s-PRGF + 0.1% NaHA (combined treatment); 0.1% NaHA; and 1% BSA as a negative control. The percentage of re-epithelialized area of RPCE cultures after 48 hr (**A**), and percentage of wells in which the defect in the monolayer had completely resolved at 24 (**B**), 36 (**C**) and 48 (**D**) hours are shown. Statistically significant differences with respect to the combined s-PRGF + NaHA treatment (#) (# $p < 0.05$; n/s, not significant. χ^2 test and Fisher's exact test).

In HCE cultures, s-PRGF treatment (alone or combined with NaHA), as well as FBS treatment, promoted faster re-epithelialization of the defect in the monolayer from 12 h of treatment onwards, showing significant differences at all times (Figure 4A). Furthermore, in the HCE cultures, no statistically significant differences were found in the mean remaining denuded area (in square millimeters) between cells treated with NaHA and control cells.

With respect to the resolution of defects in the HCE cultures, s-PRGF treatment (alone or combined), together with FBS, produced statistically significant differences in the number of wells in which the denuded area had been completely covered, compared with the control and NaHA treatments, from 24 h (Figure 4B). At 36 h, almost 100% of wounds treated with s-PRGF or s-PRGF + NaHA were completely solved, whereas none of the denuded areas had completely closed in the control and NaHA cultures (Figure 4C,D).

We conclude that s-PRGF promotes the highest re-epithelialization in RPCE primary cultures and HCE cells. Furthermore, NaHA does not favor this process, and hinders the re-epithelialization effect promoted by s-PRGF.

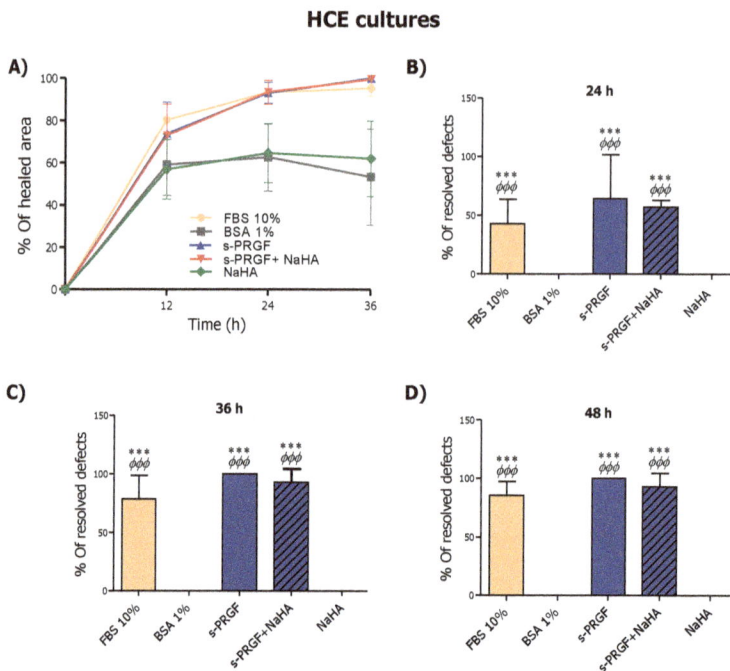

Figure 4. Effect of s-PRGF, alone or combined with NaHA, on the re-epithelialization of human corneal epithelial (HCE) cells (**A**). Cultures were exposed for 72 h to 10% FBS; 45% s-PRGF; 45% s-PRGF + 0.1% NaHA (combined treatment); 0.1% NaHA; and 1% BSA as a negative control. The percentage of re-epithelialized area of HCE cultures after 36 hr (**A**), and percentage of wells in which the defect in the monolayer had completely resolved at 24 (**B**), 36 (**C**) and 48 (**D**) hours are shown. Statistically significant differences with respect to BSA (*) or NaHA (Φ) (*** $p < 0.001$; ^{ΦΦΦ} $p < 0.001$; n/s, not significant. χ^2 test and Fisher's exact test).

2.3. In Vivo Corneal Re-Epithelialization Assay in a Rabbit Animal Model

To perform the assay, surgically induced epithelial defects were treated with 90% s-PRGF; 90% s-PRGF and 0.2% NaHA (combined treatment); 0.2% NaHA; and PBS as a control treatment.

We did not find any adverse effects, such as corneal inflammation or neovascularization, during the whole experiment. In addition, all animals were healthy and gained weight progressively.

The results showed that s-PRGF promoted faster corneal wound healing after day 2 of treatment than the other treatments. The mean time to complete the closure of the epithelial defect in the s-PRGF group was 3.11 ± 0.22 days, whereas it was 3.31 ± 0.37 days for eyes treated with any of the other treatments (Figure 5A and Table 1). Nevertheless, we did not find significant differences among treatments (Kruskal–Wallis). We also performed the Kaplan–Meier test to analyze the progression of healing of eyes at intervals of half a day. Although we again observed the marked tendency for faster epithelial closure for the s-PRGF treatment, we could not find significant differences. This fact suggests that increasing the number of analyzed animals would be advisable.

When we analyzed the number of corneal defects that had completely healed, we found that at day 3 after surgery, 78% of them had re-epithelialized in the s-PRGF treatment, while only 50% of them had healed in the eyes treated with any of the other treatments. After 3.5 days, 100% of the corneal defects had already healed with s-PRGF, compared to only 88% of the eyes treated with any of the other treatments. However, we did not find significant differences among treatments (Chi-Square test and Fisher's exact test).

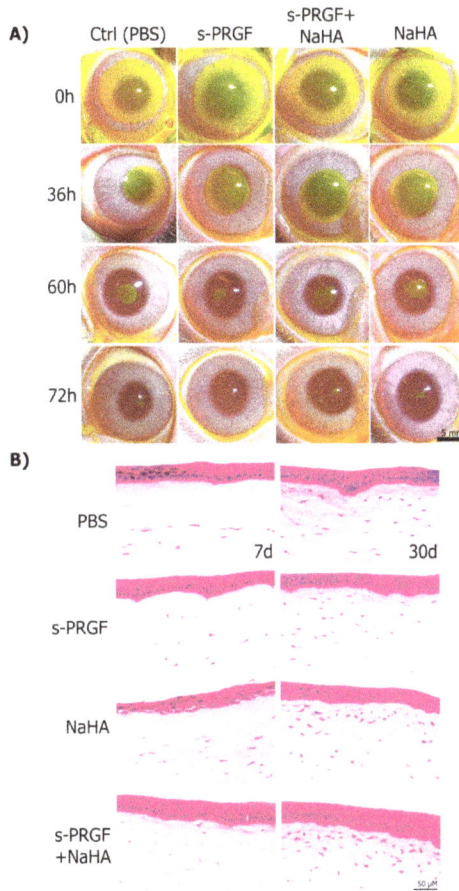

Figure 5. Re-epithelialization of corneal defects in rabbit eyes. (**A**) Evolution of the epithelial defect was monitored with fluorescein staining in eyes treated with topical s-PRGF, s-PRGF and NaHA, NaHA, or PBS as a control treatment. (**B**) Histological sections of rabbit central corneas after complete healing were stained with hematoxylin and eosin. Corneas were processed seven days after surgery or at 30 days. Scale bar: 5 mm for (**A**), 50 μm for (**B**).

Table 1. In vivo experiment assessing the progression of epithelial wound healing in rabbit eyes treated with s-PRGF, s-PRGF and NaHA, NaHA, and PBS as the control. The results are expressed as mean wound area ± standard deviation in mm^2.

Treatment	TIME (days)						
	Day 0	Day 1	Day 1.5	Day 2	Day 2.5	Day 3	Day 3.5
Control	72.32 ± 7.32	47.02 ± 4.84	33.28 ± 3.06	12.93 ± 3.36	6.12 ± 3.24	0.53 ± 0.99	0.06 ± 0.16
s-PRGF	71.91 ± 4.39	46.19 ± 4.06	30.22 ± 4.09	10.00 ± 3.15	3.65 ± 2.79	0.05 ± 0.10	0
NaHA	72.48 ± 5.13	45.32 ± 4.20	36.72 ± 7.74	12.46 ± 5.17	5.98 ± 3.69	0.65 ± 1.23	0.10 ± 0.27
s-PRGF + NaHA	72.57 ± 2.77	48.06 ± 8.97	37.44 ± 7.63	13.59 ± 5.26	6.14 ± 3.71	0.46 ± 0.76	0.02 ± 0.06

No significant differences between any treatments were found (Kruskal–Wallis test, $p \geq 0.05$).

Analysis of hematoxylin and eosin sections of the rabbit central corneas showed complete regeneration with normal histology of the epithelium in all corneas. However, we observed that corneas treated with NaHA showed a less compacted epithelium in the basal layers at day 7, suggesting that there might be adhesion deficiencies within epithelial layers, or even between the epithelium and stroma layers (Figure 5B). In addition, when euthanasia was performed 7 days after surgery, the number of keratocytes in the anterior third of the stroma was influenced by the treatment, with the s-PRGF and NaHA the only treatment that showed cells in the whole stroma. At 30 days after surgery, treatments with NaHA (alone or combined) showed the highest cell population across the anterior third of the stroma.

2.4. Immunohistochemical Analyses of the Epithelial Differentiation, Proliferation, Adhesion, and Fibrosis of the Re-Epithelialized Corneas

To assess differences in the mechanisms through which the treatments performed corneal wound healing, we used immunohistochemistry techniques to analyze cryopreserved sections of healed rabbit corneas at 7 and 30 days after surgery. We also added a healthy control (healthy rabbit cornea, which did not undergo surgery) and a wounded cornea (processed only 48 h after surgery, wound healing or W-H control). Specifically, we studied the processes of differentiation, proliferation and adhesion, the corneal barrier effect of the epithelium, and stromal fibrosis.

First, we performed a double staining for cytokeratin 3/76 (CK3), a corneal epithelium marker, and cytokeratin 15 (CK15), a stem cell marker, in both the re-epithelialized central cornea and the peripheral limbus. As we expected, we found CK3 positive staining and CK15 negative labeling in the central epithelium area of all eyes (Figure 6). At the limbal area, we found positive CK15 staining in the basal layers of all corneas (Figure 7). This staining is coherent with the presence of limbal stem/progenitor cells, and it was especially intense in the W-H control, where these cells might be specifically activated to regenerate the wounded epithelial area.

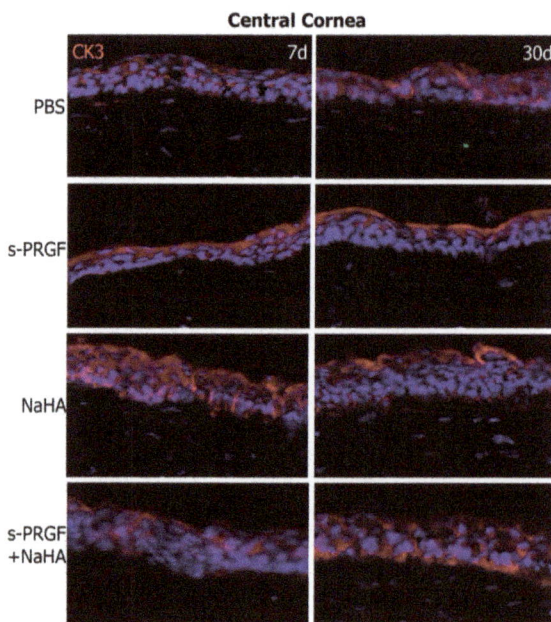

Figure 6. Fluorescent immunostaining for CK3 (red) and CK15 (green) on the regenerated central cornea of rabbit corneas after healing of the epithelial defect. Corneas were treated with s-PRGF, s-PRGF and NaHA, NaHA, or PBS (as a control) and were processed 7 and 30 days after cornea surgery. Control corresponds to a healthy rabbit cornea with no surgery. The W-H image shows a cornea processed 48 h after surgery without complete re-epithelialization. Magnification 200×.

We evaluated cell proliferation by analyzing the nuclear staining of the proliferation marker Ki76. Results showed a higher number of positive cells at 7 days after surgery than 30 days (Table 2). Interestingly, at 7 days, the nuclear staining was not confined to the epithelium but also appeared in the third anterior stroma. However, proliferation in the epithelium was significantly higher than in the stroma for all treatments, both at 7 days ($p < 0.001$) and at 30 days ($p < 0.0001$) (Wilcoxon rank sum test). Specifically, corneas treated with NaHA showed a higher number of Ki67 proliferative cells in both areas (epithelium and stroma) than corneas under the other treatments. Differences were highly significant for the epithelium (Table 2). This result is consistent with that of the proliferation study in HCE cells, in which we observed that NaHA induced higher proliferation in the short-term than the rest of the treatments under study. At 30 days after surgery, cell proliferation was lower and occurred merely in the corneal epithelium.

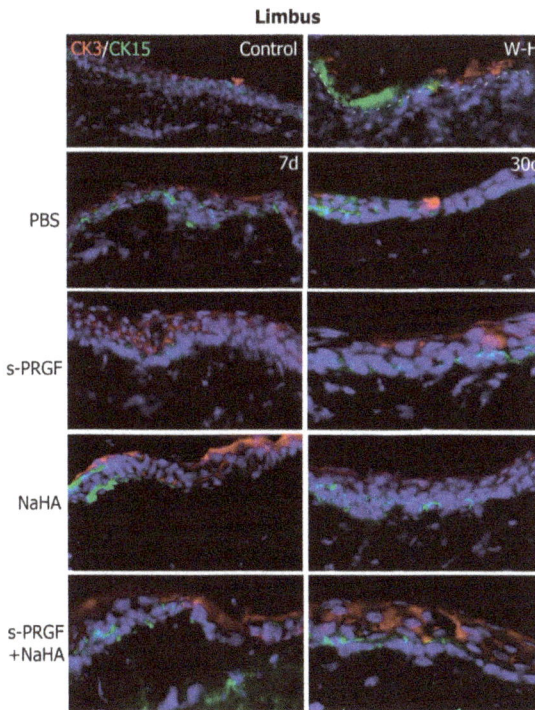

Figure 7. Fluorescent immunostaining for CK3 (red) and CK15 (green) on the limbal area of rabbit corneas after healing of the epithelial defect. Corneas were treated with s-PRGF, s-PRGF and NaHA, NaHA, or PBS (as a control) and were processed 7 and 30 days after cornea surgery. Control corresponds to a healthy rabbit cornea with no surgery. The W-H image shows a cornea processed 48 h after surgery without complete re-epithelialization. The dotted line shows the limit between the epithelium and stroma layers. Magnification 200×.

We also studied the marker of tight junctions ZO-1, in order to evaluate the recovery of the barrier effect in the regenerated corneal epithelium. We observed apical staining of the epithelium in all corneas, which was more intense at 30 days after surgery than at 7 days (Figure 8). Of note, W-H corneas, which only had a cell monolayer covering the wound area, showed a positive staining as well, meaning that the recovering of the epithelial barrier function is a priority in wound healing.

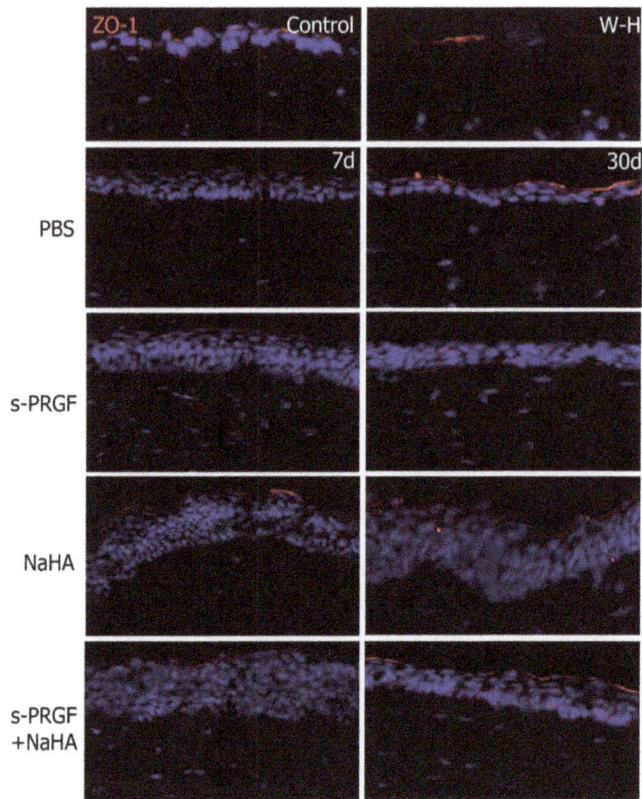

Figure 8. Fluorescent immunostaining for ZO-1 on rabbit central corneas after healing of the epithelial defect. Rabbit corneas were treated with s-PRGF, s-PRGF and NaHA, NaHA, or PBS (as a control), and were processed 7 and 30 days after cornea surgery. Control corresponds to a healthy rabbit cornea with no surgery. The W-H image shows a cornea processed 48 h after surgery without complete re-epithelialization. Magnification 200×.

In order to study the adhesion property between the regenerated epithelium and the underlying stroma, we performed immunohistochemical staining for β4 integrin, a cellular component of hemidesmosomes. Results showed that s-PRGF treatments (combined or not) had a more intense and continuous staining at 7 days (Figure 9). At 30 days after surgery, we could observe a normal staining underlying the epithelium all along the cornea in all the treatments. In W-H samples, although a fine layer of regenerated epithelium appeared, we could not detect the β4 integrin staining.

Finally, by detecting the α-SMA protein, we analyzed the differentiation process from keratocytes to myofibroblasts in the wounded area as a sign of fibrosis. We did not detect positivity in the cytoplasm of the stromal cells of the repaired tissues in any case (data not shown).

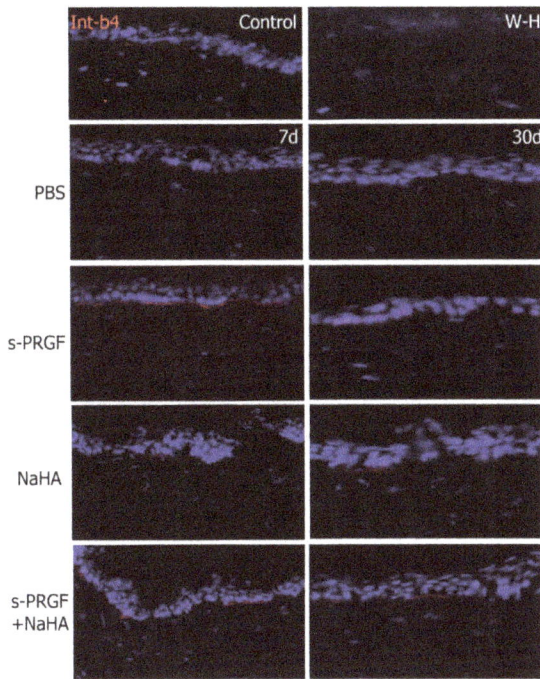

Figure 9. Fluorescent immunostaining for β4 integrin on rabbit central corneas after healing of the epithelial defect. Rabbit corneas were treated with s-PRGF, s-PRGF and NaHA, NaHA, or PBS (as a control) and were processed 7 and 30 days after cornea surgery. Control corresponds to a healthy rabbit cornea with no surgery. The W-H image shows a cornea processed 48 h after surgery without complete re-epithelialization. Magnification 200×.

Table 2. Number of Ki67 positive cells in rabbit corneas treated with s-PRGF, s-PRGF and NaHA, NaHA, and PBS as the control. The results are expressed as mean number of cells ± standard deviation in seven different areas of the central corneas at 7 and 30 days after surgery.

	Treatment			
7 Days	**PBS**	**s-PRGF**	**s-PRGF + NaHA**	**NaHA**
Epithelium	17 ± 10	4 ± 2	16 ± 15	$43 ^{***} \pm 20$
Stroma	2 ± 1	1 ± 1	2 ± 1	5 ± 4
30 days	**PBS**	**s-PRGF**	**s-PRGF + NaHA**	**NaHA**
Epithelium	12 ± 6	$5^{\Phi} \pm 2$	7 ± 3	$4^{\Phi\Phi} \pm 2$
Stroma	0.3 ± 0.5	0.3 ± 0.5	0.3 ± 0.5	0.4 ± 0.8

Statistically significant differences with respect to s-PRGF (*) or PBS (Φ) ($^{\Phi}$ $p < 0.05$; $^{\Phi\Phi}$ $p < 0,01$; *** $p < 0.001$, Kruskal–Wallis test, Dunn test with Bonferroni correction to Multiple Comparisons).

3. Discussion

It has been shown that HA improves in vitro proliferation and migration of corneal and conjunctival epithelium [44,45]. Moreover, it stabilizes the epithelial barrier of the corneal surface by binding to its corneal and conjunctiva receptor, hialadherin CD44 [46]. It has been also proven that HA helps migration and proliferation of fibroblasts [27]. In addition, it has no cytotoxicity to epithelial cells of the ocular surface, has antioxidant properties, and tends to reduce the toxic effects of preservatives [47]. However, other studies have indicated that HA specifically influences the migration of corneal epithelial cells, but not the proliferation, so that the benefit of HA in the healing of corneal wounds would be related to rapid cell migration [48].

Taking into account these results and based on the premise that HA has bioadhesive properties, we set out to assess whether the combination of the blood product s-PRGF with HA was able to increase the exposure time of the blood product to the cornea, so that the number of instillations in the treatment of the corneal epithelial defect could be reduced, thus facilitating therapeutic compliance in the case of clinical treatments. To this aim, we performed in vitro proliferation and migration assays, as well as in vivo assays in a rabbit model of an induced corneal epithelial defect.

Our proliferation results show that HA (in our case, sodium hyaluronate or NaHA) alone favors the proliferation of the human corneal epithelial line HCE, with better results than s-PRGF and the combination of both. However, the effect of NaHA on the capacity of induction of proliferation on the rabbit primary cells RPCE is similar to that of the other treatments, including the reference treatment with FBS and the negative control (BSA). On the other hand, the analysis of the Ki67 proliferation marker confirms a greater proliferative effect of NaHA on the central corneal epithelial cells (as well as on stromal keratocytes), with respect to the rest of treatments. This difference in proliferation rates according to the cell type studied may be due to the fact that the HCE are more differentiated cells and are more sensitive to certain signals in the microenvironment, while the RPCE are cells with greater intrinsic power since they contain progenitor epithelial cells. According to certain authors, the ability to stimulate proliferation on corneal epithelial cells depends on the concentration of EGF in the medium they are cultured with [13]. We observed, in the primary cultures, equivalent proliferation rates with medium containing EGF (s-PRGF treatment, combined or not combined with NaHa), or not containing EGF (NaHA and even in the BSA control treatment). Therefore, we propose that the proliferation of RPCE cells is independent, in the short term, from the medium to which they are exposed, since they have an intrinsic proliferation capacity. However, HCE epithelial cells mimic cells in the central cornea and show increased proliferation in response to HA.

On the other hand, our results suggest that a negative interaction between s-PRGF and NaHA occurs, so that the proliferative capacity of the HCE cells decreases when both are combined with respect to any of them alone. This result is supported by studies by other authors who have tested other mucoadhesive polymers, such as polyacrilic acid, combined with the platelet lysate in rabbit primary cultures, in both corneal epithelial cells and keratocytes. They show that cell proliferation is lower than when using platelet lysate alone [31].

However, the combination of HA with PRP on chondrocytes (mesodermal cells, such as corneal fibroblasts) improved cell proliferation, although not in a statistically significant manner [49], while significant changes in the expression levels of certain inflammatory markers and extracellular matrix proteins were observed. In addition, randomized controlled studies showed improvement in the clinical outcome of osteoarthritis of the knee when treated with HA and PRP with respect to PRP at three months, as well as with respect to HA at one year [50].

Considering this, we can conclude that the combination of s-PRGF and NaHA does not act synergistically in the proliferation of some kinds of cells of ectodermal origin, such as the corneal epithelium, and could even disadvantage the proliferative effect that HA has. Conversely, this combination does favor the proliferation of some kinds of mesodermal cells [43,49]. All of this suggests that the effect of the PRPs or the HA, or the combination of both, is dependent on the cell type and that it can also favor different biological functions depending on the case.

To study the effect of the combination of NaHA and s-PRGF on corneal re-epithelialization, we performed an in vitro wound healing assay in HCE cells and RPCE cells. We observed that the NaHA alone is not as good as s-PRGF alone for re-epithelialization. In fact, s-PRGF alone is the treatment that best stimulates corneal re-epithelialization. However, NaHA alone stimulates cell migration to a greater extent in primary cultures (RPCE) than in the HCE cell line. On the other hand, the combination of both did not provide any benefit in most of the assays, or was even counterproductive in the in vitro test with RPCE, in which the addition of NaHA to the blood product impairs the re-epithelialization capacity of s-PRGF.

The fact that NaHA favors, in a certain way, the epithelial closure of the RPCE could be explained by the fact that HA is an essential component of the niche matrix of limbal progenitor cells [51], so that more undifferentiated cells, such as the RPCE (which still retain the HA receptors), when in contact with HA, could migrate more actively than differentiated corneal epithelial cells (HCE).

We did not observe significant differences in the in vivo re-epithelialization capacity between any of the treatments used (s-PRGF, NaHA, both combined, or PBS as the control treatment), although s-PRGF offered a tendency to achieve better results both in the evolution of the area of the corneal defect and in the number of defects totally closed at certain times. In other in vivo studies performed on mesodermal tissues, different results have been found: Cartilage repair of better quality is achieved when PRP is combined with HA, compared to HA alone [52], and excellent results with the combination of HA and PRP in the repair of pressure ulcers and surgical wounds have also been reported [53]. However, other authors have shown equal cartilage repair capacity histologically in an in vivo model when using PRP, with respect to the combined use of PRP and HA [54].

Our histological analysis by hematoxylin and eosin staining showed correct epithelia in all cases, although those treated with NaHA were more disorganized than those undergoing other treatments or healthy controls. In addition, a greater density of fibroblast cells was observed in the anterior stroma of the corneas treated with NaHA, alone or combined with s-PRGF, at 30 days after in vivo scraping surgery. It has been described that stromal cells, possibly myofibroblasts, migrate to the superficial layers of the stroma to help close the exposed area [55]. By Ki67 cell proliferation labeling, we have demonstrated that NaHA induces proliferation in both epithelial and stromal cells, mainly in the first days after injury. The rapid initial epithelial proliferation may be the reason for the disorganization of the epithelia in the corneas under this treatment. However, the proliferation (Ki67 positive cells) obtained in the anterior stroma suggests that the accumulation of cells in that area is not only due to the cell proliferation process, but is also the result of cell migration, as other authors have described. In the case of combined treatment, s-PRGF can also contribute to this, since the histological images show the highest cell density for this treatment. In addition, we have already demonstrated through transwell-type migration experiments that s-PRGF exerts a chemotactic effect on corneal keratocytes [18].

The immunohistochemical analysis revealed similar results for the CK3 and CK15 markers, as well as for the ZO-1 protein, between the different treatments. CK15 is a marker of progenitor cells of the corneal epithelium [56], whose positivity is restricted to the basal layers of the limbal epithelium. Our results confirm the presence of these cells in the sclero-corneal limbus of all the corneas studied. When these cells divide and differentiate towards corneal epithelial cells, during their displacement of centripetal and ascending form in the cornea, they progressively express a greater labeling of the CK3 [57,58]. Similarly, the epithelial cells located in the most anterior part of the corneal epithelium express the protein belonging to the tight junction ZO-1 [59]. In all treatments, both at 7 days and 30 days after surgery, we observed a similar labeling of both proteins, demonstrating that all treatments achieve re-epithelialization of damaged corneas, generating a mature and functional corneal epithelium. It is curious to observe how the barrier function of the corneal epithelium (positivity for ZO-1) is established from the very beginning of the repair of the lesion, being observed even in those incipient epithelia formed by a single cell monolayer. Therefore, we could suggest that the establishment of the corneal barrier function is a priority in corneal healing.

Regarding the adhesion property between the newly repaired epithelium and the underlying extracellular matrix, our results show that it could be favored by treatment with s-PRGF. Thus, the β4 integrin protein is one of the components that forms part of the hemidesmosome-type junctions between the epithelium and the matrix [60], in order to achieve a compact and stable tissue. At short follow up times (7 days post-surgery), corneas treated with s-PRGF, alone or in combination, show the most intense and continuous labeling for β4 integrin, suggesting that this hemoderivative favors epithelial adhesion and that the combination with NaHA does not diminish this effect. This data is very important, since it can explain the efficacy of s-PRGF in the treatment of persistent and recurrent corneal epithelial defects [4].

4. Materials and Methods

4.1. Ethics Statements

This study was performed in accordance with the ARVO Statement for the Use of Animals in Ophthalmic and Vision Research. The procedures and experimental designs were approved by the Animal Experimentation Ethics Committee of the University of the Basque Country UPV/EHU (Permit license: CEBA/49-P03-02/2010/ANDOLLO VICTORIANO, 2011/03/11) and fulfill European and national laws.

4.2. Isolation and Expansion of Rabbit Primary Corneal Epithelial (RPCE) Cultures

To obtain RPCE cultures, 0.5×0.3 cm explants of corneas, including the limbal area, were seeded in plastic culture wells, with the corneal stroma down. We used corneas from the eyes of three 2.0–2.5 kg female New Zealand rabbits. The cells that grew from the explants were maintained at 37 °C under 5% CO_2 in DMEM: Ham's F12 mix with 2 mM L-glutamine (Lonza, Verviers, Belgium) and 1% penicillin–streptomycin (Lonza), together with 10% fetal bovine serum (FBS; Lonza). This culture medium was also supplemented with 10 ng/mL EGF (Sigma, St. Louis, MO, USA), 5 µg/mL insulin (Sigma), and 0.1 µg/mL cholera toxin (Gentaur Molecular Products, Brussels, Belgium). The positive staining for corneal epithelial markers was confirmed by immunolabeling. Cells were positive for the CK3 corneal epithelial, as well as for the CK15 and vimentin corneal epithelial stem/progenitor cell markers (Data not shown or Figure S1).

4.3. Human Corneal Epithelial (HCE) Cell Line Culture

SV-40 immortalized HCE cells were kindly provided by Dr. Araki-Sasaki et al. These cells were cultured at 37 °C under the same conditions as the RPCE cells, with the addition of the supplement 0.5% DMSO (Sigma) to the culture medium.

4.4. s-PRGF Preparation

For human s-PRGF preparation, blood was collected by venipuncture in tubes with 3.8% sodium citrate as an anticoagulant (BD Biosciences, Franklin Lakes, NJ, USA). Blood was centrifuged for 8 min at $460\times$ *g*. After collection of the complete supernatant fraction above the buffy coat, in order to induce clot formation, calcium chloride (Braun, Barcelona, Spain) was added at a final concentration of 22.8 mM. After incubation of the samples for 2 h at 36 °C, the fibrin clot was retracted and removed; the remaining fraction was the s-PRGF [61].

For rabbit s-PRGF preparation, the human protocol varied as follows: Blood was centrifuged for 8 min at 650 g. Following addition of calcium chloride, samples were incubated for 1 h at 36 °C [18].

For in vitro assays, the complement was heat inactivated in s-PRGF, and samples from several individuals pooled to obtain representative blood preparations that could provide reproducible results with minimal interindividual variability. Samples were stored at −20 °C.

For in vivo assays, autologous s-PRGF was obtained and stored at −20 °C until use.

4.5. Bioadhesive (Hyaluronic Acid) Preparation

We used an ophthalmic grade sodium hyaluronate (NaHA) with a molecular weight of 200–400 kDa (Abarán Materias Primas SL, Barcelona, Spain) in PBS (phosphate buffered saline solution).

4.6. In Vitro and In Vivo Treatments

RPCE and HCE cells were cultured under the following treatments for in vitro experiments: 1% BSA (Bovine serum albumin); 10% FBS; 45% s-PRGF; 45% s-PRGF and 0.1% NaHA; and 0.1% NaHA. The above products were diluted in supplemented culture medium (Table S1).

We used the following treatments for in vivo experiments: PBS; 90% s-PRGF; 90% s-PRGF and 0.2% NaHA; and 0.2% NaHA. The above products were diluted in PBS.

4.7. Cell Proliferation Assays

For these experiments, 3000 HCE cells (2500 in the case of RPCE cells) were seeded per well in 96-well plates. After synchronizing the cultures using DMEM:F12 with 1% BSA (Table S1) for 16 h, culture medium was substituted by the treatments to be tested (Table S1). Cell proliferation was analyzed at 0, 24, 48, and 72 h. Proliferation was described in terms of proliferation rate ± SD of viable cells, with respect to viable cells just before exposure to treatment (t = 0 h). This was measured using a 3-[4,5-dimethylthiazol-2-yl]-2,5-diphenyl tetrazolium bromide or MTT assay (Sigma-Aldrich), as previously described [61]. Optical densities at 540 nm were determined using a microplate reader (ELx800 Microplate Reader, BioTek® Instruments, Winooski, VT, USA). All experiments were performed in quadruplicate and repeated in three biological replicates.

4.8. In Vitro Wound Healing Assays

These experiments were performed as previously described [1]. Briefly, 25,000 RPCE culture cells (20,000 in the case of HCE cells) were seeded per well in 96-well plates and left to form monolayers. Once the cultures were synchronized by using DMEM:F12 with 1% BSA (Table S1) for 16 h, a circular central epithelial defect was created using a tip. Wells were divided in groups depending on the treatment (Table S1). After that, areas from which cells had been scraped away were photographed every 12 h with a phase contrast microscope (Nikon Eclipse TS 100; Nikon, Tokyo, Japan) and the images were acquired with the ProgRes CapturePro 2.6 software (Jenoptik, Jena, Germany). The size of the denuded areas was quantified using ImageJ software (developed by Wayne Rasband at the Research Services Branch, National Institute of Mental Health, Bethesda, MD). The closure rate was described in terms of the mean remaining denuded area ± SD in square millimeters. All the experiments were performed at least in quintuplicate (5 wells) and repeated in three biological replicates of RPCE and HCE cultures. For wound healing experiments in HCE cells (with high proliferation capacity), cells were previously treated with 10 μg/mL of mitomycin C for 3 h at 37 °C and washed three times with PBS after that. Afterwards, HCE cells were separated from the well by using EDTA-trypsin, and then seeded. In the case of RPCE cells, this step was not needed.

4.9. In Vivo Rabbit Corneal Re-Epithelialization Assays

Seventeen adult 2.0–2.5 kg female New Zealand white rabbits (33 eyes) were included in the study. They were under diary observation to assess their welfare. Initially, each rabbit underwent surgery in the right eye and the left eye was then operated on two to three weeks after the right eye had recovered.

The corneal epithelium inside a 9-mm corneal trephine circular mark was scraped off with an ophthalmic blade as previously described [1], without the limbal area being involved. Postoperatively, until the epithelial closure was complete, every rabbit was treated twice a day with topical dexamethasone and chloramphenicol (Deicol® ophthalmic ointment, Alcon laboratories, Barcelona, Spain), diclofenac drops (Voltaren® drops, Allergan, Irvine, CA, OSA), and with one of the treatments under study. Rabbits were randomized for each surgical intervention into one of the following four groups: (1) PBS (control), (2) 90% s-PRGF, (3) 90% s-PRGF and 0.2% NaHA, and (4) 0.2% NaHA. PBS was used for the dilution of treatments. In addition, the order in which the animals in the different experimental groups were treated was randomized.

To assess the size of the residual epithelial defect, the eyes were photographed with and without fluorescein once a day, with a ruler placed in the same plane as the ocular surface, and always at the same time of day. Wounded areas were measured using ImageJ software and results were expressed as mean wound area $\pm$ SD in mm^2. Rabbit eyes were also examined for signs of corneal inflammation and neovascularization.

4.10. Immunocytochemistry and Histochemical Analysis

The positive staining for corneal epithelial markers of primary cultures was confirmed by immunolabeling for CK3, CK15, and vimentin markers. Single cells were spin onto microscope slides using a cytospin (Cytofuge; Fisher Scientific, Houston, TX, USA). Cells were fixed with 2% paraformaldehyde (Table S2) and immunostaining was performed in the same manner as with tissue sections (see below).

After both eyes of each animal had been operated on and followed-up; that is, 7 days after surgery for the left eyes and 30 days after surgery for the right eyes, half of the corneas from each treatment were fixed in 2% paraformaldehyde and posteriorly included in paraffin to perform H-E staining. Tissue sections were observed with a phase contrast microscope (Nikon Eclipse TS 100) and images were acquired with the ProgRes CapturePro 2.6 software. We evaluated the structural integrity and histological characteristics of the cornea, as well as the regeneration of the epithelium and cell infiltration.

The other half of the corneas from each treatment were included in OCT (Optimal Cutting Temperature) compound (TissueTek®, Sakura Finetek, NL) and frozen below -80 °C. Tissue sections of 10 μm were made with a Leica CM 3050S cryostat (Leica Biosystems, Barcelona, Spain) and stored below -20 °C until immunofluorescent staining, according to conventional protocols. Briefly, sections were fixed using 2% paraformaldehyde or acetone (Table S2) and permeabilized in the former case with phosphate-buffered saline (PBS) solution containing 0.5% Triton X-100 (Sigma) for 10 min. To minimize nonspecific signals, sections were incubated for an additional hour with blocking solution, consisting of PBS containing 0.1% Triton X-100 (PBT) with 5% BSA and 10% FBS. After that, sections were incubated at 4 °C overnight with the appropriate primary antibodies at the respective dilutions in blocking solution (Table S2). After the sections were washed with phosphate-buffered saline, the samples were incubated with Alexa Fluor secondary antibodies (Invitrogen) (Table S2) for 1 h at room temperature and protected from light. The DNA specific dye DAPI (1 μg/mL, Sigma) was used to detect nuclei. Finally, the sections were mounted with Fluoromount-g (Electron Microscopy Sciences, Hatfield, PA, USA) and photographed with a fluorescence microscope (Zeiss, Göttingen, Germany).

4.11. Statistical Analysis

R program, version 3.4.0. (R Foundation for Statistical Computing, General Public License, University of Auckland, New Zealand) was used to calculate means and standard deviations and to perform statistical tests. To assess the statistical significance of two mean differences we used the Wilcoxon rank sum test. For the statistical comparison of mean differences between treatments we used the Kruskall–Wallis test and Dunn's test with Bonferroni correction to Multiple Comparisons. For qualitative variables we used the Chi-squared test and Fisher's exact test. The Kaplan–Meier estimator was also used to study the number of days that corneal epithelial defects took to heal completely. Differences were considered statistically significant when p-values were <0.05.

5. Conclusions

In summary, we must bear in mind that the use of biopolymers associated with medications in the eye has its limitations, since they can produce blurred vision after instillation for longer than usual [62,63]. In addition, we have not found additional benefit in terms of in vivo corneal epithelial wound healing when used in combination. Therefore, it is possible that the HA used in the concentrations employed in clinical practice (0.1–0.4%) creates a shield that restricts the contact of the s-PRGF components with their receptors [25], or acts by seizing growth factors, instead of as a vehicle that facilitates long-standing contact of growth factors with the ocular surface, making their combined use have a worse effect than their use alone.

It is critical when evaluating the results of the combination of HA and PRP to perform different tests in which different molecular weights and concentrations of the HA are studied (our HA has 200–400 kDa) with different concentrations and formulations of the PRP it is combined with [64]. In this sense, discrepancies are again found among authors who suggest that L-PRP (leukocyte-rich PRP) has more anti-inflammatory and anabolic effects [65] and others that affirm the opposite [66].

On the other hand, HA is a necessary component of the limbal niche. HA has a very significant role in the maintenance of the phenotype of the limbal progenitor cells [52], so damage to the HA that forms the limbal niche produces an alteration in epithelial corneal regeneration. Similarly, PRP also seems to maintain the undifferentiated phenotype of mesenchymal stem cells [67,68].

In addition, the combination of PRP and HA seems to favor the viability and proliferation of mesenchymal stem cells [69]. However, it remains to be demonstrated that the combination of PRP with HA is superior to the use of each of the treatments separately in the maintenance of the undifferentiated phenotype of the corneal scleral limbal cells.

Supplementary Materials: Supplementary materials can be found at http://www.mdpi.com/1422-0067/20/7/1655/s1.

Author Contributions: Conceptualization, N.A., J.A.D., R.H.-V., I.M. and J.E.; Methodology, J.E., C.S.-B., R.H.-M., M.d.V.-A., M.V., V.F., M.-C.M., and N.A.; Formal Analysis, C.S.-B., J.E. and N.A.; Statistical Data Analysis, A.U. and N.A.; Writing—Original Draft Preparation, J.E., C.S.-B., M.R.-A. and N.A.; Writing—Review & Editing, J.E., N.A., M.R.-A., R.H.-V., I.M., and J.A.D.; Funding Acquisition, N.A. and J.A.D.

Funding: Research study supported by grants from the University of the Basque Country UPV/EHU-Instituto Clinico Quirurgico de Oftalmologia ICQO (US16/23), and from the Basque Foundation for Health Research and Innovation BIOEF (BIO14/TP/002).

Acknowledgments: The authors thank SGIker (UPV/EHU/ ERDF, EU) for their technical and human support with animal care, imaging, and microscopy. They also gratefully acknowledge the technical support provided by Cristina Tobillas and Maria Jesus Fernandez-Martín with immunohistochemistry techniques.

Conflicts of Interest: No sponsor or funding organization had any role in the design or conduct of this research. None of the authors had any conflict of interest.

Abbreviations

HA	Hyaluronic acid
HaNA	Sodium hyaluronate
PRP	Platelet Rich Plasma
s-PRGF	Serum derived from Plasma Rich in Growth Factors
HCE	Human Corneal Epithelial
RPCE	Rabbit Primary Corneal Epithelial
PBS	Phosphate Buffered Saline
FBS	Fetal Bovine Serum
BSA	Bovine Serum Albumin
OCT	Optimal Cutting Temperature compound
MTT	3-(4,5-dimethylthiazol-2-yl)-2,5 diphenyltetrazolium bromide
DMSO	Dimethyl Sulfoxide
DAPI	4′,6-diamidino-2-phenylindole
W-H	Wound-Healing
CD	Cluster of Differentiation
CK	Cytokeratin
ZO-1	Zonula Occludens-1
α-SMA	Alpha-Smooth Muscle Actin

References

1. Freire, V.; Andollo, N.; Etxebarria, J.; Hernáez-Moya, R.; Durán, J.A.; Morales, M.C. Corneal wound healing promoted by 3 blood derivatives: An in vitro and in vivo comparative study. *Cornea* **2014**, *33*, 614–620. [CrossRef] [PubMed]

2. Tseng, S.C.G.; Tsubota, K. Important concepts for treating ocular surface and tear disorders. *Am. J. Ophthalmol.* **1997**, *124*, 825–835. [CrossRef]

3. Klenkler, B.; Sheardown, H. Growth factors in the anterior segment: Role in tissue maintenance, wound healing and ocular pathology. *Exp. Eye Res.* **2004**, *79*, 677–688. [CrossRef] [PubMed]

4. López-Plandolit, S.; Morales, M.C.; Freire, V.; Etxebarria, J.; Durán, J.A. Plasma Rich in Growth Factors as a Therapeutic Agent for Persistent Corneal Epithelial Defects. *Cornea* **2010**, *29*, 843–848. [CrossRef] [PubMed]

5. Panda, A.; Pushker, N.; Bageshwar, L.M. Lateral tarsorrhaphy: Is it preferable to patching? *Cornea* **1999**, *18*, 299–301. [CrossRef] [PubMed]

6. Rosenthal, P.; Cotter, J.M.; Baum, J. Treatment of persistent corneal epithelial defect with extended wear of a fluid-ventilated gas-permeable scleral contact lens. *Am. J. Ophthalmol.* **2000**, *130*, 33–41. [CrossRef]

7. Seitz, B.; Grüterich, M.; Cursiefen, C.; Kruse, F.E. Konservative und chirurgische therapie der neurotrophen keratopathie. *Ophthalmologe* **2005**, *102*, 15–26. [CrossRef]

8. Kruse, F.E.; Rohrschneider, K.; Völcker, H.E. Multilayer amniotic membrane transplantation for reconstruction of deep corneal ulcers. *Ophthalmology* **1999**, *106*, 1504–1511. [CrossRef]

9. Lambiase, A.; Rama, P.; Bonini, S.; Caprioglio, G.; Aloe, L. Topical Treatment with Nerve Growth Factor for Corneal Neurotrophic Ulcers. *N. Engl. J. Med.* **1998**, *338*, 1174–1180. [CrossRef]

10. Murali, S.; Hardten, D.R.; Demartelaere, S.; Olevsky, O.M.; Mindrup, E.A.; Hecht, M.L.; Karlstad, R.; Chan, C.C.; Holland, E.J. Effect of topically administered platelet-derived growth factor on corneal wound strength. *Curr. Eye Res.* **1994**, *13*, 857–862. [CrossRef]

11. Pastor, J.C.; Calonge, M. Epidermal growth factor and corneal wound healing: A multicenter study. *Cornea* **1992**, *11*, 311–314. [CrossRef] [PubMed]

12. Han, K.E.; Park, M.H.; Kong, K.H.; Choi, E.; Choi, K.-R.; Jun, R.M. Therapeutic Effects of Three Human-derived Materials in a Mouse Corneal Alkali Burn. *Cutan. Ocul. Toxicol.* **2019**, *10*, 1–24. [CrossRef] [PubMed]

13. Yamada, N.; Matsuda, R.; Morishige, N.; Yanai, R.; Chikama, T.I.; Nishida, T.; Ishimitsu, T.; Kamiya, A. Open clinical study of eye-drops containing tetrapeptides derived from substance P and insulin-like growth factor-1 for treatment of persistent corneal epithelial defects associated with neurotrophic keratopathy. *Br. J. Ophthalmol.* **2008**, *92*, 896–900. [CrossRef] [PubMed]

14. Tsubota, K.; Goto, E.; Shimmura, S.; Shimazaki, J. Treatment of persistent corneal epithelial defect by autologous serum application. *Ophthalmology* **1999**, *106*, 1984–1989. [CrossRef]

15. Alio, J.L.; Abad, M.; Artola, A.; Rodriguez-Prats, J.L.; Pastor, S.; Ruiz-Colecha, J. Use of autologous Platelet-Rich Plasma in the treatment of dormant corneal ulcers. *Ophthalmology* **2007**, *114*, 1286–1293. [CrossRef] [PubMed]

16. Geerling, G.; MacLennan, S.; Hartwig, D. Autologous serum eye drops for ocular surface disorders. *Br. J. Ophthalmol.* **2004**, *88*, 1467–1474. [CrossRef]

17. López-Plandolit, S.; Morales, M.C.; Freire, V.; Grau, A.E.; Durán, J.A. Efficacy of Plasma Rich in Growth Factors for the Treatment of Dry Eye. *Cornea* **2011**, *30*, 1312–1317. [CrossRef]

18. Etxebarria, J.; Sanz-Lázaro, S.; Hernáez-Moya, R.; Freire, V.; Durán, J.A.; Morales, M.C.; Andollo, N. Serum from plasma rich in growth factors regenerates rabbit corneas by promoting cell proliferation, migration, differentiation, adhesion and limbal stemness. *Acta Ophthalmol.* **2017**, *95*, e693–e705. [CrossRef] [PubMed]

19. Anitua, E.; de la Fuente, M.; Muruzabal, F.; Riestra, A.; Merayo-Lloves, J.; Orive, G. Plasma rich in growth factors (PRGF) eye drops stimulates scarless regeneration compared to autologous serum in the ocular surface stromal fibroblasts. *Exp. Eye Res.* **2015**, *135*, 118–126. [CrossRef]

20. Anitua, E.; Zalduendo, M.; Troya, M.; Padilla, S.; Orive, G. Leukocyte inclusion within a platelet rich plasma-derived fibrin scaffold stimulates a more pro-inflammatory environment and alters fibrin properties. *PLoS ONE* **2015**, *10*, e0121713. [CrossRef]

21. Bongiovì, F.; Di Prima, G.; Palumbo, F.S.; Licciardi, M.; Pitarresi, G.; Giammona, G. Hyaluronic Acid-Based Micelles as Ocular Platform to Modulate the Loading, Release, and Corneal Permeation of Corticosteroids. *Macromol. Biosci.* **2017**, *17*, 1700261. [CrossRef]

22. De Campos, A.M.; Sánchez, A.; Alonso, M.J. Chitosan nanoparticles: A new vehicle for the improvement of the delivery of drugs to the ocular surface. Application to cyclosporin A. *Int. J. Pharm.* **2001**, *224*, 159–168. [CrossRef]

23. Yenice, I.; Mocan, M.C.; Palaska, E.; Bochot, A.; Bilensoy, E.; Vural, I.; Irkeç, M.; Atilla Hincal, A. Hyaluronic acid coated poly-ε-caprolactone nanospheres deliver high concentrations of cyclosporine A into the cornea. *Exp. Eye Res.* **2008**, *87*, 162–167. [CrossRef]

24. Zeng, W.; Li, Q.; Wan, T.; Liu, C.; Pan, W.; Wu, Z.; Zhang, G.; Pan, J.; Qin, M.; Lin, Y.; et al. Hyaluronic acid-coated niosomes facilitate tacrolimus ocular delivery: Mucoadhesion, precorneal retention, aqueous humor pharmacokinetics, and transcorneal permeability. *Colloids Surf. B Biointerfaces* **2016**, *141*, 28–35. [CrossRef] [PubMed]

25. Lin, J.; Wu, H.; Wang, Y.; Lin, J.; Chen, Q.; Zhu, X. Preparation and ocular pharmacokinetics of hyaluronan acid-modified mucoadhesive liposomes. *Drug Deliv.* **2016**, *23*, 1144–1151. [CrossRef] [PubMed]

26. Andrés-Guerrero, V.; Vicario-de-la-Torre, M.; Molina-Martínez, I.T.; Benítez-del-Castillo, J.M.; García-Feijoo, J.; Herrero-Vanrell, R. Comparison of the in vitro tolerance and in vivo efficacy of traditional timolol maleate eye drops versus new formulations with bioadhesive polymers. *Investig. Ophthalmol. Vis. Sci.* **2011**, *52*, 3548–3556. [CrossRef] [PubMed]

27. Voigt, J.; Driver, V.R. Hyaluronic acid derivatives and their healing effect on burns, epithelial surgical wounds, and chronic wounds: A systematic review and meta-analysis of randomized controlled trials. *Wound Repair Regen.* **2012**, *20*, 317–331. [CrossRef] [PubMed]

28. Steven, P.; Scherer, D.; Krösser, S.; Beckert, M.; Cursiefen, C.; Kaercher, T. Semifluorinated Alkane Eye Drops for Treatment of Dry Eye Disease—A Prospective, Multicenter Noninterventional Study. *J. Ocul. Pharmacol. Ther.* **2015**, *31*, 498–503. [CrossRef] [PubMed]

29. Prause, J.U. Treatment of keratoconjunctivitis sicca with Lacrisert. *Scand. J. Rheumatol. Suppl.* **1986**, *61*, 261–263.

30. Ciolino, J.B.; Ross, A.E.; Tulsan, R.; Watts, A.C.; Wang, R.F.; Zurakowski, D.; Serle, J.B.; Kohane, D.S. Latanoprost-Eluting Contact Lenses in Glaucomatous Monkeys. *Ophthalmology* **2016**, *123*, 2085–2092. [CrossRef]

31. Sandri, G.; Bonferoni, M.C.; Rossi, S.; Ferrari, F.; Mori, M.; Del Fante, C.; Perotti, C.; Scudeller, L.; Caramella, C. Platelet lysate formulations based on mucoadhesive polymers for the treatment of corneal lesions. *J. Pharm. Pharmacol.* **2011**, *63*, 189–198. [CrossRef] [PubMed]

32. López-García, J.S.; García-Lozano, I.; Rivas, L.; Ramírez, N.; Raposo, R.; Méndez, M.T. Autologous serum eye drops diluted with sodium hyaluronate: Clinical and experimental comparative study. *Acta Ophthalmol.* **2014**, *92*, e22–e29. [CrossRef] [PubMed]

33. Andia, I.; Abate, M. Knee osteoarthritis: Hyaluronic acid, platelet-rich plasma or both in association? *Expert Opin. Biol. Ther.* **2014**, *14*, 635–649. [CrossRef] [PubMed]

34. Goa, K.L.; Benfield, P. Hyaluronic Acid: A Review of its Pharmacology and Use as a Surgical Aid in Ophthalmology, and its Therapeutic Potential in Joint Disease and Wound Healing. *Drugs* **1994**, *47*, 536–566. [CrossRef]

35. Choi, K.Y.; Lee, S.; Park, K.; Kim, K.; Park, J.H.; Kwon, I.C.; Jeong, S.Y. Preparation and characterization of hyaluronic acid-based hydrogel nanoparticles. *J. Phys. Chem. Solids* **2008**, *69*, 1591–1595. [CrossRef]

36. Aragona, P.; Papa, V.; Micali, A.; Santocono, M.; Milazzo, G. Long term treatment with sodium hyaluronate-containing artificial tears reduces ocular surface damage in patients with dry eye. *Br. J. Ophthalmol.* **2002**, *86*, 181–184. [CrossRef]

37. Müller, W. *Bioquímica. Fundamentos para Medicina y Ciencias de la Vida*; Ed Reverté: Barcelona, Spain, 2008; ISBN 9788429173932.

38. Waddell, D.D. Viscosupplementation with hyaluronans for osteoarthritis of the knee: Clinical efficacy and economic implications. *Drugs Aging* **2007**, *24*, 629–642. [CrossRef]

39. Prasadam, I.; Mao, X.; Shi, W.; Crawford, R.; Xiao, Y. Combination of MEK-ERK inhibitor and hyaluronic acid has a synergistic effect on anti-hypertrophic and pro-chondrogenic activities in osteoarthritis treatment. *J. Mol. Med.* **2013**, *91*, 369–380. [CrossRef] [PubMed]

40. Muto, J.; Yamasaki, K.; Taylor, K.R.; Gallo, R.L. Engagement of CD44 by hyaluronan suppresses TLR4 signaling and the septic response to LPS. *Mol. Immunol.* **2009**, *47*, 449–456. [CrossRef] [PubMed]

41. Zavan, B.; Ferroni, L.; Giorgi, C.; Calò, G.; Brun, P.; Cortivo, R.; Abatangelo, G.; Pinton, P. Hyaluronic acid induces activation of the κ-opioid receptor. *PLoS ONE* **2013**, *8*, e55510. [CrossRef] [PubMed]

42. Scheibner, K.A.; Lutz, M.A.; Boodoo, S.; Fenton, M.J.; Powell, J.D.; Horton, M.R. Hyaluronan Fragments Act as an Endogenous Danger Signal by Engaging TLR2. *J. Immunol.* **2006**, *177*, 1272–1281. [CrossRef] [PubMed]

43. Anitua, E.; Sanchez, M.; De la Fuente, M.; Zalduendo, M.M.; Orive, G. Plasma rich in growth factors (PRGF-Endoret) stimulates tendon and synovial fibroblasts migration and improves the biological properties of hyaluronic acid. *Knee Surg. Sport Traumatol. Arthrosc.* **2012**, *20*, 1657–1665. [CrossRef]

44. Calienno, R.; Curcio, C.; Lanzini, M.; Nubile, M.; Mastropasqua, L. In vivo and ex vivo evaluation of cell–cell interactions, adhesion and migration in ocular surface of patients undergone excimer laser refractive surgery after topical therapy with different lubricant eyedrops. *Int. Ophthalmol.* **2018**, *38*, 1591–1599. [CrossRef]

45. Inoue, M.; Katakami, C. The effect of hyaluronic acid on corneal epithelial cell proliferation. *Investig. Ophthalmol. Vis. Sci.* **1993**, *34*, 2313–2315.

46. Brignole, F.; Pisella, P.J.; Dupas, B.; Baeyens, V.; Baudouin, C. Efficacy and safety of 0.18% sodium hyaluronate in patients with moderate dry eye syndrome and superficial keratitis. *Graefe's Arch. Clin. Exp. Ophthalmol.* **2005**, *243*, 531–538. [CrossRef]

47. Debbasch, C.; De La Salle, S.B.; Brignole, F.; Rat, P.; Warnet, J.M.; Baudouin, C. Cytoprotective effects of hyaluronic acid and carbomer 934P in ocular surface epithelial cells. *Investig. Ophthalmol. Vis. Sci.* **2002**, *43*, 3409–3415.

48. Gomes, J.A.; Amankwah, R.; Powell-Richards, A.; Dua, H.S. Sodium hyaluronate (hyaluronic acid) promotes migration of human corneal epithelial cells in vitro. *Br. J. Ophthalmol.* **2004**, *88*, 821–825. [CrossRef] [PubMed]

49. Chen, W.H.; Lo, W.C.; Hsu, W.C.; Wei, H.J.; Liu, H.Y.; Lee, C.H.; Tina Chen, S.Y.; Shieh, Y.H.; Williams, D.F.; Deng, W.P. Synergistic anabolic actions of hyaluronic acid and platelet-rich plasma on cartilage regeneration in osteoarthritis therapy. *Biomaterials* **2014**, *35*, 9599–9607. [CrossRef] [PubMed]

50. Lana, J.F.; Weglein, A.; Sampson, S.E.; Vicente, E.F.; Huber, S.C.; Souza, C.V.; Ambach, M.A.; Vincent, H.; Urban-Paffaro, A.; Onodera, C.M.; et al. Randomized controlled trial comparing hyaluronic acid, platelet-rich plasma and the combination of both in the treatment of mild and moderate osteoarthritis of the knee. *J. Stem. Cells Regen. Med.* **2016**, *12*, 69–78.

51. Gesteira, T.F.; Sun, M.; Coulson-Thomas, Y.M.; Yamaguchi, Y.; Yeh, L.-K.; Hascall, V.; Coulson-Thomas, V.J. Hyaluronan Rich Microenvironment in the Limbal Stem Cell Niche Regulates Limbal Stem Cell Differentiation. *Investig. Ophthalmol. Vis. Sci.* **2017**, *58*, 4407–4421. [CrossRef]

52. Marmotti, A.; Bruzzone, M.; Bonasia, D.E.; Castoldi, F.; Rossi, R.; Pras, L.; Maiello, A.; Realmuto, C.; Peretti, G.M. One-step osteochondral repair with cartilage fragments in a composite scaffold. *Knee Surg. Sport Traumatol. Arthrosc.* **2012**, *20*, 2590–2601. [CrossRef] [PubMed]

53. Cervelli, V.; Lucarini, L.; Spallone, D.; Palla, L.; Colicchia, G.M.; Gentile, P.; De Angelis, B. Use of Platelet-Rich Plasma and Hyaluronic Acid in the Loss of Substance with Bone Exposure. *Adv. Skin Wound Care* **2011**, *24*, 176–181. [CrossRef] [PubMed]

54. Smyth, N.A.; Ross, K.A.; Haleem, A.M.; Hannon, C.P.; Murawski, C.D.; Do, H.T.; Kennedy, J.G. Platelet-Rich Plasma and Hyaluronic Acid Are Not Synergistic When Used as Biological Adjuncts with Autologous Osteochondral Transplantation. *Cartilage* **2017**, *9*, 321–328. [CrossRef] [PubMed]

55. Alcalde, I.; Íñigo-Portugués, A.; Carreño, N.; Riestra, A.C.; Merayo-Lloves, J.M. Efectos de nuevos agentes regenerativos biomiméticos sobre la cicatrización corneal en un modelo experimental de úlceras posquirúrgicas. *Arch. Soc. Esp. Oftalmol.* **2015**, *90*, 467–474. [CrossRef]

56. Yoshida, S.; Shimmura, S.; Kawakita, T.; Miyashita, H.; Den, S.; Shimazaki, J.; Tsubota, K. Cytokeratin 15 can be used to identify the limbal phenotype in normal and diseased ocular surfaces. *Investig. Ophthalmol. Vis. Sci.* **2006**, *47*, 4780–4786. [CrossRef] [PubMed]

57. Schlötzer-Schrehardt, U.; Kruse, F.E. Identification and characterization of limbal stem cells. *Exp. Eye Res.* **2005**, *81*, 247–264. [CrossRef] [PubMed]

58. Secker, G.A.; Daniels, J.T. *Limbal Epithelial Stem Cells of the Cornea.* StemBook; Harvard Stem Cell Institute: Cambridge, MA, USA, 2008.

Int. J. Mol. Sci. **2019**, *20*, 1655

59. Wu, Z.; Zhou, Q.; Duan, H.; Wang, X.; Xiao, J.; Duan, H.; Li, N.; Li, C.; Wan, P.; Liu, Y.; et al. Reconstruction of auto-tissue-engineered lamellar cornea by dynamic culture for transplantation: A rabbit model. *PLoS ONE* **2014**, *9*, e93012. [CrossRef] [PubMed]
60. Lauweryns, B.; Van den Oord, J.J.; Volpes, R.; Foets, B.; Missotten, L. Distribution of very late activation integrins in the human cornea: An immunohistochemical study using monoclonal antibodies. *Investig. Ophthalmol. Vis. Sci.* **1991**, *32*, 2079–2085.
61. Freire, V.; Andollo, N.; Etxebarria, J.; Durán, J.A.; Morales, M.C. In Vitro Effects of Three Blood Derivatives on Human Corneal Epithelial Cells. *Investig. Ophthalmol. Vis. Sci.* **2012**, *53*, 5571–5578. [CrossRef]
62. Calonge, M. The treatment of dry eye. *Surv. Ophthalmol.* **2001**, *45*, S227–S239. [CrossRef]
63. Johnson, M.E.; Murphy, P.J.; Boulton, M. Carbomer and sodium hyaluronate eyedrops for moderate dry eye treatment. *Optom. Vis. Sci.* **2008**, *85*, 750–757. [CrossRef] [PubMed]
64. Andia, I.; Maffulli, N. A contemporary view of platelet-rich plasma therapies: Moving toward refined clinical protocols and precise indications. *Regen. Med.* **2018**, *13*, 717–728. [CrossRef] [PubMed]
65. Carmona, J.U.; Ríos, D.L.; López, C.; Álvarez, M.E.; Pérez, J.E.; Bohórquez, M.E. In vitro effects of platelet-rich gel supernatants on histology and chondrocyte apoptosis scores, hyaluronan release and gene expression of equine cartilage explants challenged with lipopolysaccharide. *BMC Vet. Res.* **2016**, *12*, 135. [CrossRef]
66. Assirelli, E.; Filardo, G.; Mariani, E.; Kon, E.; Roffi, A.; Vaccaro, F.; Marcacci, M.; Facchini, A.; Pulsatelli, L. Effect of two different preparations of platelet-rich plasma on synoviocytes. Knee Surgery. *Sport Traumatol. Arthrosc.* **2015**, *23*, 2690–2703. [CrossRef] [PubMed]
67. Tobita, M.; Tajima, S.; Mizuno, H. Adipose tissue-derived mesenchymal stem cells and platelet-rich plasma: Stem cell transplantation methods that enhance stemness. *Stem Cell Res. Ther.* **2015**, *6*, 215. [CrossRef] [PubMed]
68. Li, H.; Usas, A.; Poddar, M.; Chen, C.W.; Thompson, S.; Ahani, B.; Cummins, J.; Lavasani, M.; Huard, J. Platelet-Rich Plasma Promotes the Proliferation of Human Muscle Derived Progenitor Cells and Maintains Their Stemness. *PLoS ONE* **2013**, *8*, e64923. [CrossRef] [PubMed]
69. Vadalà, G.; Russo, F.; Musumeci, M.; D'Este, M.; Cattani, C.; Catanzaro, G.; Tirindelli, M.C.; Lazzari, L.; Alini, M.; Giordano, R.; et al. Clinically relevant hydrogel-based on hyaluronic acid and platelet rich plasma as a carrier for mesenchymal stem cells: Rheological and biological characterization. *J. Orthop. Res.* **2017**, *35*, 2109–2116. [CrossRef]

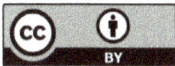

International Journal of
Molecular Sciences

MDPI

Article

Fibrin Sealant Derived from Human Plasma as a Scaffold for Bone Grafts Associated with Photobiomodulation Therapy

Karina Torres Pomini [1], Daniela Vieira Buchaim [1,2,3], Jesus Carlos Andreo [1],
Marcelie Priscila de Oliveira Rosso [1], Bruna Botteon Della Coletta [1], Íris Jasmin Santos German [4],
Ana Carolina Cestari Biguetti [1], André Luis Shinohara [1], Geraldo Marco Rosa Júnior [5,6],
João Vitor Tadashi Cosin Shindo [1], Murilo Priori Alcalde [5,7], Marco Antônio Hungaro Duarte [7],
Daniel de Bortoli Teixeira [2] and Rogério Leone Buchaim [1,2,*]

[1] Department of Biological Sciences (Anatomy), Bauru School of Dentistry, University of São Paulo (USP), Bauru 17012-901, Brazil; karinatorrespomini@gmail.com (K.T.P.); danibuchaim@usp.br (D.V.B.); jcandreo@usp.br (J.C.A.); marcelierosso@usp.br (M.P.d.O.R.); brucoletta@hotmail.com (B.B.D.C.); anacarolinacb25@gmail.com (A.C.C.B.); andreshinohara@yahoo.com.br (A.L.S.); jvshindo@gmail.com (J.V.T.C.S.)
[2] Department of Human Morphophysiology, Medical and Dentistry School, University of Marilia (UNIMAR), Marília 17525-902, Brazil; daniel.dbt@hotmail.com
[3] Department of Human Anatomy and Neuroanatomy, Medical School, University Center of Adamantina (UniFAI), Adamantina 17800-000, Brazil
[4] Department of Dentistry, Faculty of Health Science, Universidad Iberoamericana (UNIBE), Santo Domingo 10203, Dominic Republic; irish_knaan@hotmail.com
[5] Department of Health Science, University of the Sacred Heart (USC), Bauru 17011-160, Brazil; geraldomrjr@yahoo.com.br (G.M.R.J.); murilo_alcalde@hotmail.com (M.P.A.)
[6] Department of Anatomy, University of the Ninth of July (UNINOVE), Bauru 17011-102, Brazil
[7] Department of Dentistry, Endodontics and Dental Materials, Bauru School of Dentistry, University of São Paulo (USP), Bauru 17012-901, Brazil; mhungaro@fob.usp.br
* Correspondence: rogerio@fob.usp.br

Received: 14 March 2019; Accepted: 7 April 2019; Published: 10 April 2019

check for
updates

Abstract: Fibrin sealants derived from human blood can be used in tissue engineering to assist in the repair of bone defects. The objective of this study was to evaluate the support system formed by a xenograft fibrin sealant associated with photobiomodulation therapy of critical defects in rat calvaria. Thirty-six rats were divided into four groups: BC ($n = 8$), defect filled with blood clot; FSB ($n = 10$), filled with fibrin sealant and xenograft; BC^{PBMT} ($n = 8$), blood clot and photobiomodulation; FSB^{PBMT} ($n = 10$), fibrin sealant, xenograft, and photobiomodulation. The animals were killed after 14 and 42 days. In the histological and microtomographic analysis, new bone formation was observed in all groups, limited to the defect margins, and without complete wound closure. In the FSB group, bone formation increased between periods (4.3 ± 0.46 to 6.01 ± 0.32), yet with lower volume density when compared to the FSB^{PBMT} (5.6 ± 0.45 to 10.64 ± 0.97) group. It was concluded that the support system formed by the xenograft fibrin sealant associated with the photobiomodulation therapy protocol had a positive effect on the bone repair process.

Keywords: bone regeneration; bone repair; fibrin sealant; biomaterial; photobiomodulation therapy; low-level laser therapy

Int. J. Mol. Sci. **2019**, *20*, 1761; doi:10.3390/ijms20071761   26   www.mdpi.com/journal/ijms

1. Introduction

There are currently available treatment options for the repair of bone defects, but their effectiveness is limited in large defects, and the influence of extrinsic factors such as smoking and alcohol exposure are unfavourable in this process [1–3]. Annually more than two million bone grafts are performed worldwide, the second most frequent tissue transplantation, being surpassed only by blood transfusion [4,5].

Among all available types, the autologous graft is still considered the gold standard, since all the necessary properties in bone regeneration in terms of osteoconduction, osteoinduction, and osteogenesis are combined [6,7]. However, its availability is limited, and morbidity at the donor site has led to the development of new bone substitutes that restore, ameliorate, or prevent aggravation of compromised tissue function [8,9].

In order to solve this problem, tissue engineering has developed xenografts that are skeletal derivatives of other species, mainly bovine, with satisfactory osteoconductive properties and widely used in reconstructive procedures with greater scientific evidence among biomaterials [4,10].

To form a graft material mouldable to the surgical bed, facilitate its insertion and agglutination, and prevent its dispersion and collapse of soft tissue into the defect, biodegradable polymers known as scaffolds are used as three-dimensional supports for the lodging of cells and biologically active molecules, providing a favourable environment for tissue regeneration [10].

Among the scaffolds, fibrin sealants derived from human blood may have the potential to guide this process of bone remodelling, because it has compatible physiological characteristics to human tissue and thus is readily colonised by the surrounding cells. Thus, they allow surgeons to influence and improve the cellular microenvironment in vitro or in vivo, increasing the success rate of the bone graft [11].

Other attempts have been studied to minimise the time of bone healing and to reduce the chance of possible complications arising from the abnormal regeneration process. Among them, low-intensity pulsed ultrasound [12] and laser photobiomodulation therapy have been highlighted by their satisfactory effects on bone metabolism and repair, due to their possible osteogenic effect [13,14].

Laser photobiomodulation therapy is a non-invasive treatment method with relatively low cost [15]. However, there are controversies regarding the best parameters to be used to obtain an effective result in the process of bone repair of critical size defects filled with biomaterials [5].

Despite the growing interest in blood-derived biomaterials in the reconstruction of bone defects, in the literature reviewed, no studies were found on the effects of the combination of sealant with bone grafts and alternative methods such as photobiomodulation. Thus, this study evaluated the support system formed by a xenograft fibrin sealant associated with the protocol of photobiomodulation therapy in critical size defects in rats.

2. Results

2.1. Microtomographic Analysis

In microtomographic images, at 14 days, it was observed that in all the defects, the new bone formation occurred centripetally from the critical defect margins towards the centre. All groups exhibited a continuous increase of new bone formation during the analysed periods; however, in no specimen was there a complete closure of the defect, and the formed bone was restricted to the defect borders (blue arrow—Figure 1A).

In the groups where the defects were filled with fibrin sealant associated with the xenogeneic graft (FSB—Fibrin sealant with xenograft, and FSB[PBMT]—Fibrin sealant with xenograft and photobiomodulation therapy), the images showed the surgical cavity filled with the materials implanted and fine bone trabeculae adjacent to the border of the defect and under the dura mater. In animals that were biostimulated with a low-level laser, a more evident formation of the bone tissue was observed in FSB[PBMT] compared to the FSB group (Figure 1A).

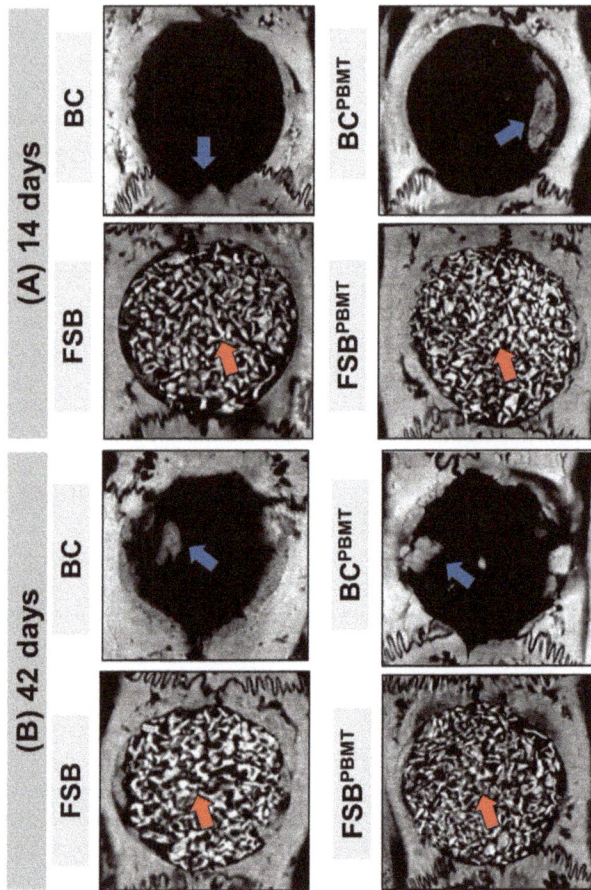

Figure 1. Microtomographic images showing the evolution of the repair of defects filled with clot and fibrin sealant plus xenograft (biomaterial) with or without low-level laser biostimulation therapy. Biomaterial particles (red arrow) and newly formed bone tissue (blue arrow). Two-dimensional trans-axial cuts at (**A**) 14 days; and (**B**) 42 days, respectively.

In the subsequent period, at 42 days, an increase in the amount of bone tissue, interweaving the biomaterial, in a more organised configuration, especially in the FSB^PBMT group was observed. The xenograft particles were still evident (red arrow), with some areas of remodelled tissue at the defect margins (Figure 1B).

2.2. Histological Evaluation

In all groups, the repair of bone defects occurred centripetally, with the absence of necrotic tissue, the presence of bone cells, osteoid matrix, and budding of new blood vessels at the site.

At 14 days, all BC (defect filled with Blood Clot without photobiomodulation therapy) and BC^PBMT (defect filled with Blood Clot with photobiomodulation therapy) animals presented incomplete bone repair both in the height and in the conformation of the newly formed bone, which was irregular along the dura mater (Figures 2A(i)–A(ii) and 3A). In the animals in the BC group, the central area of the defect was predominantly filled by loose connective tissue with small loci of new bone formation at the defect border, but in the BC^PBMT animals, the defects were filled by immature bone and more obvious blood vessels (Figures 2A(i)–A(ii) and 3A).

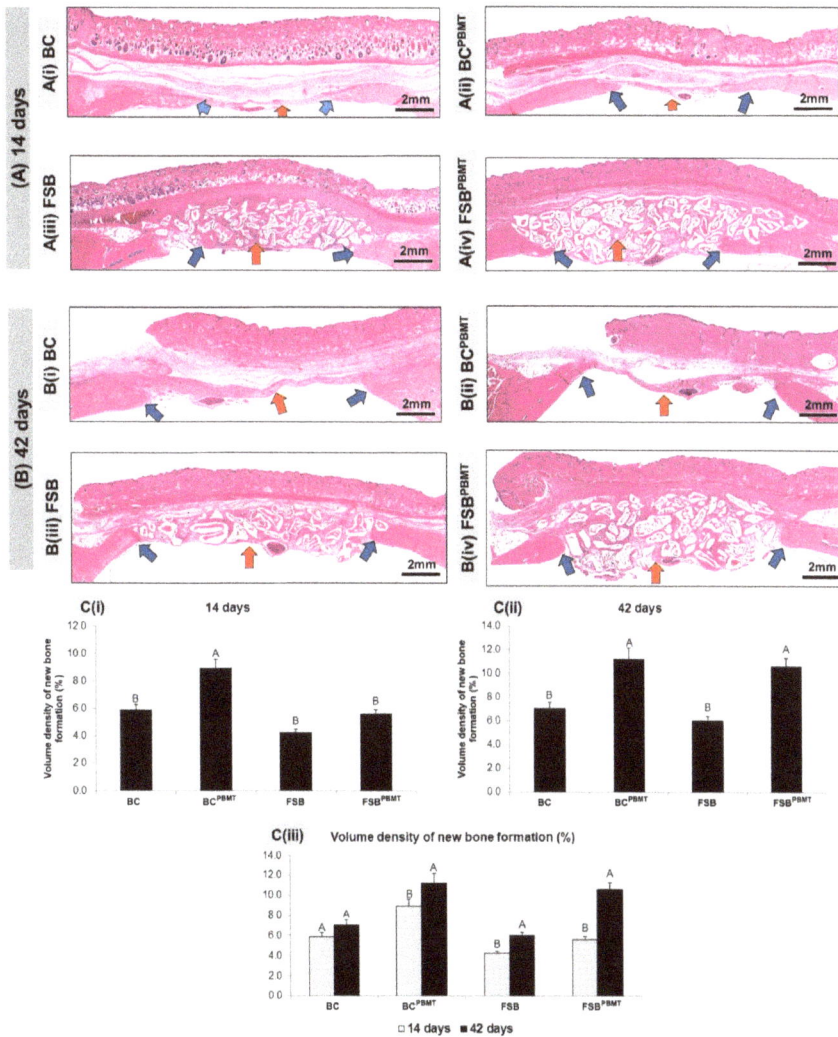

Figure 2. Panoramic histological views at (**A**) 14 days; and (**B**) 42 days, respectively; (**C**) graphs of volume density of newly formed bone in skull defects filled with a blood clot or fibrin sealant plus xenograft and with or without laser photobiomodulation therapy. (**A**) A(i)–A(ii) bone formation (blue arrows) occurring at the defect border and under the dura mater surface. A(iii)–A(iv): the defect showed trabecular bone formation (blue arrows) adjacent to the defect border, in a more advanced stage of bone maturation. (**B**) B(i)–B(ii) both groups showed similar bone formation limited to the defect border and a large region filled with fibrous connective tissue (red arrows); B(iii)–B(iv) a large part of the defect was filled by connective tissue and biomaterials (red arrows), but in the FSB^{PBMT} group, greater bone formation defect could be observed compared to the FSB group; (**C**) Graphs of newly formed bone showed smaller bone formation in the non-biostimulated group (BC and FSB) than the biostimulated group (BC^{PBMT} and FSB^{PBMT}). (BC and BC^{PBMT}: $N = 4$/group and periods), (FSB and FSB^{PBMT}: $N = 5$/group and periods). C(i) and C(ii) where different letters (A≠B) indicate a statistically significant difference between groups in the same period and C(iii) where the different letters (A≠B) indicate a statistically significant difference in the same group in the two periods analysed ($p < 0.05$). (HE; original magnification × 4; bar = 2 mm).

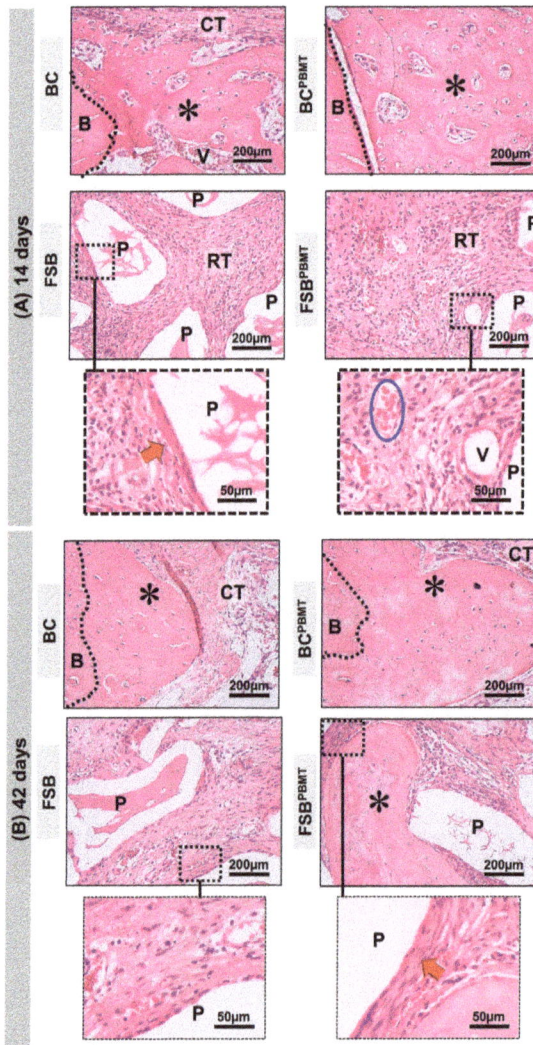

Figure 3. Details of the evolution of the bone healing of the skull defects filled with a blood clot or fibrin sealant plus xenograft (biomaterial) with or without low-level laser biostimulation therapy. (**A**) At 14 days, BC and BC^{PBMT}: the defect shows the trabecular bone formation (asterisks) adjacent to the defect border and spaces between the trabeculae filled by connective tissue. FSB: the defect was filled by particles of the biomaterial (P) surrounded by connective tissue with some inflammatory cells (RT—reactional tissue). Collagen fibres surrounding the xenograft particles (red arrow). FSB^{PBMT}: the defect was filled by particles of the biomaterial (P) surrounded by connective tissue with some inflammatory cells (RT—reactional tissue). Presence of many red blood cells (inside the blue lined area) and blood vessels (V) permeating connective tissue; (**B**) At 42 days, BC and BC^{PBMT}: the new bone shows a gradual increase in thickness of the trabeculae leading to a compact structure. FSB: the new bone formation increases, becoming compact, there is a presence of xenograft particles and a decrease in inflammatory response. In FSB^{PBMT}, the collagen fibres are arranged in more layers surrounding the particles. (HE; original magnification × 40; bar = 200 μm; and Insets, magnified images × 100; bar = 50 μm).

In all animals of the FSB and FSB[PBMT] groups, in the same experimental period, the defects presented with large amounts of the biomaterial. The new bone formation also occurred from the defect border, with trabecular conformation, being more pronounced in the FSB[PBMT] group. The presence of inflammatory infiltrate was identified in both groups, diffusely distributed in the interstitial space (Figures 2A(iii)–A(iv) and 3A).

At 42 days, in the BC group, the formed connective tissue filled the entire extent of the defect, maintaining a seemingly smaller thickness in relation to the remaining (original) bone, and the new bone formed was limited to the proximities of the injured borders. In the BC[PBMT] animals, biostimulated with low power laser, the defect was still filled by a large amount of connective tissue, exhibiting a thin layer of bone tissue (asterisk) with diploe characteristics, and in some cases partial closure of the defect, but without recovery of its height (Figures 2B(i)–B(ii) and 3B).

In the same period, in all FSB and FSB[PBMT] animals, the surgical area was almost completely filled by biomaterial particles, without any significant changes in relation to the previous period. The bone formation remained limited to the edges, but with a denser and lamellar arrangement. The tissue reaction appeared to be in the resolution phase, with the most fibrotic interstitial space. In the FSB[PBMT] group, the reduction of oedema was more evident resulting in the formation of a denser stroma with more cells and with concentric collagen fibres forming a capsule around the biomaterial (Figures 2B(iii)–(iv) and 3B).

2.3. Histomorphometric Evaluation

At 14 days of the repair process and after a quantitative evaluation of the volume density of the newly formed bone, it was observed that animals of the BC[PBMT] group presented the highest means (8.9 ± 0.64) with significant difference in relation to the other experimental groups BC, FSB, and FSB[PBMT] (5.9 ± 0.38; 4.3 ± 0.46; 5.6 ± 0.45, respectively), that were not significantly different to each other (Figure 2C(i)).

In the 42-day period, the groups biostimulated with a low-power laser (BC[PBMT] and FSB[PBMT]) presented the highest means, but without significant difference between them (11.22 ± 0.94; 10.64 ± 0.97, respectively). However, the animals in the aforementioned groups showed a significant difference when compared to the non-biostimulated animals BC and FSB (7.06 ± 0.49; 6.02 ± 0.32, respectively), but did not show any significant difference when compared to each other (Figure 2C(ii)).

The evaluation of the volume density of the newly formed bone within the same group in the two experimental periods (14 and 42 days) revealed that bone formation was higher in all groups in the 42-day period, with a significant difference between periods except for the BC group (Figure 2C(iii)).

3. Discussion

The existing scientific evidence in the field of tissue engineering indicates promising results in the treatment of bone defects with the use of fibrin sealants derived from human plasma as scaffolds for cellular development [11,16–19]. However, there is no data in the literature which reports its effect on the bone repair process when associated with xenograft and alternative therapeutic methods. Thus, the results in this study show that the association of these treatments favoured the repair process of critical bone defects in the calvaria of rats.

The bone calvarium defect rat model is the most used among others in the scientific literature since it provides a clinically relevant evaluation of regenerative therapies and bone substitute materials, allowing for more effective clinical interventions. The defect produced is perfectly reproducible, fast, and does not require fixation for stabilisation, as compared to long bones [20].

The search for noninvasive methods, such as low intensity ultrasound (LIPUS), electromagnetic fields, and laser photobiomodulation therapy, has been increasing exponentially in recent years to improve the bone healing process [12]. As a consequence, there are numerous clinical and experimental studies with low-level laser photobiomodulation therapies, but so far without consensus on the optimal parameters for the bone repair process [5].

This study used a wavelength of 830 nm, a power density of 258.6 mW/cm^2, and mode of continuous operation, corroborating previous studies that presented satisfactory results in the process of bone repair [21].

Therefore, with the knowledge that the biomodulation effects of the laser are intrinsically related to the wavelength and that the loss of intensity may compromise its function, the right choice of the spectral band has become of extreme importance in the treatment. Thus, the wavelength in the infrared spectrum became widely used due to its lower loss, which can reach up to 37% of its intensity after a depth of 2 mm [22]. Knowing previously that the pre-calvarial tissue thickness in the rat has small dimensions, it is assumed that the loss is minimal. In situations exceeding 2 mm, there may be a maximum loss of 162.92 mW for each cm^2 of tissue, with the same protocol used in this study.

In addition, the infrared spectrum, between 780 and 1100 nm, is based on non-thermal mechanisms, which do not generate a significant increase in tissue temperature (up to 37.5 °C). In excitation states, a fraction of energy is converted into heat, which causes local and transient increases in the temperature of absorbent chromophores, without heating the total cell [23].

To evaluate the potential of fibrin sealants derived from human blood, this study comprised microtomographic, histological, and histomorphometric analyses. In the microtomographic analysis, at 14 days it was possible to observe the formation of new bone at the margins of the surgical wound in all groups, probably via the stimulation of growth factors released after craniotomy. The growth remained limited to this region until the end of the experiment, as reported in other experimental studies [24,25].

In the groups where the defects were filled with the fibrin sealant associated with the xenogeneic graft (FSB and FSB^{PBMT}), the particles remained at the site of implantation without dispersion, corroborating with studies that report on the mechanical stability and the binding effects provided by the fibrin sealant to bone grafts [26,27].

Histologically, at 14 days, the BC and BC^{PBMT} groups exhibited new bone formed in the defect margins, overlapping the dura, with a trabecular and immature arrangement. This can be attributed to the action of growth factors in this region after vascular rupture due to craniotomy and the presence of the underlying periosteum, which is the main source of osteoprogenitor cells and osteoinductive factors [28]. At 42 days, the newly formed bone became lamellar and compact. These findings are generally observed in repair procedures in lesions similar to those performed in this study [3,29,30]. However, none of the defects presented complete closure, with a large part being filled by fibrous connective tissue, in agreement with studies that reported that this is a critical defect according to Gosain et al. [31], An et al. [32], and Maciel et al. [30].

In the two analysed periods, the animals biostimulated with the laser presented greater evidence of new bone formation and greater tissue organisation at the end of the experiment [33]. These results are consistent with the literature that indicates the positive photobiomodulatory effects of the laser in the initial phases of bone repair, when, among several events, there is a proliferation of osteoblasts and differentiation of mesenchymal cells [34,35].

The defects filled with fibrin and xenograft (FSB and FSB^{PBMT}) sealers showed intense angiogenesis as early as 14 days, as well as the presence of reactional tissue at 42 days of resolution [36]. The tissue reaction observed in these groups did not trigger a foreign body type granulomatous reaction, which suggests that the grafts used were biocompatible [26,37,38] and the biological response was consistent with the inflammatory process after implantation of the biomaterial [14,35,39–43].

Histomorphometric analysis of the clot-treated and biostimulated laser defects, BC^{PBMT}, revealed a gradual and significant increase in bone volume during the experimental periods (8.9 $\pm$ 0.64 to 11.22 $\pm$ 0.94) in relation to the animals of group BC (5.9 $\pm$ 0.38 to 7.06 $\pm$ 0.49) in periods of 14 to 42 days, respectively [44]. The biological mechanisms involved in improving the growth of bone tissue irradiated by a low-power laser are still not clearly understood. Studies suggest that laser energy can excite intracellular chromophores, especially the cytochromes of mitochondria, stimulating the cellular activity and consequently increasing ATP concentration, calcium, protein synthesis, and signalling pathways actively interconnected with the differentiation of stem cells into osteoblasts [45,46].

In the group with defects treated with sealant and xenograft, FSB, the bone formation was increasing between the periods (4.3 ± 0.46 to 6.01 ± 0.32), but in lower volume density compared to the animals of the FSB^{PBMT} group (5.6 ± 0.45 to 10.64 ± 0.97), supporting the positive influence of laser photobiomodulation in the repair process. Similar results were reported by De Oliveira et al. [21] in calvarial defects of autogenous graft-filled rats treated with low-power laser, in which a higher bone formation was also observed in all analysed periods.

The results obtained in this experiment provide evidence that defects filled with fibrin sealant and xenograft, and treated with low-power laser presented an evolution in the tissue repair process, with a better response compared to the other groups investigated, suggesting that there was a photobiomodulatory action in the inflammatory process, with a more organised deposition of collagen fibres in the defect area and consequently with a more homogenous bone conformation.

3.1. Strengths

The present research is a pioneer experimental study on the use of a fibrin sealant derived from human blood and xenograft associated with the protocol of photobiomodulation therapy with the use of low-power laser demonstrating effective repair of nerve and bone lesions. In addition, the association provided ease of insertion, local haemostasis, and maintenance of the implanted materials in the surgical bed, allowing the accomplishment of procedures in a shorter operative time.

3.2. Limitations

One limitation of this study is the absence of a quantitative evaluation of the microtomographic images due to the similar radiopacity between the newly formed bone and the xenograft, which makes it difficult to quantify [47].

For prospective studies requiring repair of bone defects, analysis of other fibrin sealants may be proposed, such as a promising fibrin biopolymer free of human blood components [16], and associations with complementary therapies that present osteogenic potential as pulsed ultrasound (LUPUS) and ultralaser [12].

4. Materials and Methods

4.1. Blood-Derived Biomaterials—Fibrin Sealant

Tisseel Lyo™ (Baxter Healthcare Ltd., Norfolk, United Kingdom; Ministry of Health Registration n^o: 1.0683.0182) is a two-component fibrin sealant that contains two of the proteins that make the blood clot, fibrinogen and thrombin. Tisseel Lyo is prepared as two solutions which mix when applied. When prepared, 1 mL of each solution contains human fibrinogen (as a clotting protein), 91 mg/mL in 3000 UIC/mL protein; aprotinin (synthetic) and human thrombin, 500 UI/mL, in 40 µmol/mL calcium chloride.

Initially, the vials containing lyophilised sealer protein concentrate and aprotinin solution, lyophilised human thrombin, and calcium chloride solution were preheated for approximately three minutes in a water bath at a temperature of 33–37 °C, with the aid of a mercury thermometer (Termometros Labor™, São Paulo, Brazil). Thereafter, the sealant protein concentrate was dissolved with the aprotinin solution to form the sealant solution. Simultaneously, the lyophilised human thrombin was dissolved with the calcium chloride solution to form the thrombin solution. The two solutions were kept in the water bath until use.

4.2. Biomaterial—Xenograft

The commercial demineralised bovine bone matrix (Bio-Oss™; Geistlich Pharma AG, Wolhusen, Switzerland; Ministry of Health Registration n^o: 806.969.30002) is a natural biomaterial available as granules of cancellous bone (0.25–1 mm granule size; 2.0 g vial). The highly purified osteoconductive mineral structure is produced from natural bone in a multi-stage purification process and sterilisation is carried out by γ-irradiation. Thus, it is chemically as well as structurally comparable to the mineralized human bone. Bio-Oss™ contains pores of different sizes: macropores (300–1500 μm), micropores (size of Haversian and vascular marrow canals), and intracrystalline spaces (3–26 nm), resulting in an overall porosity of 70–75% and a wide internal surface area of almost 100 m^2/g [48].

4.3. Experimental Design

Thirty-six adult male Wistar rats (*Rattus norvegicus*), 90 days old, weighing around 400 g, were obtained from the animal laboratory of the Ribeirão Preto campus of the University of São Paulo.

The animals were housed in conventional cages initially containing four animals each (alteration according to the animal weight recommended by the Animal Laboratory of Bauru School of Dentistry—University of São Paulo), with feeders and drinkers "*ad libitum*" (irradiated feed—Nuvilab rodents and filtered water), in an air-conditioned environment, air exhaustion, light-dark period 12L/12D, temperature 22 °C ± 2 °C, humidity 60% ± 10, lighting 150lux/1 m floor, maximum noise 70 dB (decibel—SPL, Sound Pressure Level). All experimental procedures in the animals were conducted with the approval of the Institutional Review Board in Animal Studies of the Bauru School of Dentistry, University of São Paulo (Protocol: CEEPA-019/2016).

Initially, the animals were randomly divided into two groups: BC, *n* = 16 (Blood Clot, the defect was filled with a blood clot) and FSB, *n* = 20 (the defect was filled with a mixture of xenograft and fibrin sealant). After the surgical procedures, four subgroups were preformatted according to the treatment: BC, *n* = 8 (the defect was filled with blood clot without photobiomodulation), BC^{PBMT}, n = 8 (the defect was filled with blood clot and photobiomodulation), FSB, *n* = 10 (the defect was filled with a mixture of fibrin sealant and biomaterial without photobiomodulation) and FSB^{PBMT}, *n* = 10 (the defect was filled with a mixture of fibrin sealant and biomaterial and photobiomodulation) (Figure 4A).

4.4. Surgical Procedures

All surgical procedures were performed at the Mesoscopic Laboratory—discipline of Anatomy (Bauru School of Dentistry, University of São Paulo, Brazil) by the same team of professionals.

The animal surgeries were performed under general anaesthesia with an intramuscular injection of Ketamine (50 mg/kg i.m. (Dopalen ™, Ceva, Paulínia, SP, Brazil) and Xylazine (10 mg/kg i.m. (Anasedan ™, Ceva, Paulínia, SP, Brazil) followed by fronto-parietal trichotomy and disinfection with 10% povidone-iodine (PI). With a scalpel blade n. 10, a half-moon incision was made in the cranial tegument and folded to expose the calvarium. Then, a defect was created in the centre of the parietal bone using an 8 mm diameter trephine bur, under continuous irrigation with saline, exposing the dura mater [20,49] (Figure 4B$_1$). The defects in the BC group were filled with 0.25 mm^3 of cardiac puncture blood [50] (Figure 4B$_2$).

In the FSB group, the defects were filled with 0.1 mm^3 of xenograft incorporated into 40 μL of the reconstituted fibrinogen solution in aprotinin and 40 μL of reconstituted human thrombin solution in sodium chloride (proportion 1:1, according to the manufacturer's recommendations) (Figure 4B$_3$–B$_4$). The amounts of xenograft and fibrin sealant used were previously established in a pilot study.

The periosteum and tegument were repositioned and sutured with nylon 5-0 (Mononylon™, Somerville S.A, NJ, USA) and silk 4-0 (Ethicon™ Johnson & Johnson Company, New Orleans, LA, USA), respectively, to provide stability to the graft, decreasing the risk of soft tissue collapse [20,51].

The postoperative care consisted of a single oral administration of acetaminophen at a dose of 200 mg/kg (Paracetamol, Medley, São Paulo, Brazil) dissolved in water, available in the cages.

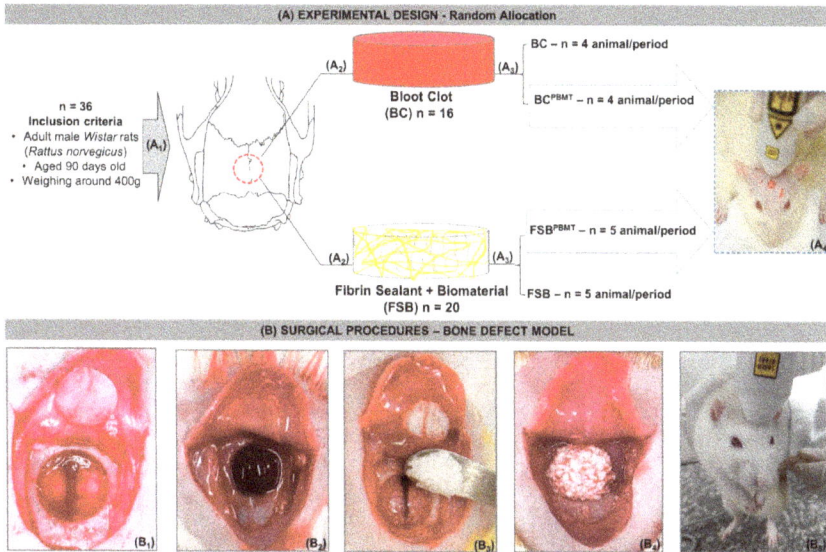

Figure 4. (**A**) Experimental design (**A$_1$**) Random allocation: Thirty-six rats were divided into two groups; (**A$_2$**) BC (*n* = 16)—Blood Clot and FSB (*n* = 20)—Fibrin Sealant + Biomaterial; (**A$_3$**) After surgical procedures, two subgroups were preformatted according to treatment: BC, *n* = 8 (Blood Clot, the defect was filled with blood clot and without photobiomodulation), BC^{PBMT}, *n* = 8 (Blood Clot, the defect was filled with blood clot and photobiomodulation), FSB, *n* = 10 (the defect was filled with a mixture of biomaterial and fibrin sealant and without photobiomodulation), and FSB^{PBMT}, *n* = 10 (the defect was filled with a mixture of biomaterial and fibrin sealant and photobiomodulation); (**A$_4$**) illustration of the four points of cross-application of the low-level laser on rat calvarium; (**B**) Surgical procedures—bone defect model; (**B$_1$**) Osteotomy using an 8 mm trephine bur with exposure of the fragment removed from the parietal bones; (**B$_2$**) defect filled with blood clot; (**B$_3$**) deposition of the mixture fibrin sealant + biomaterial in the defect; (**B$_4$**) defect filled with mixture; (**B$_5$**) low-level laser therapy (photobiostimulation).

4.5. Photobiomodulation Therapy Protocol

The animals of Groups BC^{PBMT} and FSB^{PBMT} underwent laser irradiation (Laserpulse IBRAMED, Amparo, SP, Brazil) with continuous pulse GaAlAs (gallium–aluminium–arsenide). The following parameters were used for photobiomodulation therapy [21]—Table 1 below (Figure 4A$_4$,B$_5$):

Table 1. Therapeutic parameters of the photobiomodulation therapy used in this study.

Parameter	Unit/Explanation
Optical Power	30 mW
Wavelength	830 nm
Density of Power or Irradiance	258.6 mW/cm^2
Fluency or Density of Energy or Dosimetry	6 J/cm^2
Beam Area	0.116 cm^2
Total Power	2.9 J
Type of Beam	Positioned for laser irradiation at perpendicular incidence to the skull
Emission Mode	Continuous (laser power remains constant at all times)
Form of Application	Four points surrounding the surgical area, north, south, east, and west
Duration of Irradiation	24 s/point
Total Time of each Application	96 s
Treatment Time	Immediately after surgery and three times a week until euthanasia

Laser beam emissions were self-calibrated by the device during all applications.

4.6. Collection of Samples and Histological Procedures

All animals were killed with an overdose of a Ketamine/Xylazine mixture following the guidelines of the Brazilian College of Animal Experimentation after 14 and 42 days, BC and BC^PBMT groups—4 animals/period and FSB and FSB^PBMT—5 animals/period. The cranial vaults with the lining skin were collected and fixed in 10% phosphate-buffered formalin for 48 h, and later, for examination in the microtomography.

4.7. MicroCT Scan (μ-CT)

The specimens were subjected to an X-ray beam scan in the computed microtomograph machine SkyScan 1174v2 (μ-CT—Bruker microCT, Kontich, Belgium). Initially they were packaged in an acrylic, cylindrical sample holder, (diameter 18.3 mm; height 10.9 mm), with exo- and endocranial aspects of the parietal bones in the vertical position. The images were captured with 13.76 μm voxel, 0.73° at each pace, and further reconstructed using the NRecon® v.1.6.8.0, SkyScan, 2011, Bruker microCT, with the same reconstruction parameters for all specimens. Then, the reconstructed images were realigned using the DataViewer® 1.4.4.0 software.

4.8. Histotechnical Processing

The specimens were washed in tap water for 24 h and immersed in 10% ethylenediaminetetraacetic acid (EDTA—a solution containing 4.13% Titriplex™ III Merck KGaA, Darmstadt, Germany and 0.44% sodium hydroxide Labsynth, São Paulo, Brazil), for a period of approximately 60 days [52]. Then, the collected bone fragments underwent successive standard histological staging and were finally included in Histosec™ (Merck KGaA, Darmstadt, Germany). Semi-serial coronal cuts of 5 μm thickness were performed, prioritising the centre of the circular defect and stained with haematoxylin-eosin.

4.9. Histological and Histomorphometric Evaluation of Defects Bone Healing

The histological sections were analysed by light microscopy (Olympus model BX50) at approximate magnifications of × 4, 10, and × 40 in the Histology Laboratory of the Bauru School of Dentistry, the University of São Paulo (São Paulo, Brazil). To standardise and avoid bias, a training session was performed with an experienced pathologist.

Histological analysis of sections stained with HE consisted of an evaluative description of the healing events such as inflammation, granulation tissue, new bone formation, and remodelling, and the interaction among the biomaterial bone graft and the newly formed bone.

For morphometric evaluation, two central sections stained with HE were used for quantification of newly formed bone areas using an image capture system (DP Controller 3.2.1.276—2001–2006, Olympus Corporation, Tokyo, Japan). Initially, the total area to be analysed was established as every area of the surgical defect. The limits of this area were determined from the external and internal surfaces of the original calvarium on the right and left margins of the surgical defect. Then, the drawn lines were connected following their respective curvatures. Considering the total length of the defect, its centre point, measuring from this point, was 4 mm to the right and left to the edges of the surgical wound to determine the limits of the original surgical defect.

Morphometric analysis under light microscopy allowed the determination of the volumetric density (%), defined as the volume fraction of the entire graft filled by a given component/structure (newly formed bone). The volume density (Vvi) that is equal to the area density (AAi) was determined by AxioVision Rel. 4.8 Ink (Carl Zeiss MicroImaging GmbH, Jena, Deutschland), $Vvi = AAi$ [53]. The area of graft filled by each structure (Ai) and the total area examined (A) were determined in pixels, and the volume density (Vvi) of each type of structure was calculated according to the relation $Vvi = AAi = Ai/A \times 100$.

4.10. Statistical Analysis

An analysis of variance (ANOVA) was applied to the data obtained for the percentage of newly formed bone to verify the effect of the different groups tested in each evaluated period. The homogeneity of variances and normality of residues and the necessary assumptions for the conduction of ANOVA, were tested, respectively, by the Shapiro–Wilk and Bartlett tests, both at 5% probability. Subsequently, the means were compared by the Tukey test at 5% probability. The effect of the period evaluated in each group was compared by Student's *t*-test at 5%. All analyses were conducted with R (R Core Team, 2017).

5. Conclusions

It was concluded that the support system formed by the xenograft fibrin sealant associated with the photobiomodulation therapy protocol had a positive effect on the bone repair process in critical size defects in rat calvaria.

Author Contributions: Conceptualization—K.T.P. and R.L.B.; Data collection—K.T.P.; Formal analysis—K.T.P., M.P.A., M.A.H.D. and D.d.B.T.; Methodology—K.T.P., M.P.d.O.R., D.V.B., B.B.D.C., J.V.T.C.S., I.J.S.G., A.L.S., G.M.R.J. and A.C.C.B.; Resources—J.C.A. and R.L.B.; Supervision—R.L.B.; Visualization—K.T.P., D.V.B., T.M.C. and R.L.B.; Writing of original draft—K.T.P., D.V.B. and R.L.B.; Writing, review, and editing—K.T.P. and R.L.B.

Funding: This study was financed in part by Coordenação de Aperfeiçoamento de Pessoal de Nível Superior—Brasil (CAPES)—Finance Code 001. The content is solely the responsibility of the authors and does not necessarily represent the official views of the funding agencies.

Conflicts of Interest: The authors declare no conflict of interest.

References

1. Nee, E.A.; Chrzanowski, W.; Salih, V.; Kim, H.; Knowles, J. Tissue engineering in dentistry. *J. Dent.* **2014**, *42*, 915–928. [CrossRef]
2. Buchaim, D.V.; Bueno, P.C.D.S.; Andreo, J.C.; Roque, D.D.; Roque, J.S.; Zilio, M.G.; Salatin, J.A.; Kawano, N.; Furlanette, G.; Buchaim, R.L. Action of a deproteinized xenogenic biomaterial in the process of bone repair in rats submitted to inhalation of cigarette smoke. *Acta Cir. Bras.* **2018**, *33*, 324–332. [CrossRef]
3. Pomini, K.; Cestari, M.; German, I.; Rosso, M.; Gonçalves, J.; Buchaim, D.; Pereira, M.; Andreo, J.; Júnior, G.M.R.; della Coletta, B.; et al. Influence of experimental alcoholism on the repair process of bone defects filled with beta-tricalcium phosphate. *Drug Alcohol Depend.* **2019**, *197*, 315–325. [CrossRef]
4. Campana, V.; Milano, G.; Pagano, E.; Barba, M.; Cicione, C.; Salonna, G.; Lattanzi, W.; Logroscino, G. Bone substitutes in orthopaedic surgery: From basic science to clinical practice. *J. Mater. Sci. Mater. Med.* **2014**, *25*, 2445–2461. [CrossRef] [PubMed]
5. Wang, W.; Yeung, K.W.K. Bioactive Materials Bone grafts and biomaterials substitutes for bone defect repair: A review. *Bioact. Mater.* **2017**, *2*, 224–247. [CrossRef]
6. Giannoudis, P.V.; Dinopoulos, H.; Tsiridis, E.; Jones, E.; Einhorn, T.A. Bone substitutes: An update. *Injury* **2005**, *42*, 549–550. [CrossRef]
7. Giannoudis, P.V.; Jones, E.; Einhorn, T.A. Fracture healing and bone repair. *Injury* **2011**, *42*, 549–550. [CrossRef]
8. Melek, L.N. ScienceDirect Tissue engineering in oral and maxillofacial reconstruction. *Tanta Dent. J.* **2015**, *12*, 211–223. [CrossRef]
9. Chen, F.; Liu, X. Advancing biomaterials of human origin for tissue engineering. *Prog. Polym. Sci.* **2017**, *53*, 86–168. [CrossRef] [PubMed]
10. Kim, Y.; Kim, S.; Yun, P. Autogenous teeth used for bone grafting: A comparison with tradicional grafting materials. *Oral Maxillofac. Surg.* **2014**, *117*, e39–e45. [CrossRef] [PubMed]
11. Burnouf, T.; Su, C.; Radosevich, M.; Goubran, H. Blood-derived biomaterials: Fibrin sealant. *Platelet Gel Platelet Fibrin Glue* **2009**, *4*, 136–142.
12. Pomini, K.T.; Andreo, J.C.; de Rodrigues, A.C.; de Gonçalves, J.B.O.; Daré, L.R.; German, I.J.S.; Rosa, G.M.; Buchaim, R.L. Effect of low-intensity pulsed ultrasound on bone regeneration biochemical and radiologic analyses. *J. Ultrasound Med.* **2014**, *33*, 713–717. [CrossRef] [PubMed]

13. Bayat, M.; Virdi, A.; Jalalifirouzkouhi, R.; Rezaei, F. Comparison of effects of LLLT and LIPUS on fracture healing in animal models and patients: A systematic review. *Prog. Biophys. Mol. Biol.* **2018**, *132*, 3–22. [CrossRef] [PubMed]

14. De Oliveira, L.; de Araújo, A.; Júnior, R.d.; Barboza, C.; Borges, B.; da Silva, J. Low-level laser therapy (780 nm) combined with collagen sponge scaffold promotes repair of rat cranial critical-size defects and increases TGF-b, FGF-2, OPG/RANK and osteocalcin expression. *Int. J. Exp. Pathol.* **2017**, *98*, 75–85. [CrossRef] [PubMed]

15. Kulkarni, S.; Meer, M.; George, R.; George, R. Efficacy of photobiomodulation on accelerating bone healing after tooth extraction: A systematic review. *Lasers Med. Sci.* **2018**. [CrossRef]

16. Barbizan, R.; Castro, M.; Junior, R.F.; Barraviera, B.; Oliveira, A. Long-Term Spinal Ventral Root Reimplantation, but not Bone Marrow Mononuclear Cell Treatment, Positively Influences Ultrastructural Synapse Recovery and Motor Axonal Regrowth. *Int. J. Mol. Sci.* **2014**, *15*, 19535–19551. [CrossRef] [PubMed]

17. Noori, A.; Ashrafi, S.; Vaez-Ghaemi, R.; Hatamian-Zaremi, A.; Webster, T. A review of fibrin and fibrin composites for bone tissue engineering. *Int. J. Nanomed.* **2017**, *12*, 4937–4961. [CrossRef] [PubMed]

18. Taniyama, K.; Shirakata, Y.; Yoshimoto, T.; Takeuchi, N.; Yoshihara, Y.; Noguchi, K. Bone formation using β-tricalcium phosphate/carboxymethyl-chitin composite scaffold in rat calvarial defects. *Oral Surg. Oral Med. Oral Pathol. Oral Radiol.* **2013**, *116*, e450–e456. [CrossRef]

19. Tani, A.; Chellini, F.; Giannelli, M.; Zecchi-orlandini, S.; Sassoli, C. Red (635 nm), Near-Infrared (808 nm) and Violet-Blue (405 nm) Photobiomodulation Potentiality on Human Osteoblasts and Mesenchymal Stromal Cells: A Morphological and Molecular In Vitro Study. *Int. J. Mol. Sci.* **2018**, *19*, 1946. [CrossRef]

20. Spicer, P.P.; Kretlow, J.D.; Young, S.; Jansen, J.A.; Kasper, F.K.; Mikos, A.G. Evaluation of bone regeneration using the rat critical size calvarial defect. *Nat. Protoc.* **2012**, *7*, 1918–1929. [CrossRef]

21. De Gonçalves, J.; Buchaim, D.; de Bueno, C.; Pomini, K.; Barraviera, B.; Júnior, R.; Andreo, J.; de Rodrigues, A.; Cestari, T.; Buchaim, R.L. Effects of low-level laser therapy on autogenous bone graft stabilized with a new heterologous fibrin sealant. *J. Photochem. Photobiol. B Biol.* **2016**, *162*, 663–668. [CrossRef] [PubMed]

22. Basford, J.R. Low intensity laser therapy: Still not an established clinical tool. *Lasers Surg. Med.* **1995**, *16*, 331–342. [CrossRef] [PubMed]

23. Karu, T.I.; Afanas'eva, N.I. Cytochrome c oxidase as the primary photoacceptor upon laser exposure of cultured cells to visible and near IR-range light. *Dokl Akad Nauk.* **1995**, *342*, 693–695.

24. Lappalainen, O.; Korpi, R.; Haapea, M.; Korpi, J.; Ylikontiola, L.P.; Kallio-pulkkinen, S.; Serlo, W.S.; Lehenkari, P.; Sándor, G.K. Healing of rabbit calvarial critical-sized defects using autogenous bone grafts and fibrin glue. *Child's Nerv. Syst.* **2015**, *31*, 581–587. [CrossRef] [PubMed]

25. Sawyer, A.; Song, S.; Susanto, E.; Chuan, P.; Lam, C.; Woodruff, M.; Hutmacher, D.; Cool, S. Biomaterials The stimulation of healing within a rat calvarial defect by mPCL–TCP/collagen scaffolds loaded with rhBMP-2. *Biomaterials* **2009**, *30*, 2479–2488. [CrossRef]

26. Brown, A.; Barker, T. Fibrin-based biomaterials: Modulation of macroscopic properties through rational design at the molecular level Ashley. *Acta Biomater.* **2015**, *10*, 1502–1514. [CrossRef] [PubMed]

27. Scognamiglio, F.; Travan, A.; Rustighi, I.; Tarchi, P.; Palmisano, S.; Marsich, E.; Borgogna, M.; Donati, I.; de Manzini, N.; Paoletti, S. Review Article Adhesive and sealant interfaces for general surgery applications. *J. Biomed. Mater. Res. Part B Appl. Biomater.* **2016**, *104*, 626–639. [CrossRef]

28. Ruvalcaba-Paredes, E.K.; Hidalgo-Bastida, L.A.; Sesman-Bernal, A.L.; Garciadiego-Cazares, D.; Pérez-Dosal, M.R.; Martínez-López, V.; Vargas-Sandoval, B.; Pichardo-Bahena, R.; Ibarra, C.; Velasquillo, C. Osteogenic potential of murine periosteum for critical-size cranial defects. *Br. J. Oral Maxillofac. Surg.* **2016**, *54*, 772–777. [CrossRef] [PubMed]

29. Rocha, C.A.; Cestari, T.M.; Vidotti, H.A.; de Assis, G.F.; Garlet, G.P.; Taga, R. Sintered anorganic bone graft increases autocrine expression of VEGF, MMP-2 and MMP-9 during repair of critical-size bone defects. *J. Mol. Histol.* **2014**, *45*, 447–461. [CrossRef] [PubMed]

30. Maciel, J.; Momesso, G.; Ramalho-Ferreira, G.; Consolaro, R.; de Carvalho, P.P.; Faverani, L.; Bassi, A.F.; Gosain, A.; Song, L.; Yu, P.; et al. Bone Healing Evaluation in Critical-Size Defects Treated With Xenogenous Bone Plus Porcine Collagen. *Implant Dent.* **2017**, *26*, 296–302. [CrossRef]

31. Gosain, A.; Song, L.; Yu, P.; Mehrara, B.; Maeda, C.; Gold, L.; Longaker, M. Experimental Osteogenesis in Cranial Defects: Reassessment of the Concept of Critical Size and the Expression of TGF-beta isoforms. *Plast. Reconstr. Surg.* **2000**, *106*, 360–371. [CrossRef]

32. An, Y.; Heo, Y.; Lee, J.; Jung, U.; H, C.S. Dehydrothermally Cross-Linked Collagen Membrane with a Bone Graft Improves Bone Regeneration in a Rat Calvarial Defect Model. *Materials* **2017**, *10*, 927. [CrossRef]

33. De Oliveira, A.; Castro-silva, I.; Vicentis, G.; Fernandes, O. Effectiveness and Acceleration of Bone Repair in Critical-Sized Rat Calvarial Defects Using Low-Level Laser Therapy Effectiveness and Acceleration of Bone Repair in Critical-Sized Rat Calvarial Defects Using Low-Level Laser Therapy. *Lasers Surg. Med.* **2014**, *46*, 61–67. [CrossRef]

34. Ozawa, Y.; Shimizu, N.; Kariya, G.; Abiko, Y. Low-Energy Laser Irradiation Stimulates Bone Nodule Formation at Early Stages of Cell Culture in Rat Calvarial Cells. *Bone* **1998**, *22*, 347–354. [CrossRef]

35. Marques, L.; Holgado, L.A.; Francischone, L.A.; Ximenez, J.P.B.; Okamoto, R.; Kinoshita, A. New LLLT protocol to speed up the bone healing process—Histometric and immunohistochemical analysis in rat calvarial bone defect. *Lasers Med. Sci.* **2015**, *30*, 1225–1230. [CrossRef]

36. Le Guéhennec, L.; Layrolle, P.; Daculsi, G. A review of bioceramics and fibrin sealant. *Eur. Cell Mater* **2004**, *8*, 1e11. [CrossRef]

37. Buchta, C.; Christian, H.; Macher, M. Biochemical characterization of autologous fibrin sealants produced by CryoSeal s and Vivostat s in comparison to the homologous fibrin sealant product Tissucol/Tisseel s. *Biomaterials* **2005**, *26*, 6233–6241. [CrossRef]

38. Pavel, Š.; Strnadová, M.; Urban, K. In vivo behaviour of low-temperature calcium-deficient hydroxyapatite: Comparison with deproteinised bovine bone. *Int. Orthop.* **2011**, *35*, 1553–1560. [CrossRef]

39. Aamodt, J.M.; Grainger, D.W. Extracellular matrix-based biomaterial scaffolds and the host response. *Biomaterials* **2016**, *86*, 68–82. [CrossRef]

40. De Almeida, A.L.P.F.; Medeiros, I.L.; Cunha, M.J.S.; Sbrana, M.C.; de Oliveira, P.G.F.P.; Esper, L.A. The effect of low-level laser on bone healing in critical size defects treated with or without autogenous bone graft: An experimental study in rat calvaria. *Clin. Oral Implant. Res.* **2014**, *25*, 1131–1136. [CrossRef]

41. Bosco, A.; Faleiros, P.; Carmona, L.; Garcia, V.; Theodoro, L.; de Araujo, N.; Nagata, M.; de Almeida, J. Effects of low-level laser therapy on bone healing of critical-size defects treated with bovine bone graft. *J. Photochem. Photobiol. B Biol.* **2016**, *163*, 303–310. [CrossRef]

42. Kazancioglu, H.O.; Ezirganli, S.; Aydin, M.S.; Dds, Þ. Effects of Laser and Ozone Therapies on Bone Healing in the Calvarial Defects. *J. Craniofacial Surg.* **2013**, *24*, 2141–2146. [CrossRef]

43. De Deco, C.P.; Marchini, A.M.P.d.; Marchini, L.; da Rocha, R.F. Extended Periods of Alcohol Intake Negatively Affects Osseointegration in Rats. *J. Oral Implantol.* **2015**, *41*, e44–e49. [CrossRef]

44. Moreira, G.; Henry, P.; Alves, M.; Esper, L.; Sbrana, M.; Dalben, S.; Neppelenbroek, K.; de Almeida, A. Effect of Low-Level Laser on the Healing of Bone Defects Filled with Autogenous Bone or Bioactive Glass: In Vivo Study. *Int. J. Oral Maxillofac. Implant.* **2018**, *33*, 169–174. [CrossRef]

45. Kushibiki, T.; Hirasawa, T.; Okawa, S.; Ishihara, M. Regulation of miRNA Expression by Low-Level Laser Therapy (LLLT) and Photodynamic Therapy (PDT). *Int. J. Mol. Sci.* **2013**, *14*, 13542–13558. [CrossRef]

46. Migliario, M.; Pittarella, P.; Fanuli, M.; Rizzi, M.; Renò, F. Laser-induced osteoblast proliferation is mediated by ROS production. *Lasers Med. Sci.* **2014**, *29*, 1463–1467. [CrossRef]

47. Pekkan, G.; Aktas, A.; Pekkan, K. Comparative radiopacity of bone graft materials Comparative radiopacity of bone graft materials. *J. Cranio-Maxillofacial Surg.* **2011**, *40*, e1–e4. [CrossRef]

48. Carinci, F.; Piattelli, A.; Degidi, M.; Palmieri, A.; Perrotti, V.; Scapoli, L.; Martinelli, M.; Laino, G.; Pezzetti, F. Genetic effects of anorganic bovine bone (Bio-OssW) on osteoblast-like MG63 cells. *Arch. Oral Biol.* **2006**, *51*, 154–163. [CrossRef]

49. Lee, J.; Ryu, M.; Baek, H.; Lee, K.; Seo, J.; Lee, H. Fabrication and Evaluation of Porous Beta-Tricalcium Phosphate/Hydroxyapatite (60/40) Composite as a Bone Graft Extender Using Fabrication and Evaluation of Porous Beta-Tricalcium Phosphate/Hydroxyapatite (60/40) Composite as a Bone Graft Exte. *Sci. World J.* **2013**, *481789*. [CrossRef]

50. Parasuraman, S.; Raveendran, R.; Kesavan, R. Blood sample collection in small laboratory animals. *J. Pharmacol. Pharmacother.* **2010**, *1*, 87. [CrossRef]

51. Neagu, T.P.; Ţigliş, M.; Cocoloş, I.; Jecan, C.R. The relationship between periosteum and fracture healing, *Rom. J. Morphol. Embryol.* **2016**, *57*, 1215–1220.

52. Warshawsky, H.; Moore, G. elect U41. *J. Histochem. Cytochem.* **1967**, *15*, 542–549. [CrossRef]
53. Weibel, E.R. Stereological Principles for Morphometry in Electron Microscopic Cytology. *Int. Rev. Cytol.* **1969**, *26*, 235–302. [CrossRef]

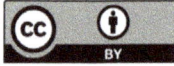

International Journal of
Molecular Sciences

MDPI

Review

Autologous Platelet Concentrates in Treatment of Furcation Defects—A Systematic Review and Meta-Analysis

Sourav Panda [1,2], Lorena Karanxha [1], Funda Goker [1], Anurag Satpathy [2], Silvio Taschieri [1,3], Luca Francetti [1,3], Abhaya Chandra Das [2], Manoj Kumar [2], Sital Panda [4] and Massimo Del Fabbro [1,3,*]

1   Department of Biomedical, Surgical and Dental Sciences, Università degli Studi di Milano, 20122 Milan, Italy; drsaurav87@gmail.com (S.P.); lorikaranxha@gmail.com (L.K.); fundagoker@yahoo.com (F.G.); silviotaschieri@gmail.com (S.T.); luca.francetti@unimi.it (L.F.)
2   Institute of Dental Science and SUM Hospital, Siksha O Anusandhan University, Bhubaneswar 751003, India; dearanurag@gmail.com (A.S.); drabhaya2011@gmail.com (A.C.D.); manojkumar@soa.ac.in (M.K.)
3   Dental Clinic, IRCCS Istituto Ortopedico Galeazzi, 20161 Milan, Italy
4   Department of Public Health, Regional Medical Research Center, Bhubaneswar 751003, India; drsheetalpanda@gmail.com
*   Correspondence: massimo.delfabbro@unimi.it; Tel.: +39-02-50319950; Fax: +39-02-50319960

check for
updates

Received: 1 February 2019; Accepted: 12 March 2019; Published: 17 March 2019

Abstract: Background: The aim of this review was to evaluate the adjunctive effect of autologous platelet concentrates (APCs) for the treatment of furcation defects, in terms of scientific quality of the clinical trials and regeneration parameters assessment. Methods: A systematic search was carried out in the electronic databases MEDLINE, SCOPUS, CENTRAL (Cochrane Central Register of Controlled Trials), and EMBASE, together with hand searching of relevant journals. Two independent reviewers screened the articles yielded in the initial search and retrieved the full-text version of potentially eligible studies. Relevant data and outcomes were extracted from the included studies. Risk of bias assessment was also carried out. The outcome variables, relative to baseline and post-operative defect characteristics (probing pocket depth (PPD), horizontal and vertical clinical attachment loss (HCAL, VCAL), horizontal and vertical furcation depth (HFD, VFD) were considered for meta-analysis. Results: Ten randomized trials were included in this review. Only one study was judged at high risk of bias, while seven had a low risk, testifying to the good level of the evidence of this review. The meta-analysis showed a favorable effect regarding all outcome variables, for APCs used in adjunct to open flap debridement ($p < 0.001$). Regarding APCs in adjunct to bone grafting, a significant advantage was found only for HCAL ($p < 0.001$, mean difference 0.74, 95% CI 0.54, 0.94). The sub-group analysis showed that both platelet-rich fibrin and platelet-rich plasma in adjunct with open flap debridement, yielded significantly favorable results. No meta-analysis was performed for APCs in combination with guided tissue regeneration (GTR) as only one study was found. Conclusion: For the treatment of furcation defects APCs may be beneficial as an adjunct to open flap debridement alone and bone grafting, while limited evidence of an effect of APCs when used in combination with GTR was found.

Keywords: autologous platelet concentrates; bone defects; bone grafting; bone regeneration; furcation defects; periodontal defects; periodontal regeneration; periodontal surgery; platelet-rich plasma; platelet-rich fibrin; plasma rich in growth factors; tissue healing

1. Introduction

Furcation involvement is defined as bone resorption and attachment loss in the inter-radicular space that results from plaque associated periodontal disease [1]. The treatment of periodontal disease associated with furcation represents a challenge for the clinician, due to the complexity in anatomy and morphology of such area. The unfavorable anatomic feature of the furcation restricts adequate instrumentation for proper debridement, thereby limiting the prognosis of the involved teeth [2].

Various treatment modalities, including surgical and non-surgical therapy, have been proposed to improve the prognosis based on the degree of furcation involvement. Several classifications have been proposed over the years (Table 1), based either on the severity of horizontal probing depth into the furcation defect or on the vertical amount of alveolar bone loss within the defect [3]. The most popular one was developed by Glickman, which divides furcation defects into four grades [4]. Non-surgical strategies such as scaling and root planing, furcation-plasty, etc. are employed to treat the furcations with Grade I initial involvement which restores the gingival health. Conversely, surgical procedures including regenerative and resective approaches, are performed for the treatment of more advanced lesions, to allow access to the internal complex areas of furcations. The traditional resective approach may negatively affect the long term prognosis of the treated teeth, however, it is considered as the treatment of choice for grade III and IV furcation lesions, aiming at facilitating maintenance of the furcation area.

Regenerative approaches are aimed at furcation closure by the formation of new bone, cementum and periodontal ligament in the involved inter-radicular space. Thorough debridement with adequate instrumentation following surgical exposure of furcation involved area, is one of the earliest and most well-documented treatment protocols to achieve regeneration in grade II furcation lesions [5]. In addition, various studies were carried out in the recent past, using bone substitutes, barrier membrane, autologous, and recombinant growth factors in order to provide evidence of improved bone fill and attachment gain in treating grade II furcation lesions [6,7].

The use of biologic agents consisting of growth and differentiation factors like rhBMP2 (recombinant human bone morphogenetic protein-2), rhPDGF (recombinant human platelet-derived growth factor), and TGF-β (transforming growth factor beta), had proven to promote osteogenic induction in cases of furcation treatment, in animal studies [8–10]. Additionally, the use of autologous platelet concentrates (APCs) is gaining popularity as a source of multiple growth factors in high concentrations, for regenerative treatments in many clinical applications. The contribution of blood-derived platelets to the bone healing process is mainly based on the growth factors stored in their granules and released upon activation. Autologous platelet concentrates are advantageously used as a cost-effective adjunct to surgical regenerative therapy, even in combination with bone grafts and barrier membranes. Several randomized controlled trials have reported on the efficacy of the use of these APCs when used alone or in combination with various regenerative strategies and other biologic agents, suggesting improvement of post-operative soft and hard tissue healing, and improved bone fill and attachment gain [6,11–17]. Different types of APCs are available, each with peculiar features, the most popular being platelet-rich plasma (PRP), along with platelet-rich fibrin (PRF), plasma rich in growth factors (PRGF) and concentrated growth factors (CGF).

A recent systematic review and meta-analysis [18], evaluating the effect of use of platelet-rich fibrin (PRF) in adjunct to open flap debridement, included two clinical trials in treatment of grade II furcation with nine month follow-up and concluded favorable results with the use of PRF in terms of clinical attachment level gain (mean difference 1.25 CI 95% [0.82, 1.65], $p = 0.07$) and bone fill (mean difference 1.52 CI 95% [1.18, 1.87], $p = 0.05$). Another systematic review [19] included two split-mouth clinical trials evaluating the effect of platelet-rich plasma and reported no consistent evidence regarding the effect of PRP in treatment of furcation defects.

The aim of this systematic review is to evaluate the adjunctive effect of APCs in treatment of furcation defects both qualitatively and quantitatively, in terms of scientific quality of the clinical trials and regeneration parameters assessment.

Table 1. Various proposed classification systems of furcation involvement.

Sl	Author	Year	Classification System
			Horizontal Component
1	Goldman, H.M [20]	1958	Grade I: Incipient lesion; Grade II: Cul-de-sac lesion; Grade III: Through-and-through lesion
2	Staffileno, H.J. [21]	1969	Class I: Furcations with a soft tissue lesion extending to furcal level but with a minor degree of osseous destruction; Class II: Furcations with a soft tissue lesion and a variable degree of osseous destruction but not a through-and-through communication through the furca; Class III: Furcations with osseous destruction with through-and-through communication
3	Glickman, I. [4]	1972	Grade I: Incipient lesion. Suprabony pocket and slight bone loss in the furcation area. Grade II: Loss of interradicular bone and pocket formation but a portion of the alveolar bone and periodontal ligament remain intact. Grade III: Through-and-through lesion. Grade IV: Through-and-through lesion with gingival recession, leading to a clearly visible furcation area.
4	Hamp, S.E. et al. [22]	1975	Degree I: Horizontal attachment loss < 3 mm; Degree II: Horizontal attachment loss > 3 mm not encompassing the width of the furcation area; Degree III: Horizontal through-and-through destruction of the periodontal tissue in the furcation area.
5	Ramjford, S.P. et al. [23]	1979	Class I: Tissue destruction < 2 mm (1/3 of tooth width) into the furcation; Class II: Tissue destruction > 2 mm (>1/3 of tooth width); Class III: Through-and-through involvement.
6	Richietti, P.A. [24]	1982	Class I: 1 mm of horizontal invasion; Class Ia. 1–2 mm of horizontal invasion; Class II: 2–4 mm of horizontal invasion; Class IIa. 4–6 mm of horizontal invasion; Class III: >6 mm of horizontal invasion.
7	Grant, D.A. et al. [25]	1988	Class I: Involvement of the flute only; Class II: Involvement partially under the roof; Class III: Through-and-through loss.
8	Goldman, H.M. et al. [26]	1988	Degree I: Involves furcation entrance; Degree II: Involvement extends under the roof of furcation; Degree III: Through-and-through involvement.
9	Basaraba, N. [27]	1990	Class I: Initial furcation involvement; Class II: Partial furcation involvement; Class III: Communicating furcation involvement.
10	Nevins, M. et al. [28]	1998	Class I: Incipient or early loss of attachment; Class II: A deeper invasion and loss of attachment that does not extend to a complete invasion; Class III: Complete loss of periodontium extending from buccal to lingual surface. Diagnosed radiographically and clinically
11	Walter, C.et al [29]	2009	Modification of the Hamp et al. classification. Degree I: Horizontal attachment loss < 1/3 of the width of the tooth; Degree II: Horizontal loss of support > 3 mm, < 6 mm; Degree II–III: Horizontal loss of support > 6 mm, but not extending completely. Degree III: Horizontal through-and-through destruction.
12	Carnevale, G. et al. [30]	2012	Degree I: Horizontal attachment loss < 1/3; Degree II: Horizontal attachment loss > 1/3; Degree III: Horizontal through-and-through destruction.
			Vertical Component
1	Tal, H. et al. [31]	1982	Furcal rating 1: Depth of the furcation is 0 mm; Furcal rating 2: Depth of the furcation is 1–2 mm; Furcal rating 3: Depth of the furcation is 3 mm; Furcal rating 4: Depth of the furcation is 4 mm or more.

Table 1. *Cont.*

Sl	Author	Year	Classification System
2	Eskow, R.N. et al. [32]	1984	Furcation involvement grade 1 is classified as: Subclass A: Vertical destruction > 1/3; Subclass B: Vertical destruction of 2/3; Subclass C: Vertical destruction beyond the apical third of interradicular height.
3	Tarnow, D. et al. [33]	1985	For each class of horizontal classification (I–III), a subclass based on the vertical bone resorption was added: Subclass A: 0–3 mm; Subclass B: 4–6 mm; Subclass C: >7 mm.
	Horizontal & Vertical Component (Combined)		
1	Easley, J.R. et al. [34]	1969	Class I: Incipient involvement, but there is no horizontal component to the furca; Class II: Type 1. Horizontal attachment loss into the furcation; Type 2. Vertical attachment loss into the furcation; Class III: Through-and-through attachment loss into the furcation; Type 1. Horizontal attachment loss into the furcation; Type 2. Vertical attachment loss into the furcation.
2	Fedi, P.F. [35]	1985	Glickman + Hamp classifications: Grades are the same as Glickman's classification (I–IV); Grade II is subdivided into degrees I and II; Degree I. Vertical bone loss 1–3 mm; Degree II. Vertical bone loss > 3 mm, but not communicate through-and-through.
3	Rosemberg, M.M. [36]	1986	Horizontal: Degree I: Probing < 4 mm; Degree II: Probing > 4 mm; Degree III: Two or three furcations classified as degree II are found. Vertical: Shallow: Slight lateral extension of an interradicular defect, from the center of the trifurcation in a horizontal direction; Deep: Internal furcation involvement but not penetrating the adjacent furcation.
4	Hou, G.L. et al. [37]	1998	Classification based on root trunk length and horizontal and vertical bone loss. Types of root trunk: • Type A: Furcation involving a cervical third of root length; • Type B: Furcation involving a cervical third and two thirds of root length; • Type C: Furcation involving a cervical two thirds of root length. Classes of furcation: • Class I: Horizontal loss of 3 mm; • Class II: Horizontal loss > 3 mm; • Class III: Horizontal "through-and-through" loss. Subclasses by radiographic assessment of the periapical view: • Sub-class 'a'. Suprabony defect; • Sub-class 'b'. Infrabony defect.

2. Results

2.1. Study Characteristics

A total of ten studies were included in this systematic review after independent screening of titles and abstracts from a pool of 153 articles retrieved from the search platforms. The systematic flow chart of the study selection process is provided in Figure 1. Out of 21 eligible studies, 11 studies were excluded with reasons provided in Table 2. The general information and the study characteristics of the included studies are detailed in Table 3.

The general comparison was between a group that received APC as an adjunct to surgical treatment (experimental group), and a group that received surgical treatment alone (control group). Three different types of comparisons were assessed, based on the treatment type. Five studies reported the comparison of open flap debridement (OFD) + APC versus OFD alone (Bajaj 2009 study evaluated the adjunctive effects of two different types of APCs in the same study, compared to OFD alone as the control group). Four studies reported the comparison of bone graft (BG) + APC versus BG alone, and only one study reported the comparison of guided tissue regeneration (GTR) + APC versus GTR alone. The results of these studies were separated for types of platelet concentrate data to facilitate subgroup meta-analysis for OFD + APC versus OFD comparison. However, it was impossible to undertake the subgroup analysis for the other two comparisons due to the lack of enough studies for sub-grouping. The risk of bias of all included studies is synthesized in Figure 2.

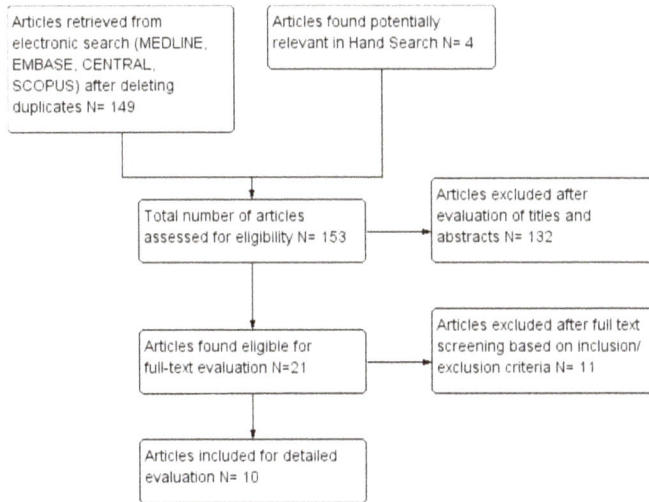

Figure 1. Flow chart depicting study selection process.

Table 2. List of excluded studies.

Study & Year	Reason for Exclusion
Mehta et al. 2018 [38]	Use of Collagen Membrane along with DFDBA in control group
Wanikar et al. 2018 [39]	Both Control and Experimental group use PRF
Kaur et al. 2018 [40]	Both Control and Experimental group use PRF
Sharma et al. 2017 [41]	Both Control and Experimental group use PRF
Asimuddin et al. 2017 [42]	Comparison between use of PRF and Allograft + GTR
Salaria et al. 2016 [43]	Case Report
Biswas et al. 2016 [44]	Comparison between PRF and Bioactive Glass.
Pradeep et al. 2016 [45]	Both Control and Experimental group uses PRF
Sandhu et al. 2015 [46]	Case Report
Mellonig et al. 2009 [47]	Histological assessment
Lekovic et al. 2003 [48]	Comparison of PRP/BPBM/GTR versus OFD alone

PRF—platelet-rich fibrin, PRP—platelet-rich plasma, DFDBA—de-mineralized freeze-dried allograft, BPBM—bovine porous bone mineral, GTR—guided tissue regeneration.

Table 3. Characteristics of included studies.

Study & Year	Study Design	RCT Type	Treatment Comparison	N. Defects Test/Control	Age Range	Gender M/F	Follow Up
Kanoriya et al. 2017 [13]	RCT	Parallel	OFD vs. OFD + PRF	26/26	30–50 (38)	36/36	9 m
Siddiqui et al. 2016 [49]	RCT	Parallel	OFD vs. OFD + PRF	17/17	30–50	24/7	6 m
Bajaj et al. 2013 [11]	RCT	Parallel	OFD vs. OFD + PRP OFD vs. OFD + PRF	27/27 27/27	39.4	22/20	9 m
Sharma et al. 2011 [17]	RCT	Split Mouth	OFD vs. OFD + PRF	18/18	34.2	10/8	9 m

Table 3. *Cont.*

Study & Year	Study Design	RCT Type	Treatment Comparison	N. Defects Test/Control	Age Range	Gender M/F	Follow Up
Pradeep et al. 2009 [6]	RCT	Split Mouth	OFD vs. OFD + PRP	20/20	42.8	10/10	6 m
Lohi et al. 2017 [14]	RCT	Parallel	BCCG + PRF vs. BCCG alone	10/10	25–65 (43.05 + 10.73)	12/4	6 m
Lafzi et al. 2013 [15]	RCT	Parallel	ABG + PRGF vs. ABG alone	15/15	NR	NR	6 m
Mansouri et al. 2012 [50]	RCT	Split Mouth	BPBM + PRGF vs. BPBM alone	7/7	44.7 + 11.2	4/3	6 m
Qiao et al. 2017 [16]	RCT	Parallel	BG + CGF vs. CGF alone	15/16	NR	15/5	12 m
Jenabian et al. 2017 [12]	RCT	Split Mouth	GTR + PRGF vs. GTR alone	8/8	NR	NR	6 m

RCT—randomized clinical trial, OFD—open flap debridement, PRF—platelet-rich fibrin, PRP—platelet-rich plasma, BCCG—bioactive ceramic composite granules, ABG—autogenous bone graft, BG—bone graft, GTR—guided tissue regeneration.

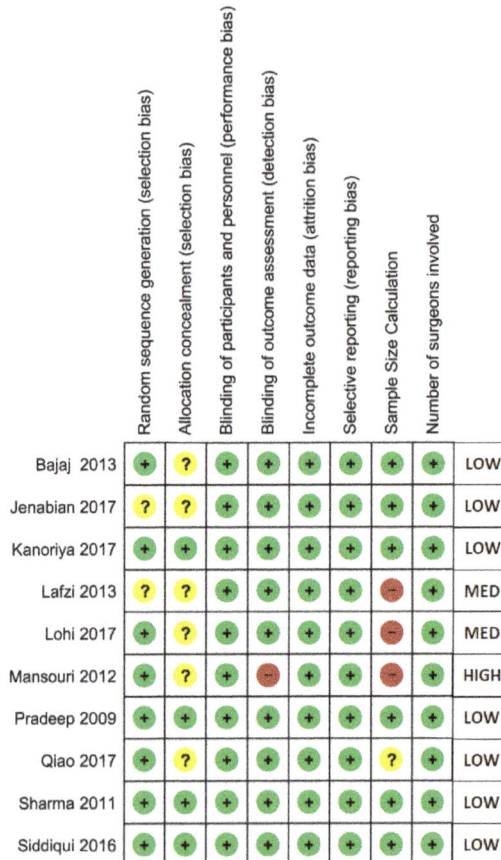

Figure 2. Risk of bias (RoB) assessment.

2.2. Meta-Analysis of Primary Outcomes

2.2.1. Probing Pocket Depth (PPD)

APC + OFD vs. OFD Alone (Figure 3)

The forest plot of the included studies evaluating the change in PPD shows evidence of an advantage of using APC in adjunct to OFD ($p < 0.001$, mean difference 1.59, 95% CI 1.38, 1.80). The subgroup analysis is also favorable for both PRF ($p < 0.001$, mean difference 1.46, 95% CI 1.22, 1.70) and PRP ($p < 0.001$, mean difference 2.09, 95% CI 1.62, 2.55).

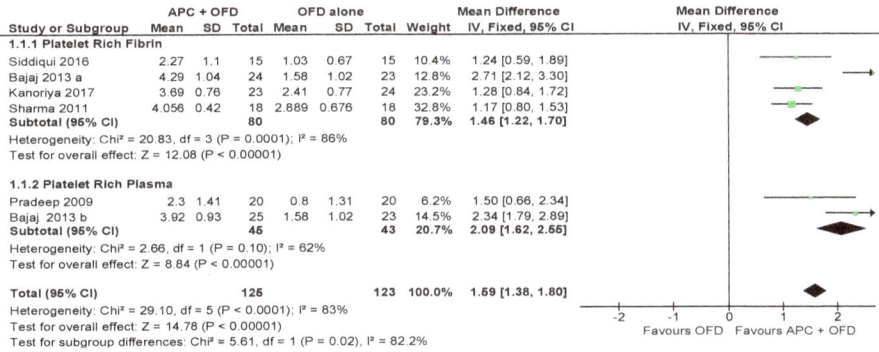

Figure 3. Forest plot showing the effect on probing pocket depth for comparison of APC + OFD versus OFD alone at end of all-follow-up (6–12 m).

APC + BG vs. BG Alone (Figure 4)

The forest plot of the included studies evaluating the change in PPD in using APC in adjunct with BG favors the use of BG alone; however, the result is not statistically significant ($p = 0.26$, mean difference -0.08, 95% CI -0.22, 0.06).

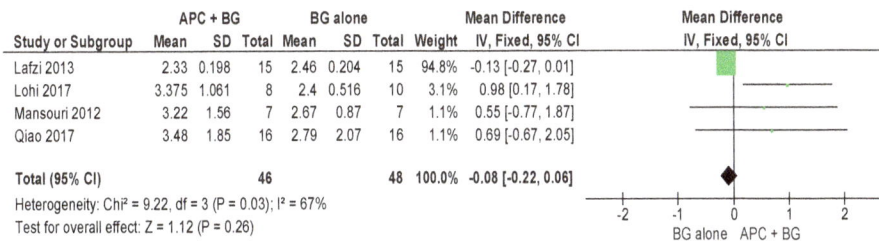

Figure 4. Forest plot showing the effect on probing pocket depth for comparison of APC + BG versus BG alone at end of all-follow-up (6–12 m).

2.2.2. Vertical Clinical Attachment Level (VCAL)

APC + OFD vs. OFD Alone (Figure 5)

The forest plot of the included studies evaluating the change in VCAL shows evidence of an advantage of using APC in adjunct to OFD ($p < 0.001$, mean difference 1.24, 95% CI 1.08, 1.40). The subgroup analysis is also favorable for both PRF ($p < 0.001$, mean difference 1.18, 95% CI 1.01, 1.36) and PRP ($p < 0.001$, mean difference 1.58, 95% CI 1.17, 2.00).

	APC + OFD			OFD alone			Mean Difference	Mean Difference
Study or Subgroup	Mean	SD	Total	Mean	SD	Total	Weight	IV, Fixed, 95% CI	IV, Fixed, 95% CI
1.2.1 Platelet Rich Fibrin									
Bajaj 2013 a	2.87	0.85	24	1.37	0.58	23	15.0%	1.50 [1.09, 1.91]	
Kanoriya 2017	3.39	0.49	23	2.33	0.48	24	33.5%	1.06 [0.78, 1.34]	
Sharma 2011	2.333	0.49	18	1.278	0.461	18	26.7%	1.06 [0.74, 1.37]	
Siddiqui 2016	2.4	0.91	15	0.93	0.46	15	9.7%	1.47 [0.95, 1.99]	
Subtotal (95% CI)			80			80	85.0%	1.18 [1.01, 1.36]	

Heterogeneity: Chi² = 4.84, df = 3 (P = 0.18); I² = 38%
Test for overall effect: Z = 13.30 (P < 0.00001)

1.2.2 Platelet Rich Plasma									
Bajaj 2013 b	2.71	1.04	25	1.37	0.58	23	11.6%	1.34 [0.87, 1.81]	
Pradeep 2009	2.5	1.64	20	0.1	1.1	20	3.4%	2.40 [1.53, 3.27]	
Subtotal (95% CI)			45			43	15.0%	1.58 [1.17, 2.00]	

Heterogeneity: Chi² = 4.44, df = 1 (P = 0.04); I² = 77%
Test for overall effect: Z = 7.49 (P < 0.00001)

Total (95% CI)			125			123	100.0%	1.24 [1.08, 1.40]	

Heterogeneity: Chi² = 12.32, df = 5 (P = 0.03); I² = 59%
Test for overall effect: Z = 15.17 (P < 0.00001)
Test for subgroup differences: Chi² = 3.04, df = 1 (P = 0.08), I² = 67.1%

Favours OFD Favours APC + OFD

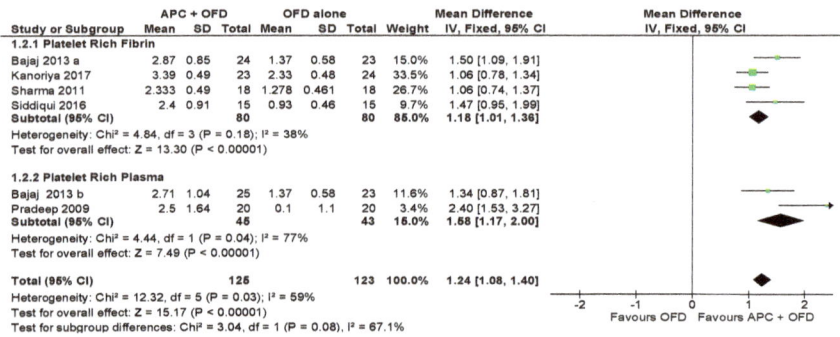

Figure 5. Forest plot showing the effect on vertical clinical attachment level for comparison of APC + OFD versus OFD alone at end of all-follow-up (6–12 m).

APC + BG vs. BG Alone (Figure 6)

The forest plot of the included studies evaluating the change in VCAL in using APC in adjunct with BG is favorable; however, the result is not statistically significant ($p = 0.62$, mean difference 0.06, 95% CI −0.18, 0.30).

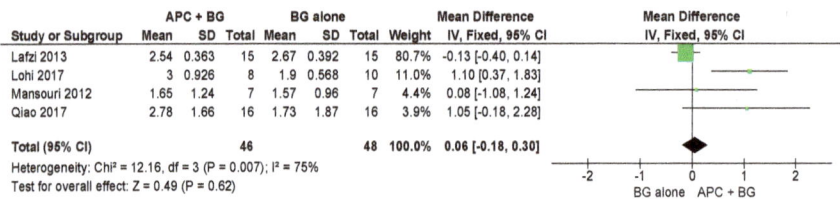

	APC + BG			BG alone			Mean Difference	Mean Difference
Study or Subgroup	Mean	SD	Total	Mean	SD	Total	Weight	IV, Fixed, 95% CI	IV, Fixed, 95% CI
Lafzi 2013	2.54	0.363	15	2.67	0.392	15	80.7%	-0.13 [-0.40, 0.14]	
Lohi 2017	3	0.926	8	1.9	0.568	10	11.0%	1.10 [0.37, 1.83]	
Mansouri 2012	1.65	1.24	7	1.57	0.96	7	4.4%	0.08 [-1.08, 1.24]	
Qiao 2017	2.78	1.66	16	1.73	1.87	16	3.9%	1.05 [-0.18, 2.28]	
Total (95% CI)			46			48	100.0%	0.06 [-0.18, 0.30]	

Heterogeneity: Chi² = 12.16, df = 3 (P = 0.007); I² = 75%
Test for overall effect: Z = 0.49 (P = 0.62)

BG alone APC + BG

Figure 6. Forest plot showing the effect on vertical clinical attachment level for comparison of APC + BG versus BG alone at end of all-follow-up (6–12 m).

2.2.3. Horizontal Clinical Attachment Level (HCAL)

APC + OFD vs. OFD Alone (Figure 7)

The forest plot of the included studies evaluating the change in HCAL shows evidence of an advantage of using APC in adjunct to OFD ($p < 0.001$, mean difference 1.01, 95% CI 0.89, 1.12). The subgroup analysis is also favorable for both PRF ($p < 0.001$, mean difference 0.93, 95% CI 0.80, 1.06) and PRP ($p < 0.001$, mean difference 1.50, 95% CI 1.18, 1.83).

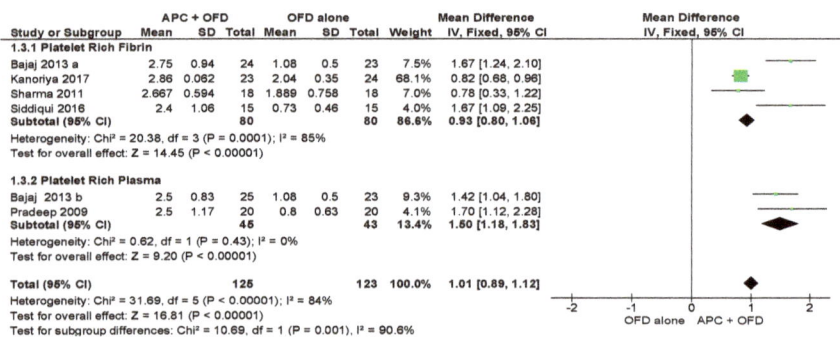

	APC + OFD			OFD alone			Mean Difference	Mean Difference
Study or Subgroup	Mean	SD	Total	Mean	SD	Total	Weight	IV, Fixed, 95% CI	IV, Fixed, 95% CI
1.3.1 Platelet Rich Fibrin									
Bajaj 2013 a	2.75	0.94	24	1.08	0.5	23	7.5%	1.67 [1.24, 2.10]	
Kanoriya 2017	2.86	0.062	23	2.04	0.35	24	68.1%	0.82 [0.68, 0.96]	
Sharma 2011	2.667	0.594	18	1.889	0.758	18	7.0%	0.78 [0.33, 1.22]	
Siddiqui 2016	2.4	1.06	15	0.73	0.46	15	4.0%	1.67 [1.09, 2.25]	
Subtotal (95% CI)			80			80	86.6%	0.93 [0.80, 1.06]	

Heterogeneity: Chi² = 20.38, df = 3 (P = 0.0001); I² = 85%
Test for overall effect: Z = 14.45 (P < 0.00001)

1.3.2 Platelet Rich Plasma									
Bajaj 2013 b	2.5	0.83	25	1.08	0.5	23	9.3%	1.42 [1.04, 1.80]	
Pradeep 2009	2.5	1.17	20	0.8	0.63	20	4.1%	1.70 [1.12, 2.28]	
Subtotal (95% CI)			45			43	13.4%	1.50 [1.18, 1.83]	

Heterogeneity: Chi² = 0.62, df = 1 (P = 0.43); I² = 0%
Test for overall effect: Z = 9.20 (P < 0.00001)

Total (95% CI)			125			123	100.0%	1.01 [0.89, 1.12]	

Heterogeneity: Chi² = 31.69, df = 5 (P < 0.00001); I² = 84%
Test for overall effect: Z = 16.81 (P < 0.00001)
Test for subgroup differences: Chi² = 10.69, df = 1 (P = 0.001), I² = 90.6%

OFD alone APC + OFD

Figure 7. Forest plot showing the effect on horizontal clinical attachment level for comparison of APC + OFD versus OFD alone at end of all-follow-up (6–12 m).

APC + BG vs. BG Alone (Figure 8)

The forest plot of the included studies evaluating the change in HCAL shows evidence of an advantage of using APC in adjunct with BG ($p < 0.001$, mean difference 0.74, 95% CI 0.54, 0.94).

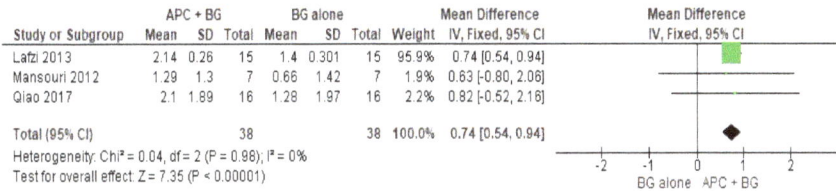

Study or Subgroup	APC + BG Mean	SD	Total	BG alone Mean	SD	Total	Weight	Mean Difference IV, Fixed, 95% CI
Lafzi 2013	2.14	0.26	15	1.4	0.301	15	95.9%	0.74 [0.54, 0.94]
Mansouri 2012	1.29	1.3	7	0.66	1.42	7	1.9%	0.63 [-0.80, 2.06]
Qiao 2017	2.1	1.89	16	1.28	1.97	16	2.2%	0.82 [-0.52, 2.16]
Total (95% CI)			38			38	100.0%	0.74 [0.54, 0.94]

Heterogeneity: Chi² = 0.04, df = 2 (P = 0.98); I² = 0%
Test for overall effect: Z = 7.35 (P < 0.00001)

Figure 8. Forest plot showing the effect on horizontal clinical attachment level for comparison of APC + BG versus BG alone at end of all-follow-up (6–12 m).

2.2.4. Vertical Furcation Depth (VFD)

APC + OFD vs. OFD Alone (Figure 9)

The forest plot of the included studies evaluating the change in VFD shows evidence of an advantage of using APC in adjunct to OFD ($p < 0.001$, mean difference 1.60, 95% CI 1.53, 1.68). The subgroup analysis is also favorable for both PRF ($p < 0.001$, mean difference 1.65, 95% CI 1.57, 1.74) and PRP ($p < 0.001$, mean difference 1.38, 95% CI 1.21, 1.56).

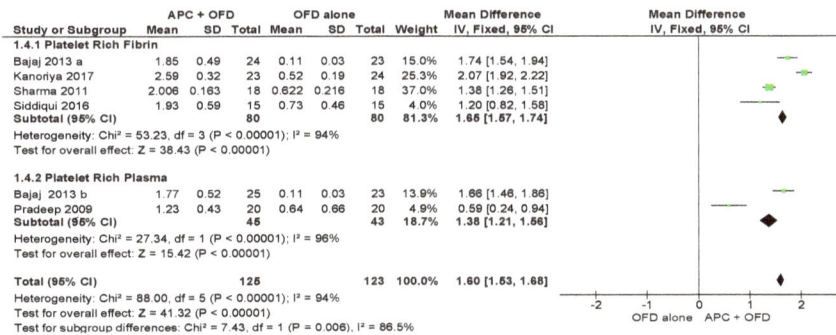

Study or Subgroup	APC + OFD Mean	SD	Total	OFD alone Mean	SD	Total	Weight	Mean Difference IV, Fixed, 95% CI
1.4.1 Platelet Rich Fibrin								
Bajaj 2013 a	1.85	0.49	24	0.11	0.03	23	15.0%	1.74 [1.54, 1.94]
Kanoriya 2017	2.59	0.32	23	0.52	0.19	24	25.3%	2.07 [1.92, 2.22]
Sharma 2011	2.006	0.163	18	0.622	0.216	18	37.0%	1.38 [1.26, 1.51]
Siddiqui 2016	1.93	0.59	15	0.73	0.46	15	4.0%	1.20 [0.82, 1.58]
Subtotal (95% CI)			80			80	81.3%	1.65 [1.57, 1.74]
Heterogeneity: Chi² = 53.23, df = 3 (P < 0.00001); I² = 94%								
Test for overall effect: Z = 38.43 (P < 0.00001)								
1.4.2 Platelet Rich Plasma								
Bajaj 2013 b	1.77	0.52	25	0.11	0.03	23	13.9%	1.66 [1.46, 1.86]
Pradeep 2009	1.23	0.43	20	0.64	0.66	20	4.9%	0.59 [0.24, 0.94]
Subtotal (95% CI)			45			43	18.7%	1.38 [1.21, 1.56]
Heterogeneity: Chi² = 27.34, df = 1 (P < 0.00001); I² = 96%								
Test for overall effect: Z = 15.42 (P < 0.00001)								
Total (95% CI)			125			123	100.0%	1.60 [1.53, 1.68]

Heterogeneity: Chi² = 88.00, df = 5 (P < 0.00001); I² = 94%
Test for overall effect: Z = 41.32 (P < 0.00001)
Test for subgroup differences: Chi² = 7.43, df = 1 (P = 0.006), I² = 86.5%

Figure 9. Forest plot showing the effect on vertical furcation depth for comparison of APC + OFD versus OFD alone at end of all-follow-up (6–12 m).

APC + BG vs. BG Alone (Figure 10)

The forest plot of the included studies evaluating the change in VFD in using APC in adjunct with BG favors the use of BG alone; however, the result is not statistically significant ($p = 0.90$, mean difference −0.02, 95% CI −0.31, 0.27).

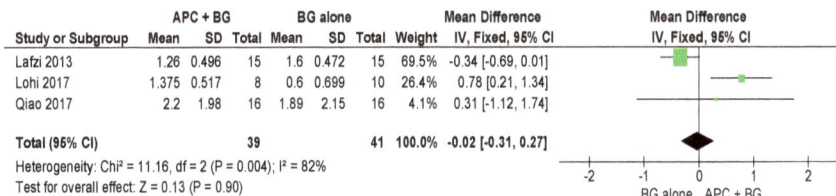

Study or Subgroup	APC + BG Mean	SD	Total	BG alone Mean	SD	Total	Weight	Mean Difference IV, Fixed, 95% CI
Lafzi 2013	1.26	0.496	15	1.6	0.472	15	69.5%	-0.34 [-0.69, 0.01]
Lohi 2017	1.375	0.517	8	0.6	0.699	10	26.4%	0.78 [0.21, 1.34]
Qiao 2017	2.2	1.98	16	1.89	2.15	16	4.1%	0.31 [-1.12, 1.74]
Total (95% CI)			39			41	100.0%	-0.02 [-0.31, 0.27]

Heterogeneity: Chi² = 11.16, df = 2 (P = 0.004); I² = 82%
Test for overall effect: Z = 0.13 (P = 0.90)

Figure 10. Forest plot showing the effect on vertical furcation depth for comparison of APC + BG versus BG alone at end of all-follow-up (6–12 m).

2.2.5. Horizontal Furcation Depth (HFD)

APC + OFD vs. OFD Alone (Figure 11)

The forest plot of the included studies evaluating the change in HFD shows evidence of an advantage of using APC in adjunct to OFD ($p < 0.001$, mean difference 1.13, 95% CI 0.85,1.41). No subgroup analysis was carried out for this outcome due to the lack of enough studies.

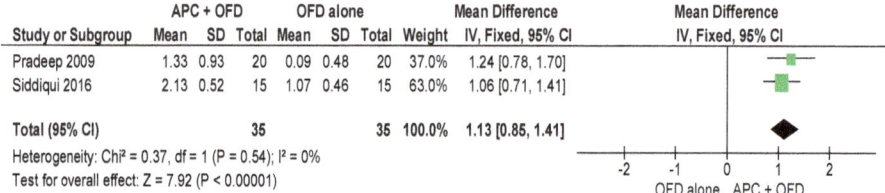

Study or Subgroup	APC + OFD Mean	SD	Total	OFD alone Mean	SD	Total	Weight	Mean Difference IV, Fixed, 95% CI	Mean Difference IV, Fixed, 95% CI
Pradeep 2009	1.33	0.93	20	0.09	0.48	20	37.0%	1.24 [0.78, 1.70]	
Siddiqui 2016	2.13	0.52	15	1.07	0.46	15	63.0%	1.06 [0.71, 1.41]	
Total (95% CI)			**35**			**35**	**100.0%**	**1.13 [0.85, 1.41]**	

Heterogeneity: Chi² = 0.37, df = 1 (P = 0.54); I² = 0%
Test for overall effect: Z = 7.92 (P < 0.00001)

-2 -1 0 1 2
OFD alone   APC + OFD

Figure 11. Forest plot showing the effect on horizontal furcation length for comparison of APC + OFD versus OFD alone at end of all-follow-up (6–12 m).

APC + BG vs. BG Alone (Figure 12)

The forest plot of the included studies evaluating the change in VFD shows evidence of an advantage of using APC in adjunct with BG ($p = 0.02$, mean difference 0.17, 95% CI 0.02, 0.31).

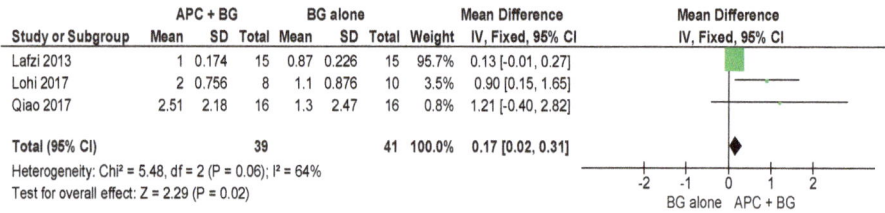

Study or Subgroup	APC + BG Mean	SD	Total	BG alone Mean	SD	Total	Weight	Mean Difference IV, Fixed, 95% CI	Mean Difference IV, Fixed, 95% CI
Lafzi 2013	1	0.174	15	0.87	0.226	15	95.7%	0.13 [-0.01, 0.27]	
Lohi 2017	2	0.756	8	1.1	0.876	10	3.5%	0.90 [0.15, 1.65]	
Qiao 2017	2.51	2.18	16	1.3	2.47	16	0.8%	1.21 [-0.40, 2.82]	
Total (95% CI)			**39**			**41**	**100.0%**	**0.17 [0.02, 0.31]**	

Heterogeneity: Chi² = 5.48, df = 2 (P = 0.06); I² = 64%
Test for overall effect: Z = 2.29 (P = 0.02)

-2 -1 0 1 2
BG alone   APC + BG

Figure 12. Forest plot showing the effect on horizontal furcation length for comparison of APC + BG versus BG alone at end of all-follow-up (6–12 m).

3. Discussion

The use of platelet concentrates to promote periodontal regeneration has gained popularity in the last 10 years, as demonstrated by the increasing number of evidence-based randomized studies and systematic reviews [19,51,52]. A recent Cochrane systematic review [53] investigated the effect of APC for the surgical treatment of infrabony defects, reporting positive effects when APC is used in combination with OFD, OFD + BG, but not with GTR and enamel matrix derivative. The latter two treatments have a predictable and well-documented efficacy, and they are since long considered the gold standard for periodontal defects, so it can be difficult for any adjunctive therapy to further enhance the clinical outcomes. Evidence-based studies on the efficacy of APC for the regeneration therapy of furcation defects are relatively scarce as compared to infrabony defects. Our systematic review published in 2011 investigated the effects of APC on infrabony defects, gingival recessions and furcation defects but found only two studies on the latter topic, both using platelet-rich plasma [19]. The present study is the first comprehensive systematic review that was aimed at exploring and comparing the effect of various APCs for enhancing furcation treatment. It was designed according to a standard protocol, aimed at selecting only the best evidence studies, so as to provide the most reliable results. Only one of the ten included studies was judged at high risk of bias [50], while seven had a low risk, testifying to the good level of the evidence of this review. The results, derived from the analysis of different clinical outcome variables, suggested that the use of APC may be beneficial for improving the regeneration of furcation defects, when associated with OFD, in line with the above findings regarding infrabony defects. Further, it may be noted that APC in adjunct to OFD + BG also showed significant improvement in HCAL and HFL. Since only one RCT evaluated the adjunctive effect of APC when using GTR for grade II furcation defects, no meta-analysis was feasible. The results of this study, suggested that the adjunct of APC produced no significant advantage as compared to GTR alone, in line with previous findings for infrabony defects.

This review has some strengths and limitations. In recent years, there has been fierce competition among companies producing different types of platelet concentrates, all claiming that their product was superior to the others. This also introduced a number of different protocols for the preparation of APC. Indeed, very few studies comparing different types of APC have been performed in the periodontal field (as well as in other fields), so that it seems difficult to indicate if there is really a superiority of some APCs over the others for specific conditions. In the present review, we were able to perform a meta-analysis with subgroups, keeping separate different APC (PRP and PRF), only in the group considering OFD alone. The outcomes using different APC was very similar as can be seen in Figures 3–6 This can be considered a strong point of the present review. However, the precise difference in effects between different APC cannot be estimated, due to a lack of direct comparisons. The same subgroup analysis could not be performed in the OFD + BG group, due to heterogeneity among studies in the type of APC used, and the insufficient number of studies using the same type of APC. Indeed, also when different studies use the same type of APC, this does not necessarily represent a warranty of homogeneity in the protocols. For example, over 20 different types of devices producing PRP are currently available on the market, and at least five different companies produce centrifuges for PRF [54]. A recent in vitro study compared the characteristics of PRF obtained using four different centrifuge systems [55]. This study found that, even though in all cases a leukocyte- and platelet-rich fibrin is obtained after centrifugation, the centrifuge characteristics and centrifugation protocols significantly impact the cell composition and distribution, the growth factors release pattern and the fibrin architecture of the final products. So, when PRF is used in different studies, one cannot be sure to refer to a product with the same features, unless the same centrifuge system is used. In spite of the above limitations, caused by lack of homogeneity in study protocols, it can be noted that all studies investigating the effect of APC as an adjunct to OFD alone, consistently reported a beneficial effect. The latter can be considered a strength point evidenced by this review.

In addition to the regenerative properties, platelet concentrates have also been demonstrated to carry further advantages in the postsurgical healing period. Evidence-based studies in different oral surgery procedures have reported that the adjunctive use of APC is associated with an improvement of patients' quality of life and pain reduction in the post-surgical period [56,57] Unfortunately, such effects were not consistently addressed in the studies included in the present review.

Finally, though specific clinical studies have not been performed so far, there is consistent preclinical evidence that APCs have an antimicrobial effect against a number of species commonly found in the oral cavity, which suggest they may potentially represent a beneficial tool for the control of postsurgical infection [58,59]. Indications for future research: There is a huge demand for conducting more evidence-based comparative studies with wide sample size (among different APC and grafting materials and versus other biological agents), to investigate patients' quality of life, to treat various grades of furcation, in order to verify the actual beneficial effects of use of APC as adjunct with wide variety of regenerative strategies.

4. Material and Methods

This systematic review and meta-analysis were carried out based on preferred reporting items for systematic reviews and meta-analysis (PRISMA) guidelines. The protocol of this systematic review was registered on the international prospective register of systematic reviews (PROSPERO) with registration number CRD42019100015.

4.1. Research Question

What is the effectiveness of autologous platelet concentrates used as an adjunct to different types of surgical techniques for the treatment of furcation defects, compared to the same surgical techniques alone?

4.2. Search Strategy

A systematic digitalized search was carried out in the following electronic databases: MEDLINE, SCOPUS, CENTRAL (Cochrane Central Register of Controlled Trials), and EMBASE, using a series of search terms combined with the Boolean Operators "AND", "OR", and "NOT". The following search string was developed with the combination of relevant keywords: "(((Furcation Defects) OR Furcation Involvement)) AND (((((((Platelet Concentrates) OR Platelet-rich plasma) OR Platelet-rich fibrin) OR Growth factors) OR PRP) OR L-PRF) OR CGF)". The last electronic search was carried out in October 2018. In addition, a hand search was performed in the following dental journals: British Dental Journal, British Journal of Oral and Maxillofacial Surgery, Clinical Implant Dentistry and Related Research, Clinical Oral Implants Research, Clinical Oral Investigations, European Journal of Oral Implantology, European Journal of Oral Sciences, Implant Dentistry, International Journal of Oral and Maxillofacial Implants, International Journal of Oral and Maxillofacial Surgery, International Journal of Periodontics and Restorative Dentistry, Journal of Clinical Periodontology, Journal of Dental Research, Journal of Dentistry, Journal of Implantology, Journal of Maxillofacial and Oral Surgery, Journal of Oral and Maxillofacial Surgery, Journal of Periodontal Research, Journal of Periodontology, and Oral Surgery, Oral Medicine, Oral Pathology, Oral Radiology. The reference citations of the eligible studies and other systematic reviews were also searched for possible additional eligible studies. Finally, the online trial registries were also searched for any ongoing studies: US National Institutes of Health Ongoing Trials Register ClinicalTrials.gov (clinicaltrials.gov; searched 20 October 2018); World Health Organization International Clinical Trials Registry Platform (apps.who.int/trialsearch; searched 20 October 2018). No language restrictions were applied.

4.3. Inclusion Criteria

The criteria for the articles to be included in this present systematic review were as follows:

- Randomized clinical trials (RCT), either of a parallel group or of a split-mouth design;
- Presence of at least one experimental group in which APCs were clinically applied as an adjunct to surgical procedures alone or in combination with bone grafting materials or GTR procedures for the therapy of furcation defects;
- Presence of an appropriate control group, in which the same therapeutic procedures as those employed in at least one experimental group were clinically applied for the treatment of furcation defects, without the adjunctive effect of APCs;
- Patients included in the RCT should present with maxillary/mandibular Grade 2 or 3 furcation defects;
- Patients included in the RCT should have no systemic diseases nor taking medications that could potentially influence the outcome of periodontal therapy;
- The follow-up period had to be at least 6 months.

4.4. Selection of Studies

Following the electronic search in all the respective databases, the records were imported into EndNote 13 software (EndNoteX3; Thomas Reuters, New York, NY, USA) and the duplicates were sorted to be removed from the pool of titles. A total of 153 titles and abstracts (if available) were independently screened by two reviewers (MDF, SP) to exclude all articles clearly not meeting the inclusion criteria. Of all the eligible articles, full texts were obtained and were thoroughly assessed.

Only articles fulfilling the inclusion criteria were considered. In cases of disagreement between the two reviewers, a third reviewer (LF) was consulted. Detailed reasons were stated for all excluded studies.

4.5. Data Extraction and Management

The relevant data of the included studies were extracted using an Excel spreadsheet (Microsoft, Radmond, WA, USA). Data were independently extracted by two review authors (MDF, FG) and recorded on predetermined spreadsheets. In case of missing or unclear information, the authors of the included studies were contacted by email for providing clarification or missing information.

The following data were recorded for each included report:

- Patients' demographic characteristics
- Study design and sample size
- Type of platelet concentrate used (PRP, PRF, PRGF, CGF)
- Follow up duration
- source of funding and study setting
- Outcome variables, relative to baseline and post-operative defect characteristics (probing pocket depth (PPD), horizontal and vertical clinical attachment loss (HCAL, VCAL), horizontal and vertical furcation depth (HFD, VFD)

4.6. Risk of Bias Assessment

Risk of Bias was assessed by two independent reviewers (ACD, AS) for all the included clinical trials and the discrepancies were resolved by discussion and in consent with a third reviewer (MK). The domains of the study were graded under high, unclear or low risk, based on the following categories: Selection bias (random sequence generation and allocation concealment), performance bias (blinding), detection bias (assessor blinding), attrition bias (incomplete outcome data), reporting bias (selective reporting), sample size calculation and number of surgeons involved. Based on the domains, the studies categorized as low risk of bias if all domains were at low risk; high risk of bias if two or more domains were at high risk; or medium risk of bias if one domain were at unclear or high risk.

4.7. Data Synthesis

Data of the various outcomes were extracted from each included study. Parallel group and split-mouth studies were combined in the meta-analysis of treatment effects. For all the outcomes, mean differences and 95% confidence interval (CI) were used to summarize the results for each included study. The meta-analysis was performed using Review Manager 5.3 software (RevMan 5.3, Version 5.3.5 Copenhagen: The Nordic Cochrane Centre, The Cochrane Collaboration, 2014) using the fixed or random effects models, as appropriate. Fixed effects meta-analysis was used when the heterogeneity was small ($i^2 < 60\%$, $p > 0.05$). When the heterogeneity was large ($i^2 > 60\%$, $p < 0.05$), a random-effects model analysis was undertaken.

5. Conclusions

In conclusion, the evidence available in the literature for the beneficial effects of platelet concentrates in periodontal furcation defects has been increasing in recent years. Platelet-rich plasma and platelet-rich fibrin may be advantageously used as an adjunct to open flap debridement alone and additional grafting procedures, while there is no evidence of an effect of APC when used in combination with GTR, for the treatment of furcation defects.

Author Contributions: S.P. (Sourav Panda), M.D.F. and L.F. designed and conducted the search strategy, M.D.F., F.G. and L.K. did the selection of studies and data extraction, S.P. (Sourav Panda) and S.P. (Sital Panda) performed and interpreted the meta-analysis, A.C.D., A.S. and M.K. carried out the risk of bias assessment. S.P. (Sourav Panda) and M.D.F. drafted the manuscript. The final version of the manuscript was read and approved by all authors.

Funding: This research received no external funding.

Acknowledgments: We would like to thank *IRCCS Istituto Ortopedico Galeazzi* for supporting us with the publication cost of this work.

Conflicts of Interest: The authors declare no conflict of interest.

Abbreviations

APCs	Autologous platelet concentrates
PPD	Probing pocket depth
HCAL	Horizontal clinical attachment loss
VCAL	Vertical clinical attachment loss
HFD	Horizontal furcation depth
VFD	Vertical furcation depth
GTR	Guided tissue regeneration
rhBMP2	Recombinant human bone morphogenetic protein-2
rhPDGF	Recombinant human platelet-derived growth factor
TGF-β	Transforming growth factor beta
PRP	Platelet-rich plasma
PRF	Platelet-rich fibrin
PRGF	Plasma rich in growth factors
CGF	Concentrated growth factors
PRISMA	Preferred reporting items for systematic reviews and meta-analysis
RCT	Randomized clinical trials
CI	Confidence interval
OFD	Open flap debridement
BG	Bone graft

References

1. Cattabriga, M.; Pedrazzoli, V.; Wilson, T.G. The conservative approach in the treatment of furcation lesions. *Periodontology 2000* **2000**, *22*, 133–153.
2. Bower, R.C. Furcation morphology relative to periodontal treatment. Furcation root surface anatomy. *J. Periodontol.* **1979**, *50*, 366–374. [CrossRef] [PubMed]
3. Pilloni, A.; Rojas, M.A. Furcation Involvement Classification: A Comprehensive Review and a New System Proposal. *Dent. J.* **2018**, *6*, 34.
4. Glickman, I. *Clinical Periodontology: Prevention, Diagnosis, and Treatment of Periodontal Disease in the Practice of General Dentistry*, 4th ed.; Saunders: Philadelphia, PA, USA, 1972; ISBN 0-7216-4137-7.
5. Martin, M.; Gantes, B.; Garrett, S.; Egelberg, J. Treatment of periodontal furcation defects. (I). Review of the literature and description of a regenerative surgical technique. *J. Clin. Periodontol.* **1988**, *15*, 227–231. [CrossRef] [PubMed]
6. Pradeep, A.R.; Pai, S.; Garg, G.; Devi, P.; Shetty, S.K. A randomized clinical trial of autologous platelet-rich plasma in the treatment of mandibular degree II furcation defects. *J. Clin. Periodontol.* **2009**, *36*, 581–588. [CrossRef] [PubMed]
7. Pontoriero, R.; Lindhe, J.; Nyman, S.; Karring, T.; Rosenberg, E.; Sanavi, F. Guided tissue regeneration in the treatment of furcation defects in mandibular molars. A clinical study of degree III involvements. *J. Clin. Periodontol.* **1989**, *16*, 170–174. [CrossRef] [PubMed]
8. Yan, X.-Z.; Ge, S.-H.; Sun, Q.-F.; Guo, H.-M.; Yang, P.-S. A pilot study evaluating the effect of recombinant human bone morphogenetic protein-2 and recombinant human beta-nerve growth factor on the healing of Class III furcation defects in dogs. *J. Periodontol.* **2010**, *81*, 1289–1298.
9. Camelo, M.; Nevins, M.L.; Schenk, R.K.; Lynch, S.E.; Nevins, M. Periodontal regeneration in human Class II furcations using purified recombinant human platelet-derived growth factor-BB (rhPDGF-BB) with bone allograft. *Int. J. Periodontics Restor. Dent.* **2003**, *23*, 213–225.

10. Synergistic Induction of Periodontal Tissue Regeneration by Binary Application of Human Osteogenic Protein-1 and Human Transforming Growth Factor-β. Available online: https://www.ncbi.nlm.nih.gov/pubmed/22142147 (accessed on 23 October 2018).

11. Bajaj, P.; Pradeep, A.R.; Agarwal, E.; Rao, N.S.; Naik, S.B.; Priyanka, N.; Kalra, N. Comparative evaluation of autologous platelet-rich fibrin and platelet-rich plasma in the treatment of mandibular degree II furcation defects: A randomized controlled clinical trial. *J. Periodontal Res.* **2013**, *48*, 573–581.

12. Jenabian, N.; Haghanifar, S.; Ehsani, H.; Zahedi, E.; Haghpanah, M. Guided tissue regeneration and platelet rich growth factor for the treatment of Grade II furcation defects: A randomized double-blinded clinical trial—A pilot study. *Dent. Res. J.* **2017**, *14*, 363–369.

13. Kanoriya, D.; Pradeep, A.R.; Garg, V.; Singhal, S. Mandibular Degree II Furcation Defects Treatment with Platelet-Rich Fibrin and 1% Alendronate Gel Combination: A Randomized Controlled Clinical Trial. *J. Periodontol.* **2017**, *88*, 250–258. [CrossRef]

14. Lohi, H.S.; Nayak, D.G.; Uppoor, A.S. Comparative Evaluation of the Efficacy of Bioactive Ceramic Composite Granules Alone and in Combination with Platelet Rich Fibrin in the Treatment of Mandibular Class II Furcation Defects: A Clinical and Radiographic Study. *J. Clin. Diagn. Res. JCDR* **2017**, *11*, ZC76–ZC80. [CrossRef] [PubMed]

15. Lafzi, A.; Shirmohammadi, A.; Faramarzi, M.; Jabali, S.; Shayan, A. Clinical Comparison of Autogenous Bone Graft with and without Plasma Rich in Growth Factors in the Treatment of Grade II Furcation Involvement of Mandibular Molars. *J. Dent. Res. Dent. Clin. Dent. Prospects* **2013**, *7*, 22–29.

16. Qiao, J.; Duan, J.Y.; Chu, Y.; Sun, C.Z. Effect of concentrated growth factors on the treatment of degree II furcation involvements of mandibular molars. *Beijing Da Xue Xue Bao* **2017**, *49*, 36–42. [PubMed]

17. Sharma, A.; Pradeep, A.R. Autologous platelet-rich fibrin in the treatment of mandibular degree II furcation defects: A randomized clinical trial. *J. Periodontol.* **2011**, *82*, 1396–1403. [PubMed]

18. Castro, A.B.; Meschi, N.; Temmerman, A.; Pinto, N.; Lambrechts, P.; Teughels, W.; Quirynen, M. Regenerative potential of leucocyte- and platelet-rich fibrin. Part A: Intra-bony defects, furcation defects and periodontal plastic surgery. A systematic review and meta-analysis. *J. Clin. Periodontol.* **2017**, *44*, 67–82. [CrossRef] [PubMed]

19. Del Fabbro, M.; Bortolin, M.; Taschieri, S.; Weinstein, R. Is platelet concentrate advantageous for the surgical treatment of periodontal diseases? A systematic review and meta-analysis. *J. Periodontol.* **2011**, *82*, 1100–1111. [CrossRef] [PubMed]

20. Goldman, H. Therapy of the incipient bifurcation involvement. *J. Periodontol.* **1958**, *29*, 112–116.

21. Staffileno, H.J. Surgical management of the furca invasion. *Dent. Clin. N. Am.* **1969**, *13*, 103–119.

22. Hamp, S.E.; Nyman, S.; Lindhe, J. Periodontal treatment of multirooted teeth. Results after 5 years. *J. Clin. Periodontol.* **1975**, *2*, 126–135.

23. Ramfjord, S.P.; Ash, M. *Periodontology and Periodontics*, 1st ed.; Saunders: Philadelphia, PA, USA, 1979; ISBN 13-978-0721674605.

24. Ricchetti, P.A. A furcation classification based on pulp chamber-furcation relationships and vertical radiographic bone loss. *Int. J. Periodontics Restor. Dent.* **1982**, *2*, 50–59.

25. Grant, D.; Stern, I.; Listgarten, M. *Periodontics*, 6th ed.; C.V. Mosby: St. Louis, IL, USA, 1988.

26. Goldman, H.; Cohen, D. *Periodontal Therapy*, 6th ed.; C.V. Mosby: St. Louis, IL, USA, 1988; ISBN 13-9780801618741.

27. Basaraba, N. Furcation invasions. In *Periodontal Diseases*; Lea and Febiger: Philadelphia, PA, USA, 1990; ISBN 13-978-0812110845.

28. Nevins, M.; Cappetta, E. Treatment of maxillary furcations. In *Periodontal Therapy—Clinical Approaches and Evidence of Success*; Nevins, M., Mellonig, J.T., Eds.; Quintessence: Chicago, IL, USA, 1998; ISBN 13-978-0867153095.

29. Walter, C.; Kaner, D.; Berndt, D.C.; Weiger, R.; Zitzmann, N.U. Three-dimensional imaging as a pre-operative tool in decision making for furcation surgery. *J. Clin. Periodontol.* **2009**, *36*, 250–257. [CrossRef] [PubMed]

30. Carnevale, G.; Pontoriero, R.; Lindhe, J. Treatment of furcation—Involved teeth. In *Clinical Periodontology and Implant Dentistry*; Lindhe, J., Lang, N.P., Karring, T., Eds.; Munksgaard: Copenhagen, Denmark, 2012; Volume 2, pp. 823–847. ISBN 978-1-118-35561-9.

31. Tal, H.; Lemmer, J. Furcal defects in dry mandibles. Part II: Severity of furcal defects. *J. Periodontol.* **1982**, *53*, 364–367. [CrossRef] [PubMed]

32. Eskow, R.N.; Kapin, S.H. Furcation invasions: Correlating a classification system with therapeutic considerations. Part I. Examination, diagnosis, and classification. *Compend. Contin. Educ. Dent.* **1984**, *5*, 479–483, 487. [PubMed]

33. Tarnow, D.; Fletcher, P. Classification of the vertical component of furcation involvement. *J. Periodontol.* **1984**, *55*, 283–284. [CrossRef]

34. Easley, J.R.; Drennan, G.A. Morphological classification of the furca. *J. Can. Dent. Assoc.* **1969**, *35*, 104–107. [PubMed]

35. Fedi, P., Jr. *The Periodontal Syllabus*, 2nd ed.; Lea and Febiger: Philadelphia, PA, USA, 1985; ISBN 13-978-0781779722.

36. Rosenberg, M. Management of osseous defects, furcation involvements, and periodontal-pulpal lesions. In *Clinical Dentistry, Periodontal and Oral Surgery*; Clark, J.W., Ed.; Harper and Row: Philadelphia, PA, USA, 1986.

37. Hou, G.L.; Chen, Y.M.; Tsai, C.C.; Weisgold, A.S. A new classification of molar furcation involvement based on the root trunk and horizontal and vertical bone loss. *Int. J. Periodontics Restor. Dent.* **1998**, *18*, 257–265.

38. Mehta, D.B.; Deshpande, N.C.; Dandekar, S.A. Comparative evaluation of platelet-rich fibrin membrane and collagen membrane along with demineralized freeze-dried bone allograft in Grade II furcation defects: A randomized controlled study. *J. Indian Soc. Periodontol.* **2018**, *22*, 322–327.

39. Wanikar, I.; Rathod, S.; Kolte, A.P. Clinico-radiographic evaluation of 1% Alendronate gel as an adjunct and smart blood derivative platelet rich fibrin in grade II furcation defects. *J. Periodontol.* **2019**, *90*, 52–60. [CrossRef]

40. Kaur, J.; Bathla, S.C. Regenerative potential of autologous platelet-rich fibrin with and without amnion membrane in the treatment of Grade-II furcation defects: A clinicoradiographic study. *J. Indian Soc. Periodontol.* **2018**, *22*, 235–242.

41. Sharma, P.; Grover, H.S.; Masamatti, S.S.; Saksena, N. A clinicoradiographic assessment of 1% metformin gel with platelet-rich fibrin in the treatment of mandibular grade II furcation defects. *J. Indian Soc. Periodontol.* **2017**, *21*, 303–308. [CrossRef]

42. Asimuddin, S.; Koduganti, R.R.; Panthula, V.N.R.; Jammula, S.P.; Dasari, R.; Gireddy, H. Effect of Autologous Platelet Rich Fibrin in Human Mandibular Molar Grade II Furcation Defects- A Randomized Clinical Trial. *J. Clin. Diagn. Res. JCDR* **2017**, *11*, ZC73–ZC77. [PubMed]

43. Salaria, S.K.; Ghuman, S.K.; Kumar, S.; Sharma, G. Management of localized advance loss of periodontal support associated Grade II furcation and intrabony defect in chronic periodontitis patient through amalgamation of platelet-rich fibrin and hydroxyapatite bioactive glass composite granules. *Contemp. Clin. Dent.* **2016**, *7*, 405–408. [CrossRef]

44. Biswas, S.; Sambashivaiah, S.; Kulal, R.; Bilichodmath, S.; Kurtzman, G.M. Comparative Evaluation of Bioactive Glass (Putty) and Platelet Rich Fibrin in Treating Furcation Defects. *J. Oral Implantol.* **2016**, *42*, 411–415. [CrossRef] [PubMed]

45. Pradeep, A.R.; Karvekar, S.; Nagpal, K.; Patnaik, K.; Raju, A.; Singh, P. Rosuvastatin 1.2 mg In Situ Gel Combined with 1:1 Mixture of Autologous Platelet-Rich Fibrin and Porous Hydroxyapatite Bone Graft in Surgical Treatment of Mandibular Class II Furcation Defects: A Randomized Clinical Control Trial. *J. Periodontol.* **2016**, *87*, 5–13. [PubMed]

46. Sandhu, G.K.; Khinda, P.K.; Gill, A.S.; Kalra, H.S. Surgical re-entry evaluation of regenerative efficacy of bioactive Gengigel® and platelet-rich fibrin in the treatment of grade II furcation: A novel approach. *Contemp. Clin. Dent.* **2015**, *6*, 570–573. [CrossRef] [PubMed]

47. Mellonig, J.T.; del Pilar Valderrama, M.; Cochran, D.L. Histological and clinical evaluation of recombinant human platelet-derived growth factor combined with beta tricalcium phosphate for the treatment of human Class III furcation defects. *Int. J. Periodontics Restor. Dent.* **2009**, *29*, 169–177.

48. Lekovic, V.; Camargo, P.M.; Weinlaender, M.; Vasilic, N.; Aleksic, Z.; Kenney, E.B. Effectiveness of a combination of platelet-rich plasma, bovine porous bone mineral and guided tissue regeneration in the treatment of mandibular grade II molar furcations in humans. *J. Clin. Periodontol.* **2003**, *30*, 746–751. [CrossRef]

49. Siddiqui, Z.R.; Jhingran, R.; Bains, V.K.; Srivastava, R.; Madan, R.; Rizvi, I. Comparative evaluation of platelet-rich fibrin versus beta-tri-calcium phosphate in the treatment of Grade II mandibular furcation defects using cone-beam computed tomography. *Eur. J. Dent.* **2016**, *10*, 496–506.

50. Mansouri, S.S.; Ghasemi, M.; Darmian, S.S.; Pourseyediyan, T. Treatment of Mandibular Molar Class II Furcation Defects in Humans with Bovine Porous Bone Mineral in Combination with Plasma Rich in Growth Factors. *J. Dent. Tehran Iran* **2012**, *9*, 41–49.

51. Del Fabbro, M.; Lolato, A.; Panda, S.; Corbella, S.; Satpathy, A.; Das, A.C.; Kumar, M.; Taschieri, S. Methodological Quality Assessment of Systematic Reviews on Autologous Platelet Concentrates for the Treatment of Periodontal Defects. *J. Evid. Based Dent. Pract.* **2017**, *17*, 239–255. [CrossRef] [PubMed]

52. Panda, S.; Doraiswamy, J.; Malaiappan, S.; Varghese, S.S.; Del Fabbro, M. Additive effect of autologous platelet concentrates in treatment of intrabony defects: A systematic review and meta-analysis. *J. Investig. Clin. Dent.* **2016**, *7*, 13–26. [PubMed]

53. Del Fabbro, M.; Karanxha, L.; Panda, S.; Bucchi, C.; Nadathur Doraiswamy, J.; Sankari, M.; Ramamoorthi, S.; Varghese, S.; Taschieri, S. Autologous platelet concentrates for treating periodontal infrabony defects. *Cochrane Database Syst. Rev.* **2018**, *11*, CD011423. [CrossRef]

54. Mozzati, M.; Muzio, G.; Del Fabbro, M.; Pol, R.; D'Antico, S.; Mortellaro, C. *Autologous Haemocomponents as Stimulators of Tissue Healing. (Emocomponenti Autologhi Come Stimolanti Della Guarigione Dei tessuti [Italian])*, 1st ed.; Tueor Servizi SRL: Torino, Italy, 2017; ISBN 978-88-940334-9-6.

55. Dohan Ehrenfest, D.M.; Pinto, N.R.; Pereda, A.; Jiménez, P.; Corso, M.D.; Kang, B.-S.; Nally, M.; Lanata, N.; Wang, H.-L.; Quirynen, M. The impact of the centrifuge characteristics and centrifugation protocols on the cells, growth factors, and fibrin architecture of a leukocyte- and platelet-rich fibrin (L-PRF) clot and membrane. *Platelets* **2018**, *29*, 171–184. [CrossRef] [PubMed]

56. Del Fabbro, M.; Corbella, S.; Ceresoli, V.; Ceci, C.; Taschieri, S. Plasma Rich in Growth Factors Improves Patients' Postoperative Quality of Life in Maxillary Sinus Floor Augmentation: Preliminary Results of a Randomized Clinical Study. *Clin. Implant Dent. Relat. Res.* **2015**, *17*, 708–716. [PubMed]

57. Del Fabbro, M.; Ceresoli, V.; Lolato, A.; Taschieri, S. Effect of platelet concentrate on quality of life after periradicular surgery: A randomized clinical study. *J. Endod.* **2012**, *38*, 733–739. [CrossRef] [PubMed]

58. Fabbro, M.D.; Bortolin, M.; Taschieri, S.; Ceci, C.; Weinstein, R.L. Antimicrobial properties of platelet-rich preparations. A systematic review of the current pre-clinical evidence. *Platelets* **2016**, *27*, 276–285. [PubMed]

59. Drago, L.; Bortolin, M.; Vassena, C.; Taschieri, S.; Del Fabbro, M. Antimicrobial activity of pure platelet-rich plasma against microorganisms isolated from oral cavity. *BMC Microbiol.* **2013**, *13*, 47.

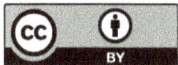

International Journal of
Molecular Sciences

MDPI

Article

Platelet-Rich Fibrin Extract: A Promising Fetal Bovine Serum Alternative in Explant Cultures of Human Periosteal Sheets for Regenerative Therapy

Tomoyuki Kawase [1,*], **Masaki Nagata** [2], **Kazuhiro Okuda** [3], **Takashi Ushiki** [4], **Yoko Fujimoto** [4], **Mari Watanabe** [4], **Akira Ito** [5] and **Koh Nakata** [4]

[1] Division of Oral Bioengineering, Institute of Medicine and Dentistry, Niigata University, Niigata 951-8514, Japan
[2] Division of Oral Surgery, Institute of Medicine and Dentistry, Niigata University, Niigata 951-8514, Japan; nagatam@dent.niigata-u.ac.jp
[3] Division of Periodontology, Institute of Medicine and Dentistry, Niigata University, Niigata 951-8514, Japan; okuda@dent.niigata-u.ac.jp
[4] Bioscience Medical Research Center, Niigata University Medical and Dental Hospital, Niigata 951-8520, Japan; tushiki@med.niigata-u.ac.jp (T.U.); yfujimoto@med.niigata-u.ac.jp (Y.F.); mwatanabe@med.niigata-u.ac.jp (M.W.); radical@med.niigata-u.ac.jp (K.N.)
[5] Kohjin Bio Co., Ltd., Sakado 350-0214, Japan; a.ito@kohjin-bio.co.jp
*   Correspondence: kawase@dent.niigata-u.ac.jp; Tel.: +81-25-262-7559

Received: 24 January 2019; Accepted: 25 February 2019; Published: 28 February 2019

check for updates

Abstract: In 2004, we developed autologous periosteal sheets for the treatment of periodontal bone defects. This regenerative therapy has successfully regenerated periodontal bone and augmented alveolar ridge for implant placement. However, the necessity for 6-week culture is a limitation. Here, we examined the applicability of a human platelet-rich fibrin extract (PRFext) as an alternative to fetal bovine serum (FBS) for the explant culture of periosteal sheets in a novel culture medium (MSC-PCM) originally developed for maintaining mesenchymal stem cells. Small periosteum tissue segments were expanded in MSC-PCM + 2% PRFext for 4 weeks, and the resulting periosteal sheets were compared with those prepared by the conventional method using Medium199 + 10% FBS for their growth rate, cell multilayer formation, alkaline phosphatase (ALP) activity, and surface antigen expression (CD73, CD90, and CD105). Periosteal sheets grew faster in the novel culture medium than in the conventional medium. However, assessment of cell shape and ALP activity revealed that the periosteal cells growing in the novel medium were relatively immature. These findings suggest that the novel culture medium featuring PRFext offers advantages by shortening the culture period and excluding possible risks associated with xeno-factors without negatively altering the activity of periosteal sheets.

Keywords: periosteal sheet; platelet-rich fibrin; growth; differentiation; bone grafting material

---

1. Introduction

Abundant growth factors and cytokines stored in platelet granules are released from activated platelets in response to tissue injury. These soluble factors are involved in wound healing and tissue repair [1]. In the 1990s, this essential role of platelets was exploited for regenerative therapy [2] and since then, therapies using platelet concentrates have been widely applied in various fields of regenerative medicine. In parallel with or even a little ahead of this therapeutic strategy, platelet lysates (PLs) have been used as a substitute for fetal bovine serum (FBS) [3] for in vitro cell expansion to reproducibly maintain cell proliferation [1]. Finding a possible alternative to FBS was strongly motivated by two major reasons: (1) limitation of the variability of FBS owing to the increased demands and decreased production ability; and (2) wide variability between batches that may affect end-product reproducibility, risks of pathogen contaminations, and ethical issues [1]. The quality of PLs also varied by source; however, shortage and risks of unexpected contamination could be avoided with the use of autologous platelets.

We have previously demonstrated a regenerative therapy with autologous periosteal sheets exhibiting osteogenic properties [4] for alveolar bone regeneration in more than 120 clinical cases [5–7] over the past 14 years on the basis of the evidence that osteogenicity, as well as osteoinductivity and osteoconductivity, are maintained in this grafting material [4,8]. Periosteal sheets are routinely expanded in vitro from small segments of alveolar periosteal tissues in the conventional medium supplemented with 10% FBS. Although no adverse events related to xeno-factors have been observed as a result of extensive washing with phosphate-buffered saline (PBS) prior to implantation, other aforementioned concerns, such as availability and efficacy of FBS, still pose difficulties. Furthermore, the requirement of a 6-week expansion period reduces the operational efficiency of cell-processing facilities, thereby increasing the economic burden. Therefore, we aimed to develop a xeno-free culture medium that may significantly shorten the period of expansion.

In a preceding study, we modified a chemically defined novel culture medium originally developed for the maintenance of mesenchymal stem cells suitable for human adult periosteal cells. This was accomplished by the addition of basic fibroblast growth factor (bFGF), platelet-derived growth factor (PDGF), and dexamethasone. Additionally, we adopted the extract of platelet-rich fibrin (PRFext) prepared from human peripheral blood samples to replace FBS. As the expansion of periosteal sheets necessitates only a limited amount of FBS replacement and as this supplement should be prepared in-house, we chose a more convenient way to obtain platelets and plasma instead of using the protocol of PL preparation. We confirmed that this novel complete medium facilitated the growth of periosteal sheets without causing genetic instability, as evident from karyotype testing. To test compatibility, we compared cell growth and fundamental characteristics of periosteal sheets prepared using the conventional culture medium (Medium199 + 10% FBS) and the newly modified stem cell medium supplemented with 2% PRFext.

2. Results

2.1. Growth of Periosteal Sheets

Figure 1 shows the onset of cell outgrowth, which indicates the days required for the migration of the first cell out of the original periosteum tissue segments. Some minor differences were reported depending on individual samples; however, no statistical difference was observed between groups. Cell outgrowth commonly occurred at 6–10 days of culture on average.

Figure 2 shows the photomicrographs of the periosteal cells that migrated out from the isolated periosteum tissue segments. The cell density was maximum in the central region in cultures with MSC-PCM + 2% PRFext (C), while the lowest density was observed in the cultures with conventional Medium199 + 10% FBS (A). Differences in cell shape were observed in the peripheral region. The majority of periosteal cells showed a typical spindle shape in the conventional medium, while their shape was relatively branched in type, indicative of their immature phenotype [9–11]. These findings are consistent with the results observed with MesenPRO-RS medium [8].

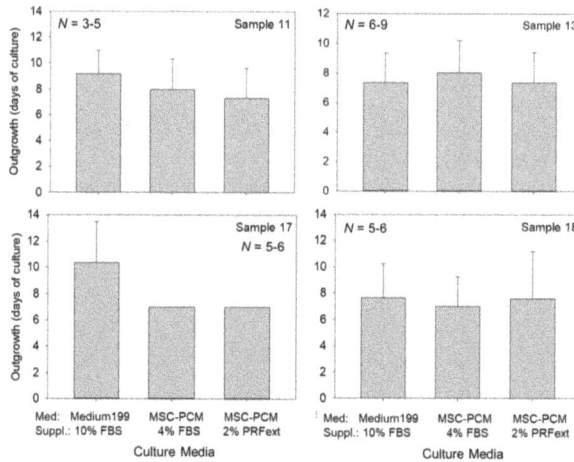

Figure 1. Effects of different culture media on the onset of periosteal cell outgrowth. The data obtained from periosteum samples derived from four independent donors are shown. *X*-axis: types of culture media. Statistical analysis was performed by Kruskal–Wallis one-way analysis of variance, followed by Steel–Dwass multiple comparison test. No significant difference was observed between the groups. $N = 3, 4, 5, 6$, or 9 replicates.

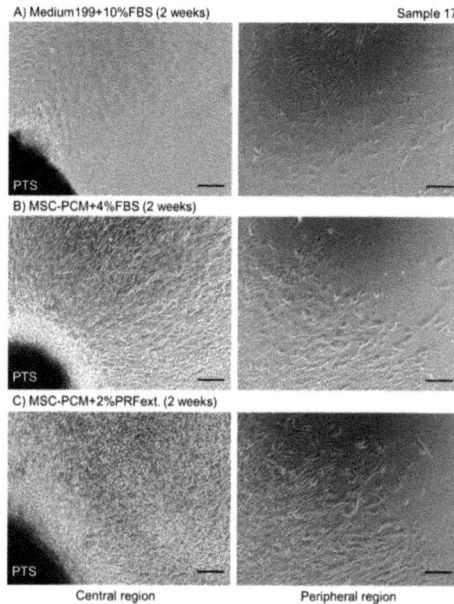

Figure 2. Photomicrographs of periosteal cells in the central and peripheral regions of periosteal sheets cultured in different culture media. (**A**) Medium199 + 10% fetal bovine serum (FBS), (**B**) MSC-PCM + 4% FBS, (**C**) MSC-PCN + 2% platelet-rich fibrin extract (PRFext). Bar = 50 μm. PTS: periosteum tissue segment.

Figure 3 shows the growth curves of periosteal sheets. Some individual differences were observed; however, overall these data indicate that MSC-PCM + 2% PRFext was the most effective of all media.

MSC-PCM + 4% FBS was equal or less effective than MSC-PCM + 2% PRFext, while the conventional medium delayed the growth of periosteal sheets.

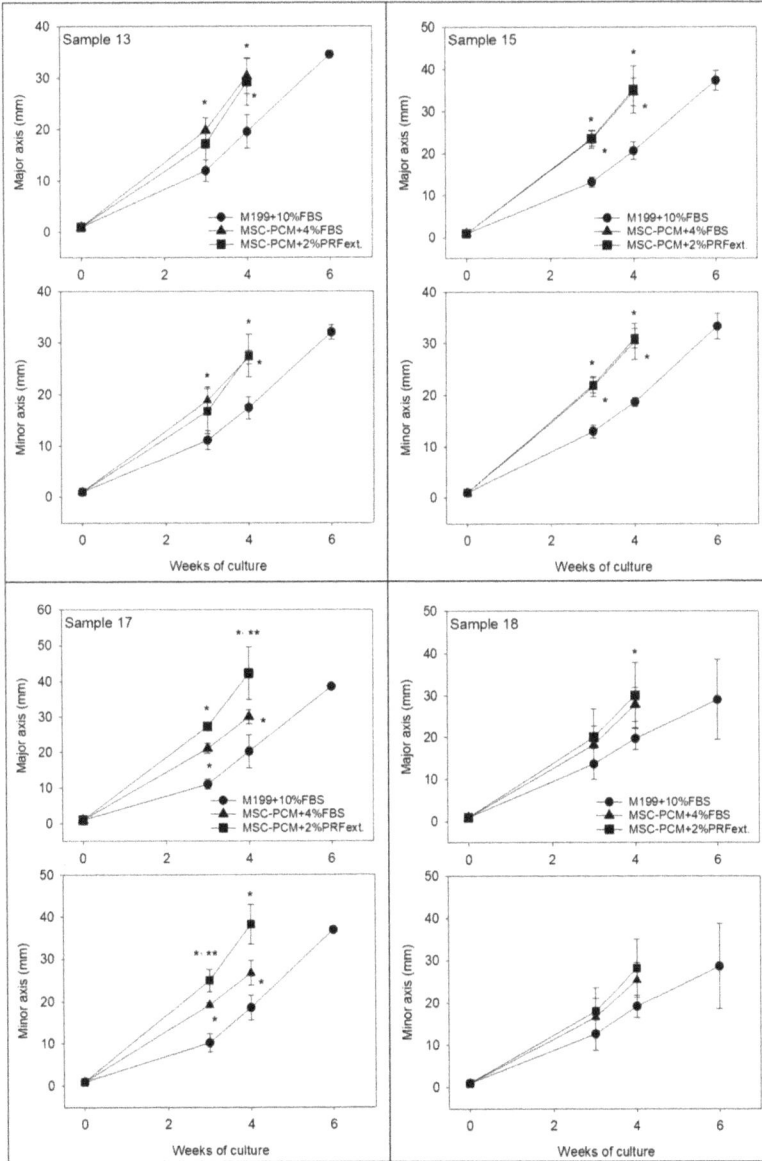

Figure 3. Effects of different culture media on the growth of periosteal sheets. The data obtained from periosteum samples derived from four independent donors are shown. X-axis: time periods (weeks) of explant culture. $N = 2$ (6 weeks), 3 (6 weeks), 4, 5, or 7 replicates. Statistical analysis was performed by Kruskal–Wallis one-way analysis of variance, followed by Steel–Dwass multiple comparison test. * $p < 0.05$ as compared with the control group (Medium199 + 10% FBS) at same time points. ** $p < 0.05$ as compared with the other experimental group (MSC-PCM + 4% FBS) at same time points.

2.2. Phenotype of Periosteal Sheets

Figure 4 shows alkaline phosphatase (ALP) activity, a representative phenotypic marker of differentiated osteoblasts, in fixed periosteal sheets. Safranin-O staining indicated the size of individual samples. As the cell multilayer formation varied with different types of media, it is difficult to compare ALP activity among groups.

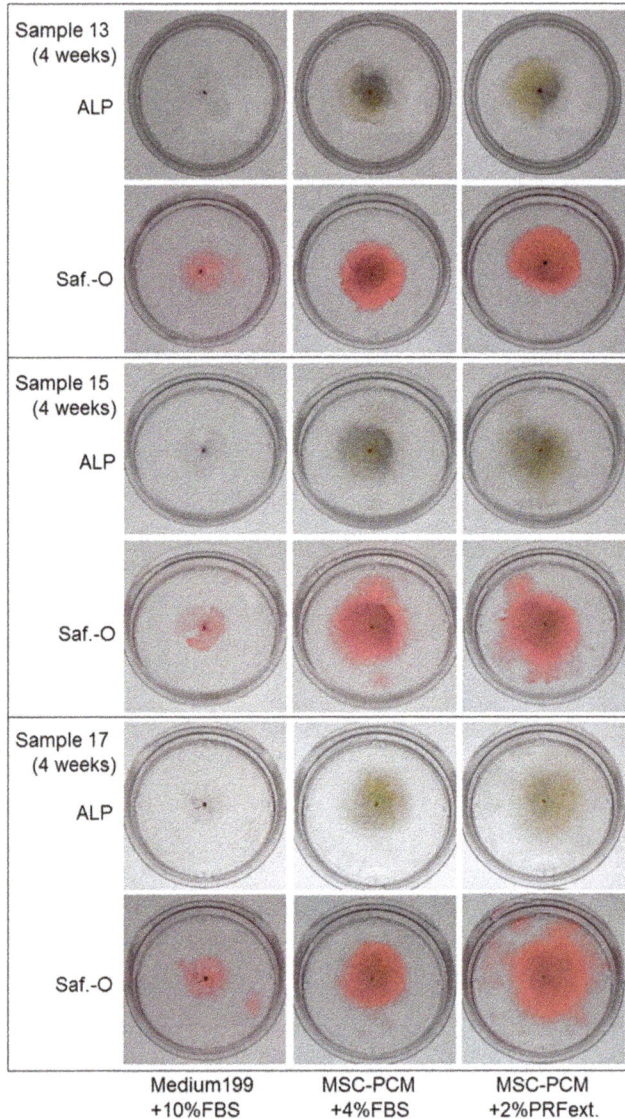

Figure 4. Effects of different culture media on the alkaline phosphatase (ALP) activity and size of periosteal sheets. Fixed individual periosteal sheets were first stained for ALP activity (positive: dark blue-purple) and subsequently treated with Safranin-O (Saf.-O) for the evaluation of their sizes. We used 60 mm culture dishes.

Figure 5 shows cell multilayers and calcium deposit formation in the sagittal section of periosteal sheets. The thickness of outgrown cell sheets varied in the presence of different types of culture media. MSC-PCM + 2% PRFext was the most effective medium for cell multilayer formation. Although cell growth in a horizontal plane is fundamentally different from cell growth in multiple layers, the observed effect was, to some extent, consistent with the growth rate results shown in Figure 3. By contrast, although calcium deposit formation largely relies on the nature of the original periosteum tissue segments, the conventional medium generally induced diffused mineralization, whereas MSC-PCM medium reduced it in limited regions.

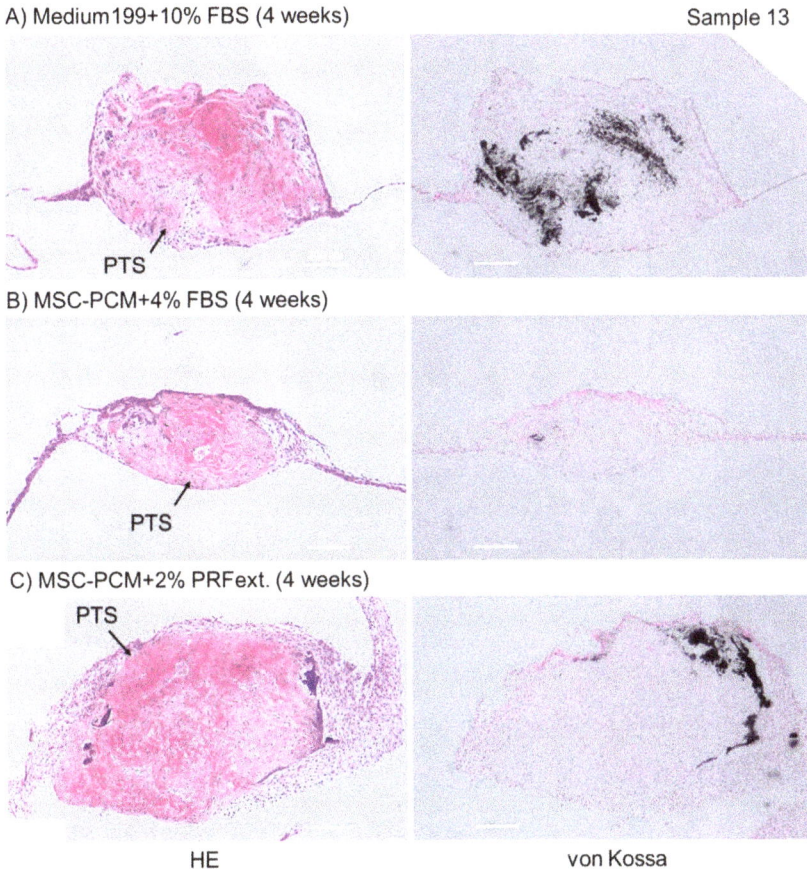

A) Medium199+10% FBS (4 weeks)   Sample 13

PTS

B) MSC-PCM+4% FBS (4 weeks)

PTS

C) MSC-PCM+2% PRFext. (4 weeks)

PTS

HE   von Kossa

Figure 5. Effects of different culture media on the thickness of periosteal sheets. In von Kossa staining, calcium deposits were stained black. These data are representative of five independent experiments. hematoxylin and eosin (HE) staining. Bar = 200 μm.

Figure 6 shows the distribution of PDGF-B, transforming growth factor beta 1 (TGFβ1), and collagen type I in the outgrown cell sheets. PDGF-B or antigenically similar proteins were not detected in any groups in Figure 6. The expression of TGFβ1 or similar proteins was slightly positive in the periosteal sheets expanded in the conventional medium. However, collagen type I was detected in all groups. As MSC-PCM + 2% PRFext produced the thickest cell multilayers, the volume of collagen type I matrix was the most abundant in the periosteal sheets expanded in this culture medium.

A) PDGF-B

B) TGFβ1

C) Col-I

| Medium199+10% FBS | MSC-PCM+4% FBS | MSC-PCM+2% PRFext. |

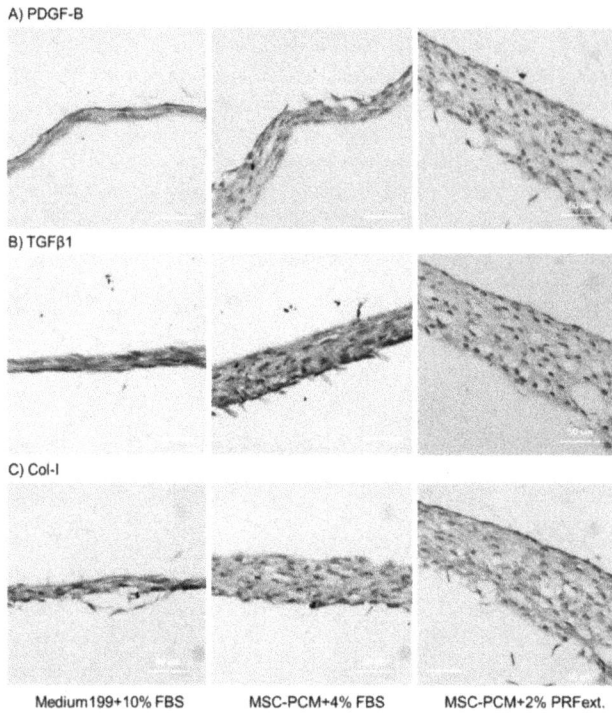

Figure 6. Effects of different culture media on the expression of platelet-derived growth factor-B (PDGF-B), transforming growth factor beta 1 (TGFβ1), and collagen type I in the central region of periosteal sheets (outgrowth area). Immunohistochemical staining with visualization using 3′-diaminobenzidine (DAB) (positive: dark brown). These data are representative of five independent experiments. Bar = 50 μm.

Figure 7 shows the expression of the basic markers of mesenchymal stem cells, CD73, CD90, and CD105, in the cells growing in periosteal sheets. Comparison was performed only between two groups; namely, the conventional medium and MSC-PCM + 2% PRFext. Expression of CD105 was lower in the newly developed medium than that in the conventional medium; however, no statistical differences were observed.

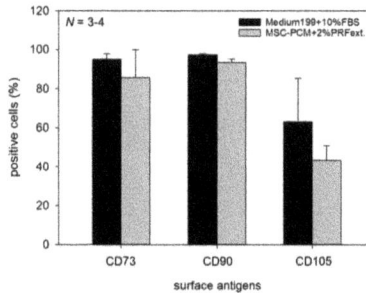

Figure 7. Effects of different culture media on the expression of surface antigens. Only periosteal sheets cultured with MSC-PCM + 2% PRFext were compared with the control sheets (Sample 21). *X*-axis: type of surface antigens. Statistical analysis was performed using the Mann–Whitney rank-sum test and no significant difference was observed between the two groups. *N* = 3 or 4 replicates.

3. Discussion

FBS is still considered a "magical" supplement for the successful cultivation of cells, although the associated disadvantages are well known. To improve the quality of the resulting cell-based products and their therapies, animal-derived factors should be completely eliminated from culture media. Several efforts have been directed toward the development of a chemically defined medium suitable for adherent cell cultures. In the initial phase of our project, we aimed to develop such a chemically defined medium or a medium free of animal components suitable for the cultivation of periosteal sheets. In comparison with single cell cultures, however, periosteal tissues require stronger adhesion systems that cannot be achieved by simply adding sufficient amounts of recombinant human adhesion molecules, such as fibronectin and vitronectin, as evident from our preliminary studies. Instead, such systems may be reproduced with the use of animal or human-derived sera. Therefore, we modified our aim to develop a xeno-free medium.

At the beginning of the second phase, we developed and patented a new expansion method using stocked human platelet-rich plasma (PRP) along with recombinant human bFGF to allow the growth of periosteal sheets [12]. This method provides a consistent source of fully confluent periosteal sheets in 100 mm dishes within 4 weeks. However, a thin fibrin membrane also forms, covering periosteal sheets that may cause easy detachment of periosteal sheets upon medium exchange. Thus, in the preliminary study, we attempted to evaluate alternative ways to utilize the factors from platelet concentrates.

In industry, it may be convenient and economical to use pooled allogeneic PRP, although complicated and costly extraction methods have to be introduced into the manufacturing process. For the preparation of small-scale homemade autologous PRP extracts, by contrast, the preparation protocol needs to be simple and cost-effective. The first choice is definitely platelet-rich fibrin (PRF) exudate or releasate. However, as various major adhesion molecules were found to be adsorbed on fibrin fibers in a preliminary experiment [Kawase et al., manuscript in submission], we homogenized the minced PRF preparations to release these adhesion molecules and used the obtained supernatant supplemented with small debris of fibrin fragments. This preparation protocol is fast, less labor-intensive, and produced better results during the initial adhesion and growth of periosteal sheets, even after reducing the content of PRFext to 2% (*v/v*).

The rapid growth induced by PRFext was not associated with the initial cell outgrowth, but was related to the acceleration of cell proliferation after outgrowth. As illustrated in Figure 8 and previously demonstrated [13], most periosteal cells are dead in the initial phase of culture, and the surviving cells actively replicate and migrate out to form periosteal sheets. Our results indicate that the added PRFext acted on cell outgrowth and subsequent cell proliferation, but not on cell turnover. The shortening of the cell turnover phase may allow further reduction in the period of periosteal sheet preparation to less than 3 weeks in the near future.

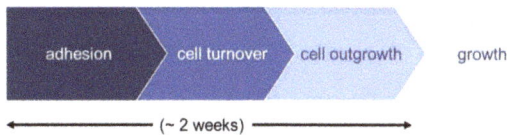

Figure 8. Phases in the process of periosteal sheet cultures.

As rapid proliferation needs to be balanced against genetic, phenotypic, and functional stability [1], we examined the compatibility of periosteal sheets prepared using the new culture medium in the validation stage of this study. Regarding genetic stability, the source of periosteal sheets, i.e., the cells from alveolar periosteum, is at a relatively late stage of differentiation compared to mesenchymal stem cells. In general, the genetic instability of cells correlates with their pluripotency and multipotency [14,15]; therefore, the majority of periosteal cells may be relatively genetically stable during expansion. In support of this speculation, we have previously demonstrated the least probability of cell transformation in X-ray-irradiated periosteal cells [16]. Furthermore, the qualitative analysis of a limited number of cells in karyotype testing (preliminary study) revealed no abnormality in the chromosomes from periosteal sheet samples at the end of the expansion period.

Regarding the rest of the criteria, the type of culture medium failed to have any significant influence on the expression of the conventional surface markers of mesenchymal stem cells, i.e., CD73, CD90, and CD105 [17]. ALP expression and calcium phosphate deposition were, to some extent, influenced by culture media. The addition of PRFext suppressed the spontaneous increase in ALP activity and consequent calcium deposit formation observed in the periosteal sheets expanded in Medium199 + 10% FBS. By contrast, MSC-PCM increased the accumulation of collagen around periosteal cells and consequently increased the thickness of periosteal sheets with an increase in growth rate. MSC-PCM induced maximum effects on sheet thickness in combination with PRFext.

Similar observations were recorded in a previous study using another stem cell medium, MesenPRO-RS medium supplemented with 2% FBS [8]. Although the ALP activity and the ability to form calcium deposits in vitro were lower, the periosteal sheets prepared with this medium showed potent osteogenesis similar to that achieved with the conventional medium upon subcutaneous implantation in animal models. Taken together with the evidence that collagen provides a platform for mineral deposition [18], the periosteal sheets prepared with MSC-PCM + 2% PRFext may possibly exhibit compatible osteogenesis.

The shortening of the preparation period is beneficial for both clinics serving this regenerative therapy and patients receiving this therapy, in terms of cost, operation efficiency, and treatment schedule. However, compatibility must be predefined and tested to ensure safety and efficacy of the resulting periosteal sheets [1] prior to clinical application. As expected, the present study demonstrates that the critical qualities of the periosteal sheet prepared with MSC-PCM + 2% PRFext are not negatively influenced during the process of expansion. The process of blood collection from patients can be estimated to be relatively low on the basis of predicted consumption as mentioned: for a medium size (2−3 tooth width) alveolar ridge augmentation, approximately 30 periosteal sheets are usually prepared. When 60 mm culture dishes are used, approximately 600 mL of the culture medium and approximately 12 mL PRFext are required for the 4-week culture. Since a 10 mL whole-blood sample, including 1 mL Acid Citrate Dextrose Formula-A (ACD-A), produces approximately 2.5 mL PRFext, approximately 45 mL peripheral blood should be collected as a sufficient starting volume prior to the explant culture. However, in case of smaller bone defects, such as periodontal bone defect, the volume of blood required for the culture can be reduced to between one-fifth and one-tenth.

In addition, this xeno-free medium minimizes the risk of unknown pathogen contamination. The newly developed MSC-PCM medium is exceptionally more expensive than the conventional Medium199, but the total cost may be markedly reduced by choosing MSC-PCM + 2% PRFext. Therefore, we proposed that this complete xeno-free medium may serve as a promising replacement medium for the conventional FBS-containing medium in the preparation of periosteal sheets.

4. Materials and Methods

4.1. Preparation of PRFext

Blood was collected from six healthy and non-smoking volunteers aged 24–44 years (three females and three males) using butterfly needles (21G 3/400; NIPRO, Osaka, Japan) and Vacutainer tubes (Japan Becton, Dickinson and Company, Tokyo, Japan). To prepare the PRFext, the blood samples were immediately (within approximately 2 min from blood collection) centrifuged by a Medifuge centrifugation system (Silfradent S. r. l., Santa Sofia, Italy) [19,20]. The red thrombus (the fraction of red blood cells) was eliminated with scissors and the resulting PRF preparations were minced using scissors, followed by homogenization with sterile BioMasher (Nippi, Tokyo, Japan), as illustrated in Figure 9 and as described previously [21]. The homogenized samples were centrifuged at maximum speed to exclude fibrin matrix fragments. The resulting supernatant was stored at −80 °C until use.

Approximately 2.5 mL PRFext can be prepared from 10 mL whole-blood sample, including 1 mL ACD-A. The levels of PDGF-BB in the resulting samples usually ranged from 25 to 50 ng/mL [21].

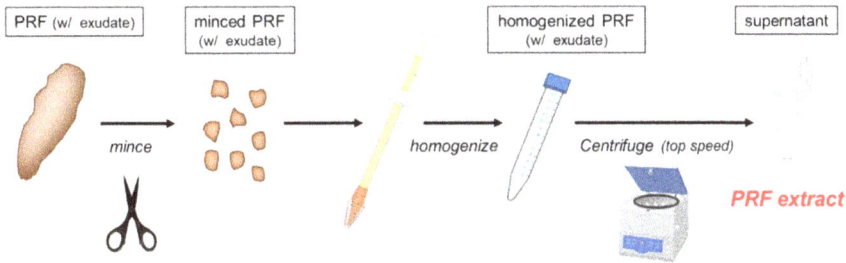

Figure 9. Graphic summary of preparation of platelet-rich fibrin (PRF) extract.

The study design and consent forms for all the procedures (project identification code: 2015-2143) were approved by the Ethics Committee for Human Subjects of the Niigata University School of Medicine (Niigata, Japan) on 12 June, 2017, in accordance with the Helsinki Declaration of 1964 as revised in 2013.

4.2. Explant Culture of Periosteum Tissue Segments to Form Periosteal Sheets

Six patients aged 20–44 years (four females and two males) in need of wisdom tooth extraction participated in this study after providing written informed consent. Aliquots of periosteum tissues were aseptically dissected from the buccal side of the retromolar region in the mandible of healthy donors, washed thrice in Dulbecco's PBS without Ca^{2+} and Mg^{2+}, cut into small segments (~1 × 1 mm), and plated on 60 mm dishes. After incubation for 15–20 min under dry conditions in a CO_2 incubator, the conventional medium (Medium199 supplemented with 10% FBS), MSC-PCM medium (Kohjin Bio, Sakado, Japan) supplemented with 4% FBS, or MSC-PCM medium supplemented with 2% PRFext was added to cover the bottom surface of the dish. All media were commonly supplemented with 25 µg/mL of L-ascorbic acid, 100 U/mL of penicillin G, 100 µg/mL of streptomycin, and 0.25 µg/mL of amphotericin B (Invitrogen, Carlsbad, CA, USA). The volume of media was increased in a stepwise manner as cell outgrowth proceeded.

4.3. Evaluation of Cell Outgrowth and Growth Rate

The onset of cell outgrowth, which indicates days required for the migration of the first cell out of the original periosteum tissue segments, was evaluated using an inverted microscope once every 3 days. Frequent examination of cell outgrowth can sometimes lead to detachment of periosteum tissue segments; hence, we did not perform a daily evaluation.

The growth rate was determined by measuring the lengths of the long (major) axis and short (minor) axis. Periosteal sheets were plated on a light box and measured by a caliper.

4.4. Histological Determination of ALP Activity

For ALP staining, periosteal sheets were fixed with 10% neutralized formalin on dishes and directly treated with an ALP staining kit (Muto Chemicals, Tokyo, Japan) for 4 h, followed by counterstaining with Safranin-O [4].

4.5. Histological and Immunohistochemical Examination for Calcium Deposition, Growth Factor Expression, and Collagen Accumulation

Periosteal sheets were gently detached using a cell scraper and immediately fixed with 10% formaldehyde in 0.1 M phosphate buffer, pH 7.4, overnight. Fixed samples were dehydrated using an ethanol series (70%−100%) and xylene and embedded in paraffin. The samples were sagittally sectioned at a thickness of 6 μm [4].

As previously described [20], the deparaffinized sections were subjected to antigen retrieval with Liberate Antibody Binding Solution (Polysciences, Inc., Warrington, PA, USA) and blocked with Block-Ace (Sumitomo Dainippon Pharma., Osaka, Japan) solution in 0.1% Tween-20-containing PBS. The sections were probed with a rabbit polyclonal anti-collagen type I antibody (1:400; Bioss Inc., Boston, MA, USA), anti-TGFβ1 antibody (1:200; Santa Cruz Biotechnology, Inc., Santa Cruz, CA, USA), or anti-PDGF-B (1:200; Santa Cruz) diluted in ImmunoShot Mild (Cosmo Bio, Tokyo, Japan) overnight at 4 °C, followed by incubation in horseradish peroxidase (HRP)-conjugated anti-rabbit IgG (Cell Signaling Technology, Danvers, MA, USA). Immunoreactive proteins were visualized with a 3,3′-diaminobenzidine (DAB) substrate solution (Kirkegaard & Perry Laboratories, Inc., Gaithersburg, MD, USA).

The sections were alternatively stained with hematoxylin and eosin (HE) or silver nitrate (von Kossa staining). For von Kossa staining, the sections were faintly counterstained with Kernechtrot solution to provide a background stain [4].

4.6. Flow Cytometric Evaluation of CD73-, CD90-, and CD105-Positive Periosteal Cells

Cells were dispersed from cultured periosteal sheets with 0.05% trypsin + 0.53 mM ethylenediaminetetraacetic acid (EDTA) solution (Invitrogen), washed twice with PBS, and suspended in 0.1 mL PBS containing 0.1% bovine serum albumin (BSA) at a density of 1×10^6 cells/mL. The cells were probed for 30 min at 4 °C with 5 μL of the following mouse monoclonal antibodies: anti-CD73-fluorescein isothiocyanate (FITC) (IgG1) (BioLegend, San Diego, CA, USA), anti-CD90-phycoerythrin (PE)/Cy5 (IgG1) (BioLegend), and anti-CD105-PE (IgG1) (BioLegend). After being washed twice with PBS, the cells were analyzed by flow cytometry (Navios; Beckman Coulter, Miami, FL, USA). Data analysis and histogram overlay were performed using Navios Software (Beckman Coulter). For isotype controls, individual corresponding antibodies (all from BioLegend) were used [8].

4.7. Statistical Analysis

The data were expressed as mean ± standard deviation (SD). For multigroup comparisons, statistical analyses were performed to compare the mean values by Kruskal–Wallis one-way analysis of variance, followed by Steel–Dwass multiple comparison test (BellCurve for Excel version 3.00; Social Survey Research Information Co., Ltd., Tokyo, Japan). For two group comparisons, statistical differences were tested using the Mann-Whitney rank-sum test (SigmaPlot 12.5; Systat Software, Inc., San Jose, CA, USA). Differences with P values of less than 0.05 were considered statistically significant.

5. Conclusions

This preclinical study successfully validated the applicability of PRFext for FBS replacement in explant cultures of periosteum tissue segments to form periosteal sheets. These findings were established using the samples donated by healthy volunteers. For therapeutic use, however, autologous periosteum tissue and PRFext must be employed for the preparation of periosteal sheets. Thus, the efficacy of PRFext and the responsiveness of periosteum tissue may vary with individual samples, and more careful measures should be adopted while evaluating the quality of periosteal sheets prepared by this protocol.

Author Contributions: Conceptualization, T.K., A.I. and K.N.; methodology, T.K., M.N. and K.O.; formal analysis, T.K., T.U. and K.N.; investigation, T.K., T.U., Y.F., M.W. and A.I.; data curation, Y.F., M.W., A.I. and K.N.; Supervision, T.K., A.I. and K.N.; writing—original draft preparation, T.K.; writing—review and editing, M.N, K.O., T.U., A.I. and K.N.

Funding: This study is financially supported by the budget provided by Kojin Bio, Co., Ltd. for the collaborative research investigation.

Acknowledgments: Kojin Bio, Co., Ltd. modified the stem cell medium suitable for the explant culture of human periosteum tissue in response to our requests and provided it by free of charge.

Conflicts of Interest: A.I. who is an employee of Kohjin Bio, Co., Ltd. was involved in the collection, analyses and interpretation of data. Author T.K., M.N., K.O., T.U., Y.F., M.W. and K.N. state that there are no conflicts of interest. The funders had no role in the design of the study; in the collection, analyses, or interpretation of data; in the writing of the manuscript, or in the decision to publish the results.

Abbreviations

PRF	platelet-rich fibrin
PRFext	platelet-rich fibrin extract
PRP	platelet-rich plasma
bFGF	basic fibroblast growth factor
ALP	alkaline phosphatase
Saf.-O	Safranin-O
IgG	immunoglobulin
HRP	horseradish peroxidase
DAB	3,3′-diaminobenzidine tetrahydrochloride
PDGF-B	Platelet-derived growth factor-B
TGFβ1	Transforming growth factor beta 1
EDTA	Ethylenediaminetetraacetic acid

References

1. Karnieli, O.; Friedner, O.M.; Allickson, J.G.; Zhang, N.; Jung, S.; Fiorentini, D.; Abraham, E.; Eaker, S.S.; Yong, T.K.; Chan, A.; et al. A consensus introduction to serum replacements and serum-free media for cellular therapies. *Cytotherapy* **2017**, *19*, 155–169. [CrossRef] [PubMed]

2. Marx, R.E.; Carlson, E.R.; Eichstaedt, R.M.; Schimmele, S.R.; Strauss, J.E.; Georgeff, K.R. Platelet-rich plasma: Growth factor enhancement for bone grafts. *Oral Surg. Oral Med. Oral Pathol. Oral Radiol. Endodontics* **1998**, *85*, 638–646. [CrossRef]

3. Burnouf, T.; Strunk, D.; Koh, M.B.; Schallmoser, K. Human platelet lysate: Replacing fetal bovine serum as a gold standard for human cell propagation? *Biomaterials* **2016**, *76*, 371–387. [CrossRef] [PubMed]

4. Kawase, T.; Okuda, K.; Kogami, H.; Nakayama, H.; Nagata, M.; Nakata, K.; Yoshie, H. Characterization of human cultured periosteal sheets expressing bone-forming potential: In vitro and in vivo animal studies. *J. Tissue Engin. Regener. Med.* **2009**, *3*, 218–229. [CrossRef] [PubMed]

5. Yamamiya, K.; Okuda, K.; Kawase, T.; Hata, K.; Wolff, L.F.; Yoshie, H. Tissue-engineered cultured periosteum used with platelet-rich plasma and hydroxyapatite in treating human osseous defects. *J. Periodontol.* **2008**, *79*, 811–818. [CrossRef] [PubMed]

6. Nagata, M.; Hoshina, H.; Li, M.; Arasawa, M.; Uematsu, K.; Ogawa, S.; Yamada, K.; Kawase, T.; Suzuki, K.; Ogose, A.; et al. A clinical study of alveolar bone tissue engineering with cultured autogenous periosteal cells: Coordinated activation of bone formation and resorption. *Bone* **2012**, *50*, 1123–1129. [CrossRef] [PubMed]

7. Ogawa, S.; Hoshina, H.; Nakata, K.; Yamada, K.; Uematsu, K.; Kawase, T.; Takagi, R.; Nagata, M. High-Resolution Three-Dimensional Computed Tomography Analysis of the Clinical Efficacy of Cultured Autogenous Periosteal Cells in Sinus Lift Bone Grafting. *Clin. Implant Dent. Relat. Res.* **2016**, *18*, 707–716. [CrossRef] [PubMed]

8. Uematsu, K.; Kawase, T.; Nagata, M.; Suzuki, K.; Okuda, K.; Yoshie, H.; Burns, D.M.; Takagi, R. Tissue culture of human alveolar periosteal sheets using a stem-cell culture medium (MesenPRO-RS): In vitro expansion of CD146-positive cells and concomitant upregulation of osteogenic potential in vivo. *Stem cell Res.* **2013**, *10*, 1–19. [CrossRef] [PubMed]

9. Lavenus, S.; Berreur, M.; Trichet, V.; Pilet, P.; Louarn, G.; Layrolle, P. Adhesion and osteogenic differentiation of human mesenchymal stem cells on titanium nanopores. *Eur. Cells Mater.* **2011**, *22*, 84–96. [CrossRef]

10. Lavenus, S.; Pilet, P.; Guicheux, J.; Weiss, P.; Louarn, G.; Layrolle, P. Behaviour of mesenchymal stem cells, fibroblasts and osteoblasts on smooth surfaces. *Acta Biomater.* **2011**, *7*, 1525–1534. [CrossRef] [PubMed]

11. Olivares-Navarrete, R.; Hyzy, S.L.; Hutton, D.L.; Erdman, C.P.; Wieland, M.; Boyan, B.D.; Schwartz, Z. Direct and indirect effects of microstructured titanium substrates on the induction of mesenchymal stem cell differentiation towards the osteoblast lineage. *Biomaterials* **2010**, *31*, 2728–2735. [CrossRef] [PubMed]

12. Kawase, T.; Okuda, K. Method for culturing human periosteum. U.S. Patent 8,420,392B2, 16 April 2013.

13. Kawase, T.; Kogami, H.; Nagata, M.; Uematsu, K.; Okuda, K.; Burns, D.M.; Yoshie, H. Manual cryopreservation of human alveolar periosteal tissue segments: Effects of pre-culture on recovery rate. *Cryobiology* **2011**, *62*, 202–209. [CrossRef] [PubMed]

14. Catalina, P.; Cobo, F.; Cortes, J.L.; Nieto, A.I.; Cabrera, C.; Montes, R.; Concha, A.; Menendez, P. Conventional and molecular cytogenetic diagnostic methods in stem cell research: A concise review. *Cell Biol. Int.* **2007**, *31*, 861–869. [CrossRef] [PubMed]

15. Mohn, F.; Schubeler, D. Genetics and epigenetics: Stability and plasticity during cellular differentiation. *Trends Genet.* **2009**, *25*, 129–136. [CrossRef] [PubMed]

16. Kawase, T.; Kamiya, M.; Hayama, K.; Nagata, M.; Okuda, K.; Yoshie, H.; Burns, D.M.; Tsuchimochi, M.; Nakata, K. X-ray and ultraviolet C irradiation-induced gamma-H2AX and p53 formation in normal human periosteal cells in vitro: Markers for quality control in cell therapy. *Cytotherapy* **2015**, *17*, 112–123. [CrossRef] [PubMed]

17. Dominici, M.; Le Blanc, K.; Mueller, I.; Slaper-Cortenbach, I.; Marini, F.; Krause, D.; Deans, R.; Keating, A.; Prockop, D.; Horwitz, E. Minimal criteria for defining multipotent mesenchymal stromal cells. The International Society for Cellular Therapy position statement. *Cytotherapy* **2006**, *8*, 315–317. [CrossRef] [PubMed]

18. Williams, D.C.; Frolik, C.A. Physiological and pharmacological regulation of biological calcification. *Int. Rev. Cytol.* **1991**, *126*, 195–292. [PubMed]

19. Masuki, H.; Okudera, T.; Watanebe, T.; Suzuki, M.; Nishiyama, K.; Okudera, H.; Nakata, K.; Uematsu, K.; Su, C.Y.; Kawase, T. Growth factor and pro-inflammatory cytokine contents in platelet-rich plasma (PRP), plasma rich in growth factors (PRGF), advanced platelet-rich fibrin (A-PRF), and concentrated growth factors (CGF). *Int. J. Implant Dent.* **2016**, *2*, 19. [CrossRef] [PubMed]

20. Kobayashi, M.; Kawase, T.; Horimizu, M.; Okuda, K.; Wolff, L.F.; Yoshie, H. A proposed protocol for the standardized preparation of PRF membranes for clinical use. *Biologicals* **2012**, *40*, 323–329. [CrossRef] [PubMed]

21. Tsukioka, T.; Hiratsuka, T.; Nakamura, M.; Watanabe, T.; Kitamura, Y.; Isobe, K.; Okudera, T.; Okudera, H.; Azuma, A.; Uematsu, K.; et al. An on-site preparable, novel bone-grafting complex consisting of human platelet-rich fibrin and porous particles made of a recombinant collagen-like protein. *J. Biomed. Mater. Res. B Appl. Biomater.* **2018**. [CrossRef] [PubMed]

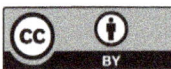

International Journal of
Molecular Sciences

MDPI

Article

Short-Term Outcomes of Percutaneous Trephination with a Platelet Rich Plasma Intrameniscal Injection for the Repair of Degenerative Meniscal Lesions. A Prospective, Randomized, Double-Blind, Parallel-Group, Placebo-Controlled Study

Rafal Kaminski [1],*[ID], Marta Maksymowicz-Wleklik [1], Krzysztof Kulinski [1], Katarzyna Kozar-Kaminska [2], Agnieszka Dabrowska-Thing [3] and Stanislaw Pomianowski [1]

[1] Department of Musculoskeletal Trauma Surgery and Orthopaedics, Centre of Postgraduate Medical Education, Professor A. Gruca Teaching Hospital, Konarskiego 13, 05-400 Otwock, Poland; maksymowicz.mm@gmail.com (M.M.-W.); k.kulinski@o2.pl (K.K.); spom@spskgruca.pl (S.P.)

[2] Department of Medical Biology, The Stefan Cardinal Wyszynski Institute of Cardiology, ul. Alpejska 42, 04-628 Warsaw, Poland; k.kozar@ikard.pl

[3] Departament of Radiology, Centre of Postgraduate Medical Education in Warsaw, ul. Konarskiego 13, 05-400 Otwock, Poland; dabrowska@poczta.fm

* Correspondence: rkaminski@spskgruca.pl

check for
updates

Received: 28 January 2019; Accepted: 12 February 2019; Published: 16 February 2019

Abstract: Meniscal tears are the most common orthopaedic injuries, with chronic lesions comprising up to 56% of cases. In these situations, no benefit with surgical treatment is observed. Thus, the purpose of this study was to investigate the effectiveness and safety of percutaneous intrameniscal platelet rich plasma (PRP) application to complement repair of a chronic meniscal lesion. This single centre, prospective, randomized, double-blind, placebo-controlled study included 72 patients. All subjects underwent meniscal trephination with or without concomitant PRP injection. Meniscal non-union observed in magnetic resonance arthrography or arthroscopy were considered as failures. Patient related outcome measures (PROMs) were assessed. The failure rate was significantly higher in the control group than in the PRP augmented group (70% vs. 48%, $P = 0.04$). Kaplan-Meyer analysis for arthroscopy-free survival showed significant reduction in the number of performed arthroscopies in the PRP augmented group. A notably higher percentage of patients treated with PRP achieved minimal clinically significant difference in visual analogue scale (VAS) and Knee injury and Osteoarthritis Outcome Score (KOOS) symptom scores. Our trial indicates that percutaneous meniscal trephination augmented with PRP results in a significant improvement in the rate of chronic meniscal tear healing and this procedure decreases the necessity for arthroscopy in the future (8% vs. 28%, $P = 0.032$).

Keywords: meniscus; meniscus repair; meniscus tear; trephination; platelet-rich plasma; PRP; chronic meniscal lesion; horizontal meniscal tear

1. Introduction

The menisci are known to play a pivotal role during normal functioning of the knee joint. Their unique and complex chondral structure, as well as their biology, make treatment and repair very challenging. The menisci increase joint stability, distribute load, absorb shock and provide lubrication and nutrition to the remaining joint elements.

Meniscal tears are considered the most common orthopaedic diagnoses. For many years, arthroscopy was regarded as a "gold standard" in therapy with almost 4 million arthroscopies for meniscus pathologies performed annually all over the world, thus representing a serious socio-economic concern with relevant Health Care System costs [1]. Interestingly, more than 50% of these surgeries are conducted in patients older than 45 years with degenerative meniscal lesions [2]. This type of injury is a slowly progressing phenomenon, typically involving horizontal cleavage of the meniscal body with prevalence in the population reaching up to 56%. Interestingly, 61% of those tears have no clinical symptoms of meniscal pathology (pain, aching, stiffness or oedema) [2]. These data provided the background for studies analysing the efficacy of arthroscopy in chronic meniscal lesion therapy. Several randomized clinical trials were performed and demonstrated no additional benefit of partial meniscectomy to sham surgery [3]. These data introduced doubt into the current practice and resulted in making clinical decisions more challenging. Additionally, meniscectomy or partial meniscectomy results in rapid deterioration of articular cartilage and the development of arthritis [4]. Despite the trend of meniscus tear repair and maintaining as much vital tissue as possible [5] there is an inability amongst surgeons to restore anatomical and functional roles of the repaired meniscus. Simultaneously, osteoarthritis progressively develops. These rationales shifted the treatment protocols of chronic meniscal tears into the non-operative manner and motivated the search for new therapeutic strategies.

There are several clinical trials that have provided evidence for the use of blood or bone marrow derived products in the surgical treatment of meniscal pathology: the fibrin clot technique [6,7], platelet-rich plasma (PRP) [8,9] or the bone marrow venting procedure [10,11]. There is, however, no data in the literature evaluating the effect of blood derived products on healing of chronic meniscal tears. Thus we designed a prospective, randomized, double-blind, parallel-group, placebo-controlled study to investigate the effectiveness and safety of minimally invasive (percutaneous) intrameniscal PRP application to complement repair of a symptomatic chronic meniscal lesion. We hypothesized that intrameniscal injection of PRP with concomitant meniscal trephination would result in both an improved healing rate and better functional outcomes.

2. Results

Follow-up ended on 15 January 2019. The median follow-up lasted for 92 weeks (54–157 weeks). 1 patient was lost to follow-up and 2 additional patients were excluded from analysis due to additional procedures (ligament surgery and radio synovectomy) (Figure 1). All remaining patients were functionally assessed at 3, 6, 12 months after the initial procedure. Patients undergoing arthroscopy due to unacceptable quality of life were excluded from analysis of the PROMs. There were no significant differences in baseline characteristics between the groups (Table 1).

Table 1. Baseline characteristics of study patients in the control and PRP-treated groups.

	Control Group (*n* = 30)	PRP-Treated Group (*n* = 42)	*P*-Value
Age (years)	46 (27–68)	44 (18–67)	*P* = 0.31
Sex (M:F)	19:11	22:20	*P* = 0.25
BMI (range)	28 (21–36)	27 (19–37)	*P* = 0.27
Kellgren-Lawrence scale (0 grade:1 grade:2 grade)	23:7:0	30:12:0	*P* = 0.79
PRP (PLT $\times\ 10^3/\mu$L)	732 (220–1586)	823 (320–1659)	*P* = 0.16
Meniscus (MM:ML)	30:0	41:1	*P* = 0.58

Data are presented as median (range) or mean ± standard error (confidence interval (CI) 95%) unless otherwise indicated. BMI, body mass index; PRP, platelet rich plasma; PLT, platelets; MM—medial meniscus; ML—lateral meniscus.

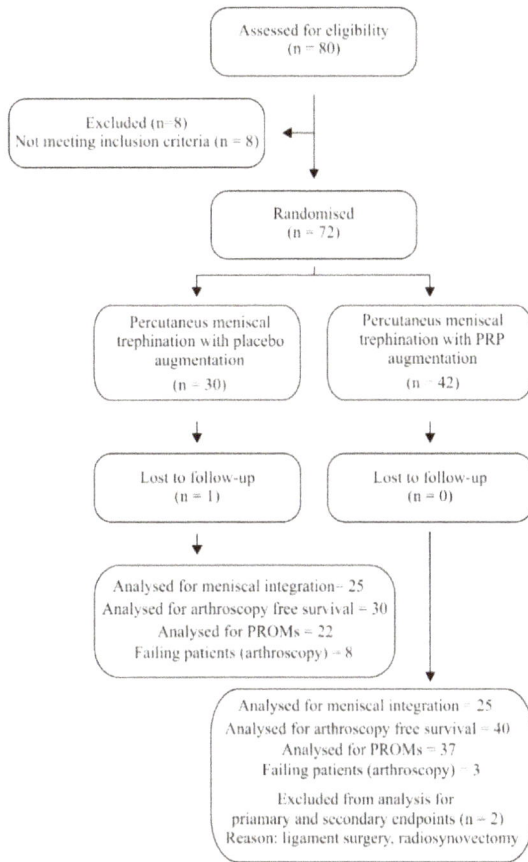

Figure 1. Flow diagram of the trial.

2.1. Primary Outcome

Assessment of meniscal healing on MR arthrography was performed at week 33 (13–78) in both groups (Table 2). Induction of the healing process within the meniscus was observed. The healing rate of the meniscal tear, although not significant, was superior in the PRP augmented percutaneous trephination repair group (11 fully and 4 partially healed menisci out of 25 assessed, 60%) than in the control group (7 fully and 4 partially healed menisci out of 26 assessed). When considering cumulative failure rate (arthroscopy and arthrography MRI), the success ratio was significantly better in PRP augmented percutaneous trephination group ($P = 0.04$) (Table 2). In case of 10 patients (8 in the control group and 2 in the PRP augmented group) subsequent arthroscopic meniscectomy or meniscal repair was performed due to unacceptable clinical symptoms. The survival of the PRP injected meniscus (arthroscopy free survival) was superior versus the control group ($P = 0.032$, Figure 2). No significant influence of the number of injected platelets or fold increase in the number of platelets in PRP on meniscal healing was detected.

Table 2. Primary outcome assessment.

Cumulative Outcome (Assessed Using MRI and Arthroscopy) ($P = 0.04$)		
Outcome	PRP-treated group (*n* of menisci)	Control group (*n* of menisci)
Healed	10	5
Partially healed	4	3
Failed	13	19
MRI ($P = 0.41$)		
Outcome	PRP-treated group (*n* of menisci)	Control group (*n* of menisci)
Healed	11	7
Partially healed	4	4
Failed	10	15

MRI, magnetic resonance imaging; PRP, platelet-rich plasma.

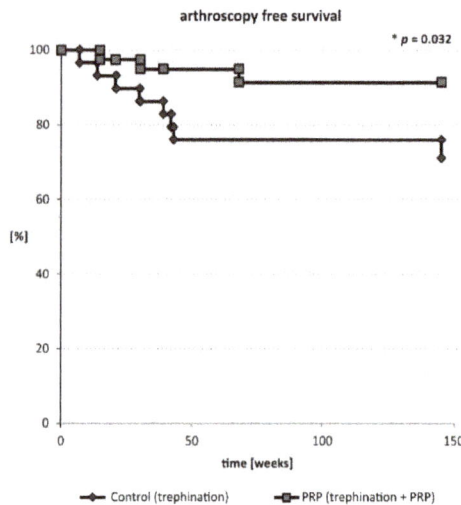

Figure 2. Arthroscopy free survival of patients undergoing trephination of the meniscus with or without PRP augmentation.

2.2. Secondary Outcomes-Pain

Baseline pain characteristics (VAS and KOOS-pain) of the patients did not differ significantly between groups (Table 3). All patients presented an improvement in pain scores. The changes in VAS and KOOS-pain exceeded minimal clinically important difference (MCID) value in majority of patients (Table 4). We detected a significant difference level in the percentage of patients who benefited by at least MCID in VAS score (39% vs. 65%, $P = 0.046$). No other significant changes were detected.

2.3. Secondary Outcomes-Function

Functional outcomes were measured with the IKDC subjective scale, WOMAC and the KOOS subscales (symptoms, function in daily living [ADL], sport/recreation and knee related quality of life [QOL]). Each parameter improved over time in both groups, exceeding the MCID values in vast majority of patients. A significant difference in the percentage of patients who benefited by at least the MCID value in the KOOS Symptoms subscale was detected (48% vs. 76%, $P = 0.028$). We noted that the remaining KOOS subscales, IKDC score and WOMAC score were improved in both groups (Tables 3 and 4).

2.4. Complications

No peri- or post- procedure complications were noted among patients who participated in the final follow-up.

Table 3. Patient-reported outcome measures (pain: VAS and KOOS-pain; function: IKDC, WOMAC, KOOS: symptom, ADL, sport/recreation and QOL).

PROM	Control Group		PRP Group		p [a]
	Pre-Procedure	Post Trephination	Pre-Procedure	Post Trephination	
VAS	4.40 ± 0.07 (3.55–5.25)	2.05 ± 0.08 (1.27–2.82)	5.38 ± 0.05 (4.77–5.99)	1.97 ± 0.05 (1.40–2.55)	0.39
IKDC	54.92 ± 0.54 (49.08–60.77)	88.12 ± 0.89 (79.97–96.28)	51.99 ± 0.34 (47.62–56.36)	85.98 ± 0.52 (79.79–92.16)	0.36
WOMAC	28.93 ± 0.61 (22.42–35.45)	7.50 ± 0.59 (2.06–12.94)	34.36 ± 0.35 (29.90–38.82)	9.72 ± 0.32 (5.95–13.48)	0.21
KOOS					
Pain	65.30 ± 0.54 (59.51–71.10)	89.00 ± 0.63 (83.19–94.81)	57.48 ± 0.30 (57.18–57.78)	87.24 ± 0.36 (82.99–91.48)	0.22
Symptoms	69.86 ± 0.62 (63.18–76.54)	90.42 ± 0.56 (85.26–95.58)	63.53 ± 0.39 (63.23–63.83)	92.03 ± 0.27 (88.80–95.26)	0.27
ADL	68.42 ± 0.66 (61.33–75.50)	92.38 ± 0.61 (86.80–97.95)	63.70 ± 0.37 (63.40–64.00)	89.36 ± 0.36 (85.07–93.64)	0.25
S/R	33.50 ± 0.62 (26.84–40.16)	78.98 ± 1.10 (68.83–89.12)	35.83 ± 0.51 (35.53–36.14)	69.52 ± 0.77 (60.29–78.74)	0.11
QoL	35.00 ± 0.49 (29.73–40.27)	68.18 ± 1.08 (58.28–78.08)	37.90 ± 0.26 (37.59–38.20)	67.06 − 0.55 (60.56–73.56)	0.42

[a] For the control group vs. PRP group; Data are presented as mean ± standard error (CI 95%) unless otherwise indicated. PROM, patient related outcome measures; VAS, visual analogue scale; WOMAC, Western Ontario and McMaster Universities Osteoarthritis Index; IKDC, International Knee Documentation Committee; KOOS, Knee injury and Osteoarthritis Outcome Score; ADL, activities of daily living; S/R, sport/recreation; QOL, quality of life.

Table 4. Patient-reported outcome measures (pain: VAS and KOOS-pain; function: IKDC, WOMAC, KOOS: symptom, ADL, sport/recreation and QOL).

PROM	MCID	Control Group		PRP Group		$p^{\,a}$	$p^{\,b}$
		Mean Change	Improved by at Least MCID [%]	Mean Change	Improved by at Least MCID [%]		
VAS	2 [12]	2.36 ± 0.0.09 (3.86–5.20)	39	3.62 ± 0.07 (2.82–4.43)	65	0.027	0.046
IKDC	16.7 [13]	33.66 ± 0.84 (25.95–41.36)	83	34.74 ± 0.55 (28.17–41.31)	78	0.48	0.48
WOMAC	11.5 [14]	21.77 ± 0.67 (15.65–27.90)	65	24.77 ± 0.37 (20.40–29.14)	86	0.16	0.053
KOOS							
Pain	16.7 [13]	24.95 ± 0.62 (19.24–30.66)	65	29.50 ± 0.45 (24.18–34.81)	73	0.17	0.36
Symptoms	17.4 [13]	18.38 ± 0.82 (10.81–25.95)	48	27.93 ± 0.42 (22.89–32.96)	76	0.016	0.028
ADL	18.4 [13]	24.61 ± 0.74 (17.79–31.43)	57	26.27 ± 0.39 (21.67–30.87)	76	0.18	0.1
S/R	12.5 [13]	43.75 ± 1.12 (33.43–54.07)	83	34.65 ± 0.76 (25.57–43.74)	70	0.12	0.22
QoL	15.6 [13]	32.67 ± 1.06 (22.93–42.41)	70	28.43 ± 0.52 (22.23–34.64)	76	0.29	0.41

[a] For mean changes; [b] for % of patients improved by at least MCID. Data are presented as mean ± standard error (CI 95%) unless otherwise indicated. PROM, patient related outcome measures; VAS, visual analogue scale; WOMAC, Western Ontario and McMaster Universities Osteoarthritis Index; IKDC, International Knee Documentation Committee; KOOS, Knee injury and Osteoarthritis Outcome Score; ADL, activities of daily living; S/R, sport/recreation; QOL, quality of life; MCID, Minimal Clinically Important Difference.

3. Discussion

Meniscal healing has always been a major challenge for orthopaedic surgeons. All types of meniscectomies can lead to an increase in the risk of osteoarthritis [15] and evidence comparing the results of total and partial meniscectomy provide data on the beneficial effects of meniscus preservation [16]. The rising problem in meniscal injury treatment is the substantial number of chronic meniscal lesions. Recent studies comparing non-operative and arthroscopic treatment showed no benefit of surgical treatment in large cohorts of patients [3,17]. Data provided by the European Society of Sports Traumatology, Knee Surgery and Arthroscopy [18] or the guidelines published in the British Medical Journal [19] showed no or poor clinical benefit of arthroscopy in the case of degenerative meniscal lesions. In fact, arthroscopy was titled "the last resort" of treatment and applicable due to failure of conservative management.

The most significant finding of this study was that percutaneous trephination with or without a PRP boost induced the healing response of chronic meniscus tears. The process was augmented in the PRP – treated group. Interestingly, our results also demonstrated that no full meniscal integrity is necessary to obtain a clinically important difference in respect to PROMs. Additionally, we found that the functional outcomes (KOOS Symptoms) and pain levels (VAS) scored higher in patients treated with PRP-augmentation than in the control group.

For this study we used leukocyte- and platelet-rich plasma (L-PRP). Its fluid like state enables delivery to the target site by needle injection. Once activated, L-PRP forms a gel and releases most of the growth factors in the first few hours post injection until fully dissolved within 3 days [20]. It supports growth factors to act as an assembly of platelets and leukocytes in a complex matrix. Although leukocyte and platelet rich fibrin (L-PRF), was shown to slowly release growth factors over a period of about 7 days [21] providing optimal kinetics of a release, it forms a 3D matrix that cannot be delivered via a minimally invasive way (e.g., intra-articular injection)

PRP has been shown to influence not only the process of meniscal healing in vitro and in vivo [22,23] but also the treatment of other musculoskeletal injuries [24,25]. Some evidence has been provided for the use of PRP in meniscal repair [8,9]. The authors found that clinical outcomes and healing rates were better with the introduction of PRP into the lesion at the end of surgery. Griffin et al. performed a retrospective chart review with a minimum of 2 year follow-up and failed to show any benefit of PRP augmentation [26]. However, the study was underpowered for the primary and secondary outcomes. Another Study by Strümper, R. et al. demonstrated that intra-articular autologous conditioned serum injection might be an effective treatment option for knee pain associated with meniscal lesions [27]. The authors showed that surgery was avoided during the 6-month observation period and the Oxford Knee Score improved significantly from 29.1–44.3 in 83% of patients. Interestingly, the structural findings on MRI, measured by Boston Leeds Osteoarthritis Knee Score, also showed significant improvement. The limitations of the study were its retrospective character and lack of control group analysis. We believe that an additional weak point of this study was connected to not addressing perimeniscal capillary plexus (PCP) while performing the joint injection. Trephination is a known technique usually employed during arthroscopy [28,29]. It involves the formation of vascular access channels from the meniscus periphery (PCP) to the tear. This process initiates bleeding into the meniscal lesion and subsequent tissue repair response. This simple technique was showed to increase the meniscal healing rate while applied during a surgical procedure [30], most probably by providing the injury site with both growth factors and mesenchymal stem cells.

The results of experimental studies support the hypothesis that PRP may improve meniscal healing through activation of fibrochondrocytes present within the meniscus [31]. The process also involves the activity of mesenchymal stem cells, which seem to be necessary for the repair of meniscal lesions [23]. The PRP itself releases the "cytokine cocktail" of the healing cascade [25]. The main growth factors are: platelet derived growth factor, platelet derived endothelial growth factor, vascular endothelial growth factor, insulin like growth factor, platelet derived angiogenesis factor, transforming growth factor-b, hepatocyte growth factor and others [32]. This release initiates the chemotaxis of immunocompetent cells, inflammation, angiogenesis and as a consequence the process of synthesis of the extracellular matrix and tissue remodelling. The PRP works at various levels for joint homeostasis. Studies have shown that PRP application decreases catabolism while increasing anabolic activity and observations have been made that catabolic activity in meniscus chondral tissue helps identify patients who are at risk for progression of osteoarthritis [33]. Other processes, such as chondral remodelling is promoted by PRP administration. Higher production of collagen II, matrix molecules and prostaglandin has been observed in hyaline cartilage [34,35]. On the contrary, Lee et al. showed on a rabbit model of a circular meniscal defect that PRP treatment failed to enhance the production of meniscus cartilage. Additionally, it accelerated fibrosis and increased catabolic processes [36]. However, findings from in vivo and in vitro studies cannot be directly translated to clinical practice.

Increasing data provide evidence for the necessity of mesenchymal stem cells in delivering the positive effect of PRP on healing of meniscal and hyaline cartilage defects [23,37] and the process of chondrocyte differentiation [38]. PRP has been shown to enhance proliferation of stromal stem cells [39] as well as their adhesion and migration [40]. This phenomenon is probably dependent on the release of a growth factor cocktail and triggering of synovial tissue to create a more balanced intra-articular environment. Recent studies link the synovium-derived stem cells to chondral regeneration, as they possess chondrogenic potential and encouraging results have been shown for cartilage repair purposes in experimental studies [41].

We hypothesize, that trephination, by creating multiple wounds and inducing intrameniscal bleeding, starts the process of tissue repair with activation of synovial and blood derived stem cells, which—in our study—are stimulated by addition of PRP. The combination of those two processes allows for efficient meniscal tissue regeneration.

3.1. Strengths

This is the first study to employ percutaneous trephination of a chronic meniscal lesion with or without PRP augmentation. The second strength is the study design itself, the randomized and blinded nature of this study and being adequately powered to detect differences in healing rates. Lastly, independent evaluators were used for assessing of the outcomes.

3.2. Limitations

We acknowledge some limitations in this study. The study group was small, increasing the risk of type II error. Additionally, some patients refused MRI arthrography due to its interventional character, still their comfort of life improved significantly. Also, calculation of the primary outcome might have been influenced by factors that could affect MRI images and their interpretation. There is also the issue of heterogeneity within groups. Localization of the tear in medial or lateral compartments may influence the primary outcome, as the biology of those menisci might differ. We find no statistically significant differences between these groups but in the literature the results are mixed [42]. Additionally, PROMs data have partially overlapping 95% confidence intervals, increasing the risk of type II error. Moreover, it is still unknown which of the factors are solely responsible for the improved outcomes in the PRP group. The rehabilitation protocol was uniform in all patients but we could not control those differences that might have occurred in patients being treated in multiple outpatient centres. Lastly, the observation period in this study allowed only for a short-term analysis.

4. Materials and Methods

4.1. Trial Design and Informed Consent

This was a parallel-group, superiority trial with equal randomization. The study protocol was approved by an appropriate Institutional Review Board and was publicly accessible before enrolment of the first patient. We performed the study in accordance with the ethical standards outlined in the 2013 revision of 1975 Declaration of Helsinki and we report the results according to the 2010 CONSORT statement. The potential benefits and risks of meniscal trephination, PRP injection and follow-up were explained to each study patient. All patients provided written informed consent for participation in this study and no patient declined to participate. Clinical Trial Registration: The study protocol was approved by Bioethics Committee at Centre of Postgraduate Medical Education (36/PB/2013 approved on 29.05.2013) and was publicly accessible before enrolment of the first participant. The clinical trial databases at cmkp.edu.pl-36/PB/2013, clinicaltrials.gov-NCT03066583.

4.2. Eligibility Criteria

Patients were recruited from a single public knee clinic at a tertiary care, university health centre between 2016 and 2018 (Figure 1). 72 patients with chronic (horizontal) meniscal lesions were enrolled: 30 were randomized to undergo percutaneous trephination (control group) and 42 were randomized to undergo percutaneous trephination with PRP injection at the repair site. Detailed inclusion and exclusion criteria are presented in Table 5.

Table 5. Inclusion and exclusion criteria.

Inclusion Criteria	Exclusion Criteria
skeletally mature patients aged 18–70 years	arthritic changes (Kellgren-Lawrence scale >2)
chronic horizontal tears on MRI	discoid meniscus
tear located in the vascular/avascular portion of the meniscus	axial leg deformity (valgus > 6 deg)- concomitant chondral defects (> 2 ICRS)
single tear of the medial and/or lateral meniscus	Inflammatory diseases (rheumatoid arthritis)
	chondral defects above ICRS 2 on MRI

MRI, magnetic resonance imaging.

4.3. PRP and Thrombin Preparation

PRP and its activator (thrombin) was prepared as in Reference [9]. In this study we used Red-L-PRPIIB-1 according to the new classification system [43]. PRP was prepared by a dedicated laboratory assistant in the BL2 facility. Briefly, the PRP preparation procedure involved drawing of 120 mL of venous blood and centrifuging the blood using a refrigerated centrifuge in a two-step process. First, the PRP layer was isolated, including a "buffy coat" and a small fraction of underlying red blood cells (900 rpm × 9 min). Additional centrifugation and isolation of PRP was then applied (3200 rpm × 15 min). The preparation was packed into sterile vials labelled with the patient ID. In the study group, 6–8 mL of PRP solution was used, while in the control group, 6–8 mL of sterile 0.9% saline was applied. Right before application, PRP was activated using 20 mM $CaCl_2$ (Teva, Basel, Israel) and 25 IU/mL autologous thrombin. It was then injected into the tear site of the meniscus with a double chamber syringe. Platelets and leukocyte concentration were assessed for each sample.

4.4. Procedures

All procedures were performed by the same senior orthopaedic surgeon under ultrasound guidance (R.K.) in the outpatient department. In brief, the PRP or control solution was prepared as described above. Local anaesthetic was used. After identification of a horizontal tear via ultrasound, the needle was introduced into the tear lesion (passing through the PCP, red zone, red-white zone and white zone) with continuous injection of studied solutions (starting while in the PCP). 5–10 separate needle introductions through all layers were performed. After discharge, patients were referred to outpatient physiotherapy units and encouraged to follow a unified rehabilitation protocol. In short, all patients wore a hinged knee brace for 4 weeks. Exercises with a range of motion from 0 to 90 degrees for 6 weeks were encouraged. Weight bearing as tolerated was allowed - beginning from day 1. Early quadricep muscle activation was initiated. At 6 weeks post procedure, a low-resistance stationary bicycle and one-quarter body weight leg presses were initiated. Additional increases in low-impact knee exercises were permitted as tolerated starting at 12 weeks post procedure.

4.5. Outcomes

The primary outcome was meniscus healing assessed using 1.5T magnetic resonance imaging (MRI) arthrography with a dedicated knee coil (Siemens, Erlangen, Germany). Meniscus healing was evaluated by two independent attending radiology consultants, who were blinded to the patient allocation. We did not notice any intra-observer bias. Complete healing was considered when full meniscus integrity was noted during MR arthrography (no intrameniscal contrast media). Partial healing was considered with contrast media filling a defect between 1–3 mm. Healing failure was considered when contrast media was detected within the meniscal body. Additionally, failure was defined as performing arthroscopic meniscectomy or meniscal repair. Arthroscopy free survival was analysed.

Secondary outcomes (patient reported outcome measures–PROMS) included pain assessment with the visual analogue scale (VAS) and functional outcome assessment with the Knee injury and Osteoarthritis Outcome Score (KOOS), Western Ontario and McMaster Universities Osteoarthritis Index (WOMAC) and International Knee Documentation Committee Subjective Knee Evaluation (IKDC) [12,44,45]. All secondary outcomes were assessed before the procedure and at 3, 6, 12, 24 months post injection. Minimally clinical important difference (MCID) was assessed for PROMs [13,14,46,47]. Patients were closely monitored for complications. There were no changes to the protocol during study duration.

4.6. Randomization

The randomization list for allocating patients to the study groups was generated using the "simple randomization" function on the StatSoft GraphPad QuickCalcs web site (http://www.graphpad.com/quickcalcs) [48]. We used sequentially numbered, opaque, sealed envelopes to conceal the allocation. Patients were consecutively enrolled and assigned to the study groups. Intervention assignment was performed during PRP preparation.

4.7. Blinding

The patients, the data collectors and the assessors were blinded to the intervention type.

4.8. Statistical Analysis

We used the R statistical package (www.rproject.org) for statistical analyses [49]. Differences in meniscus healing rates were assessed through analysis of a contingency table using Fisher's exact test. All categorical data were analysed using Fisher's exact test. The VAS score, KOOS, WOMAC and IKDC score were analysed using the two-tailed Mann-Whitney U test or unpaired t-test (after assessment for parametric or non-parametric distribution using the Shapiro-Wilk test) [50]. Arthroscopy-free survival was analysed using Kaplan Meyer plot and log-rank testing for statistical significance. Results were considered statistically significant at a P-value < 0.05. Sample size was calculated for the primary outcome (meniscus healing), with a two-tailed significance level at alpha $= 0.05$ and beta $= 0.8$, assuming a difference in the meniscus healing rate of 15% between the study groups according to the method described in Reference [51] and based on previous studies [52,53]. Minimum recruitment level was estimated to be 28 patients per group. Assuming an attrition or non-compliance rate of 10% during the study, we aimed to recruit at least 30 patients per group.

5. Conclusions

Our blinded, prospective, randomized, controlled trial on the role of PRP and percutaneous trephination of the chronically torn meniscal tissue indicates that percutaneous trephination of the meniscal tissue is an effective technique improving meniscal integrity as well as PROMs. The augmentation of this technique with PRP results in a significant improvement in the rate of meniscal healing (52% vs. 30%, $P = 0.04$). Importantly, this simple procedure seems to decrease the necessity for arthroscopy in the future (8% vs. 28%, $P = 0.032$). This study showed that PRP augmentation could provide significant and clinically important benefits. Further studies in this field are encouraged. The risk of adverse events related to percutaneous trephination with augmentation with PRP is very low.

Author Contributions: Conceptualization, R.K. and K.K.-K.; Data curation, R.K. and K.K.-K.; Formal analysis, R.K. and S.P.; Funding acquisition, R.K. and S.P.; Investigation, R.K., M.M.-W., K.K. and A.D.-T.; Methodology, R.K., K.K.-K., A.D.-T. and S.P.; Project administration, M.M.-W.; Resources, R.K., M.M.-W. and A.D.-T.; Software, R.K.; Supervision, R.K.; Validation, R.K., M.M.-W., K.K.-K. and A.D.-T.; Visualization, R.K.; Writing—original draft, R.K. and K.K.-K.; Writing—review & editing, R.K., M.M.-W., K.K., K.K.-K. and S.P.

Funding: This research was funded by Postgraduate Center for Medical Education Grant, grant number 501–1–07–18–14.

Conflicts of Interest: The authors declare no conflict of interest.

References

1. Hawker, G. Knee Arthroscopy in England and Ontario: Patterns of Use, Changes Over Time and Relationship to Total Knee Replacement. *J. Bone Jt. Surg. Am.* **2008**, *90*, 2337. [CrossRef] [PubMed]
2. Englund, M.; Guermazi, A.; Gale, D.; Hunter, D.J.; Aliabadi, P.; Clancy, M.; Felson, D.T. Incidental meniscal findings on knee MRI in middle-aged and elderly persons. *N. Engl. J. Med.* **2008**, *359*, 1108–1115. [CrossRef] [PubMed]
3. Sihvonen, R.; Paavola, M.; Malmivaara, A.; Itälä, A.; Joukainen, A.; Nurmi, H.; Kalske, J.; Järvinen, T.L.N. Arthroscopic Partial Meniscectomy versus Sham Surgery for a Degenerative Meniscal Tear. *N. Engl. J. Med.* **2013**, *369*, 2515–2524. [CrossRef]
4. Fairbank, T.J. Knee joint changes after meniscectomy. *J. Bone Jt.Surg. Br.* **1948**, *30B*, 664–670. [CrossRef]
5. Noyes, F.R.; Barber-Westin, S.D. Repair of complex and avascular meniscal tears and meniscal transplantation. *J. Bone Jt.Surg. Am.* **2010**, *92*, 1012–1029.
6. Henning, C.E.; Lynch, M.A.; Yearout, K.M.; Vequist, S.W.; Stallbaumer, R.J.; Decker, K.A. Arthroscopic meniscal repair using an exogenous fibrin clot. *Clin. Orthop.* **1990**, 64–72. [CrossRef]

7. Van Trommel, M.F.; Simonian, P.T.; Potter, H.G.; Wickiewicz, T.L. Arthroscopic meniscal repair with fibrin clot of complete radial tears of the lateral meniscus in the avascular zone. *Arthrosc. J. Arthrosc. Relat. Surg. Off. Publ. Arthrosc. Assoc. N. Am. Int. Arthrosc. Assoc.* **1998**, *14*, 360–365. [CrossRef]

8. Pujol, N.; Tardy, N.; Boisrenoult, P.; Beaufils, P. Long-term outcomes of all-inside meniscal repair. *Knee Surg. Sports Traumatol. Arthrosc.* **2015**, *23*, 219–224. [CrossRef]

9. Kaminski, R.; Kulinski, K.; Kozar-Kaminska, K.; Wielgus, M.; Langner, M.; Wasko, M.K.; Kowalczewski, J.; Pomianowski, S. A Prospective, Randomized, Double-Blind, Parallel-Group, Placebo-Controlled Study Evaluating Meniscal Healing, Clinical Outcomes and Safety in Patients Undergoing Meniscal Repair of Unstable, Complete Vertical Meniscal Tears (Bucket Handle) Augmented with Platelet-Rich Plasma. *BioMed Res. Int.* **2018**, *2018*, 9315815.

10. Kaminski, R.; Kulinski, K.; Kozar-Kaminska, K.; Wasko, M.K.; Langner, M.; Pomianowski, S. Repair augmentation of unstable, complete vertical meniscal tears with bone marrow venting procedure. A prospective, randomized, double-blind, parallel-group, placebo-controlled study. *Arthrosc. J. Arthrosc. Relat. Surg.* **2018**, *2018*, 9315815.

11. Ahn, J.-H.; Kwon, O.-J.; Nam, T.-S. Arthroscopic Repair of Horizontal Meniscal Cleavage Tears With Marrow-Stimulating Technique. *Arthrosc. J. Arthrosc. Relat. Surg.* **2015**, *31*, 92–98. [CrossRef] [PubMed]

12. Katz, N.P.; Paillard, F.C.; Ekman, E. Determining the clinical importance of treatment benefits for interventions for painful orthopedic conditions. *J. Orthop. Surg.* **2015**, *10*, 24. [CrossRef] [PubMed]

13. Harris, J.D.; Brand, J.C.; Cote, M.P.; Faucett, S.C.; Dhawan, A. Research Pearls: The Significance of Statistics and Perils of Pooling. Part 1: Clinical Versus Statistical Significance. *Arthrosc. J. Arthrosc. Relat. Surg.* **2017**, *33*, 1102–1112. [CrossRef] [PubMed]

14. Greco, N.J.; Anderson, A.F.; Mann, B.J.; Cole, B.J.; Farr, J.; Nissen, C.W.; Irrgang, J.J. Responsiveness of the International Knee Documentation Committee Subjective Knee Form in comparison to the Western Ontario and McMaster Universities Osteoarthritis Index, modified Cincinnati Knee Rating System and Short Form 36 in patients with focal articular cartilage defects. *Am. J. Sports Med.* **2010**, *38*, 891–902. [PubMed]

15. Delos, D.; Rodeo, S.A. Enhancing meniscal repair through biology: Platelet-rich plasma as an alternative strategy. *Instr. Course Lect.* **2011**, *60*, 453–460. [PubMed]

16. Paxton, E.S.; Stock, M.V.; Brophy, R.H. Meniscal Repair Versus Partial Meniscectomy: A Systematic Review Comparing Reoperation Rates and Clinical Outcomes. *Arthrosc. J. Arthrosc. Relat. Surg.* **2011**, *27*, 1275–1288. [CrossRef]

17. Katz, J.N.; Brophy, R.H.; Chaisson, C.E.; de Chaves, L.; Cole, B.J.; Dahm, D.L.; Donnell-Fink, L.A.; Guermazi, A.; Haas, A.K.; Jones, M.H.; et al. Surgery versus Physical Therapy for a Meniscal Tear and Osteoarthritis. *N. Engl. J. Med.* **2013**, *368*, 1675–1684. [CrossRef]

18. Beaufils, P.; Becker, R.; Kopf, S.; Englund, M.; Verdonk, R.; Ollivier, M.; Seil, R. Surgical management of degenerative meniscus lesions: The 2016 ESSKA meniscus consensus. *Knee Surg. Sports Traumatol. Arthrosc.* **2017**, *25*, 335–346. [CrossRef]

19. Siemieniuk, R.A.C.; Harris, I.A.; Agoritsas, T.; Poolman, R.W.; Brignardello-Petersen, R.; Van de Velde, S.; Buchbinder, R.; Englund, M.; Lytvyn, L.; Quinlan, C.; et al. Arthroscopic surgery for degenerative knee arthritis and meniscal tears: A clinical practice guideline. *BMJ* **2017**, *357*, j1982. [CrossRef]

20. Crisci, A.; Crescenzo, U.D.; Crisci, M. Platelet-rich concentrates (L-PRF, PRP) in tissue regeneration: Control of apoptosis and interactions with regenerative cells. *J. Clin. Mol. Med.* **2018**, *1*, 1–2. [CrossRef]

21. Dohan Ehrenfest, D.M.; Bielecki, T.; Jimbo, R.; Barbé, G.; Del Corso, M.; Inchingolo, F.; Sammartino, G. Do the fibrin architecture and leukocyte content influence the growth factor release of platelet concentrates? An evidence-based answer comparing a pure platelet-rich plasma (P-PRP) gel and a leukocyte- and platelet-rich fibrin (L-PRF). *Curr. Pharm. Biotechnol.* **2012**, *13*, 1145–1152. [CrossRef] [PubMed]

22. Ishida, K.; Kuroda, R.; Miwa, M.; Tabata, Y.; Hokugo, A.; Kawamoto, T.; Sasaki, K.; Doita, M.; Kurosaka, M. The Regenerative Effects of Platelet-Rich Plasma on Meniscal Cells In Vitro and Its In Vivo Application with Biodegradable Gelatin Hydrogel. *Tissue Eng.* **2007**, *13*, 1103–1112. [CrossRef] [PubMed]

23. Zellner, J.; Mueller, M.; Berner, A.; Dienstknecht, T.; Kujat, R.; Nerlich, M.; Hennemann, B.; Koller, M.; Prantl, L.; Angele, M.; et al. Role of mesenchymal stem cells in tissue engineering of meniscus. *J. Biomed. Mater. Res. A* **2010**, *94*, 1150–1161. [CrossRef] [PubMed]

24. Andia, I.; Maffulli, N. New biotechnologies for musculoskeletal injuries. *Surg. J. R. Coll. Surg. Edinb. Irel.* **2018**. [CrossRef] [PubMed]

25. Andia, I.; Maffulli, N. A contemporary view of platelet-rich plasma therapies: Moving toward refined clinical protocols and precise indications. *Regen. Med.* **2018**, *13*, 717–728. [CrossRef] [PubMed]

26. Griffin, J.W.; Hadeed, M.M.; Werner, B.C.; Diduch, D.R.; Carson, E.W.; Miller, M.D. Platelet-rich Plasma in Meniscal Repair: Does Augmentation Improve Surgical Outcomes? *Clin. Orthop. Relat. Res.* **2015**, *473*, 1665–1672. [CrossRef] [PubMed]

27. Strümper, R. Intra-Articular Injections of Autologous Conditioned Serum to Treat Pain from Meniscal Lesions. *Sports Med. Int. Open* **2017**, *1*, E200–E205. [CrossRef] [PubMed]

28. Doral, M.N.; Bilge, O.; Huri, G.; Turhan, E.; Verdonk, R. Modern treatment of meniscal tears. *EFORT Open Rev.* **2018**, *3*, 260–268. [CrossRef]

29. Ghazi Zadeh, L.; Chevrier, A.; Farr, J.; Rodeo, S.A.; Buschmann, M.D. Augmentation Techniques for Meniscus Repair. *J. Knee Surg.* **2018**, *31*, 99–116. [CrossRef]

30. Fox, J.M.; Rintz, K.G.; Ferkel, R.D. Trephination of incomplete meniscal tears. *Arthrosc. J. Arthrosc. Relat. Surg. Off. Publ. Arthrosc. Assoc. N. Am. Int. Arthrosc. Assoc.* **1993**, *9*, 451–455. [CrossRef]

31. Tumia, N.S.; Johnstone, A.J. Platelet derived growth factor-AB enhances knee meniscal cell activity in vitro. *The Knee* **2009**, *16*, 73–76. [CrossRef] [PubMed]

32. Cozma, C.N.; Raducu, L.; Jecan, C.R. Platelet Rich Plasma- mechanism of action and clinical applications. *J. Clin. Investig. Surg.* **2016**, *1*, 41–46. [CrossRef]

33. Brophy, R.H.; Rai, M.F.; Zhang, Z.; Torgomyan, A.; Sandell, L.J. Molecular analysis of age and sex-related gene expression in meniscal tears with and without a concomitant anterior cruciate ligament tear. *J. Bone Jt.Surg. Am.* **2012**, *94*, 385–393. [CrossRef] [PubMed]

34. Dhillon, M.S.; Patel, S.; John, R. PRP in OA knee—Update, current confusions and future options. *SICOT-J* **2017**, *3*, 27. [CrossRef] [PubMed]

35. Pereira, R.C.; Scaranari, M.; Benelli, R.; Strada, P.; Reis, R.L.; Cancedda, R.; Gentili, C. Dual Effect of Platelet Lysate on Human Articular Cartilage: A Maintenance of Chondrogenic Potential and a Transient Proinflammatory Activity Followed by an Inflammation Resolution. *Tissue Eng. Part A* **2013**, *19*, 1476–1488. [CrossRef] [PubMed]

36. Lee, H.-R.; Shon, O.-J.; Park, S.-I.; Kim, H.-J.; Kim, S.; Ahn, M.-W.; Do, S.H. Platelet-Rich Plasma Increases the Levels of Catabolic Molecules and Cellular Dedifferentiation in the Meniscus of a Rabbit Model. *Int. J. Mol. Sci.* **2016**, *17*, 120. [CrossRef] [PubMed]

37. Haleem, A.M.; Singergy, A.A.E.; Sabry, D.; Atta, H.M.; Rashed, L.A.; Chu, C.R.; Shewy, M.T.E.; Azzam, A.; Aziz, M.T.A. The Clinical Use of Human Culture–Expanded Autologous Bone Marrow Mesenchymal Stem Cells Transplanted on Platelet-Rich Fibrin Glue in the Treatment of Articular Cartilage Defects: A Pilot Study and Preliminary Results. *CARTILAGE* **2010**, *1*, 253–261. [CrossRef]

38. Jeyakumar, V.; Niculescu-Morzsa, E.; Bauer, C.; Lacza, Z.; Nehrer, S. Redifferentiation of Articular Chondrocytes by Hyperacute Serum and Platelet Rich Plasma in Collagen Type I Hydrogels. *Int. J. Mol. Sci.* **2019**, *20*, 316. [CrossRef]

39. Lucarelli, E.; Beccheroni, A.; Donati, D.; Sangiorgi, L.; Cenacchi, A.; Del Vento, A.M.; Meotti, C.; Bertoja, A.Z.; Giardino, R.; Fornasari, P.M.; et al. Platelet-derived growth factors enhance proliferation of human stromal stem cells. *Biomaterials* **2003**, *24*, 3095–3100. [CrossRef]

40. Rubio-Azpeitia, E.; Sánchez, P.; Delgado, D.; Andia, I. Adult Cells Combined with Platelet-Rich Plasma for Tendon Healing: Cell Source Options. *Orthop. J. Sports Med.* **2017**, *5*, 232596711769084. [CrossRef]

41. Kubosch, E.J.; Lang, G.; Furst, D.; Kubosch, D.; Izadpanah, K.; Rolauffs, B.; Sudkamp, N.P.; Schmal, H. The Potential for Synovium-derived Stem Cells in Cartilage Repair. *Curr. Stem Cell Res. Ther.* **2018**, *13*, 174–184. [CrossRef] [PubMed]

42. Dean, C.S.; Chahla, J.; Matheny, L.M.; Mitchell, J.J.; LaPrade, R.F. Outcomes After Biologically Augmented Isolated Meniscal Repair with Marrow Venting Are Comparable with Those After Meniscal Repair With Concomitant Anterior Cruciate Ligament Reconstruction. *Am. J. Sports Med.* **2017**, *45*, 1341–1348. [CrossRef] [PubMed]

43. Harrison, P. The Subcommittee on Platelet Physiology The use of platelets in regenerative medicine and proposal for a new classification system: Guidance from the SSC of the ISTH. *J. Thromb. Haemost.* **2018**, *16*, 1895–1900. [CrossRef] [PubMed]

44. Roos, E.M.; Roos, H.P.; Lohmander, L.S.; Ekdahl, C.; Beynnon, B.D. Knee Injury and Osteoarthritis Outcome Score (KOOS)—Development of a self-administered outcome measure. *J. Orthop. Sports Phys. Ther.* **1998**, *28*, 88–96. [CrossRef]

45. Bellamy, N. WOMAC: A 20-year experiential review of a patient-centered self-reported health status questionnaire. *J. Rheumatol.* **2002**, *29*, 2473–2476. [PubMed]

46. Crawford, K.; Briggs, K.K.; Rodkey, W.G.; Steadman, J.R. Reliability, validity and responsiveness of the IKDC score for meniscus injuries of the knee. *Arthrosc. J. Arthrosc. Relat. Surg. Off. Publ. Arthrosc. Assoc. N. Am. Int. Arthrosc. Assoc.* **2007**, *23*, 839–844. [CrossRef] [PubMed]

47. Roos, E.M.; Lohmander, L.S. The Knee injury and Osteoarthritis Outcome Score (KOOS): From joint injury to osteoarthritis. *Health Qual. Life Outcomes* **2003**, *1*, 64. [CrossRef]

48. Suresh, K. An overview of randomization techniques: An unbiased assessment of outcome in clinical research. *J. Hum. Reprod. Sci.* **2011**, *4*, 8. [CrossRef]

49. R Development Core Team. *R: A Language and Environment for Statistical Computing*; R Foundation for Statistical Computing: Vienna, Austria, 2008.

50. Malavolta, E.A.; Gracitelli, M.E.C.; Ferreira Neto, A.A.; Assuncao, J.H.; Bordalo-Rodrigues, M.; de Camargo, O.P. Platelet-Rich Plasma in Rotator Cuff Repair: A Prospective Randomized Study. *Am. J. Sports Med.* **2014**, *42*, 2446–2454. [CrossRef]

51. Van der Tweel, I.; Askie, L.; Vandermeer, B.; Ellenberg, S.; Fernandes, R.M.; Saloojee, H.; Bassler, D.; Altman, D.G.; Offringa, M.; van der Lee, J.H.; et al. Standard 4: Determining adequate sample sizes. *Pediatrics* **2012**, *129* (Suppl. S3), S138–S145. [CrossRef]

52. Stein, T.; Mehling, A.P.; Welsch, F.; von Eisenhart-Rothe, R.; Jäger, A. Long-term outcome after arthroscopic meniscal repair versus arthroscopic partial meniscectomy for traumatic meniscal tears. *Am. J. Sports Med.* **2010**, *38*, 1542–1548. [CrossRef] [PubMed]

53. Järvelä, S.; Sihvonen, R.; Sirkeoja, H.; Järvelä, T. All-Inside Meniscal Repair with Bioabsorbable Meniscal Screws or with Bioabsorbable Meniscus Arrows: A Prospective, Randomized Clinical Study with 2-Year Results. *Am. J. Sports Med.* **2010**, *38*, 2211–2217. [CrossRef] [PubMed]

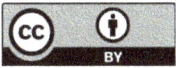

International Journal of
Molecular Sciences

MDPI

Article

Single Injection of High Volume of Autologous Pure PRP Provides a Significant Improvement in Knee Osteoarthritis: A Prospective Routine Care Study

Caroline Guillibert [1], Caroline Charpin [1], Marie Raffray [1], Annie Benmenni [1], Francois-Xavier Dehaut [2], Georges El Ghobeira [3], Roch Giorgi [4], Jeremy Magalon [5,*] and Denis Arniaud [1]

[1]   Rheumatology Department, Hôpital Saint Joseph, 13008 Marseille, France;
      cguillibert@hopital-saint-joseph.fr (C.G.); ccharpin@hopital-saint-joseph.fr (C.C.);
      mraffray@hopital-saint-joseph.fr (M.R.); anbenmenni@hopital-saint-joseph.fr (A.B.);
      darniaud@hopital-saint-joseph.fr (D.A.)
[2]   Radiology Department, Hôpital Saint Joseph, 13008 Marseille, France; fxdehaut@hopital-saint-joseph.fr
[3]   Physical Therapy Department, Hôpital Saint Joseph, 13008 Marseille, France;
      gelghobeira@hopital-saint-joseph.fr
[4]   Aix Marseille Univ, APHM, INSERM, IRD, SESSTIM, Sciences Economiques et Sociales de la Santé &
      Traitement de l'Information Médicale, Hop Timone, BioSTIC, Biostatistique et Technologies de l'Information
      et de la Communication, 13005 Marseille, France; Roch.GIORGI@ap-hm.fr
[5]   Cell Therapy Department, Hôpital de la Conception, AP-HM, INSERM CIC BT 1409, 13005 Marseille, France
*   Correspondence: jeremy.magalon@ap-hm.fr; Tel.: +33-4-91-38-14-86; Fax: +33-4-91-38-36-85

Received: 15 February 2019; Accepted: 14 March 2019; Published: 15 March 2019

check for updates

Abstract: Background: Evidence is growing regarding the ability of platelet-rich plasma (PRP) injections to enhance functional capacity and alleviate pain in knee osteoarthritis (OA). However, heterogeneity in common practice regarding PRP preparation and biological content makes the initiation of this activity in a hospital complex. The aim of this study was to document the efficacy of a single PRP injection to treat knee OA and validate a routine care procedure. Methods: Fifty-seven patients with symptomatic knee OA received a single injection of large volume of very pure PRP. They were assessed at baseline and after one, three and six months, by measuring Knee Injury and Osteoarthritis Score (KOOS), Observed Pain after a 50-foot walk test and Visual Analog Scale (VAS) assessments. Magnetic Resonance Imaging (MRI) analysis was performed at baseline and six months after the procedure. The objective was to recover 50% of responders three months after the procedure using OMERACT-OARSI criteria. Results: A single administration of high volume pure PRP provided significant clinical benefit for 84.2% of the responders, three months after the procedure. The KOOS total score significantly increased from 43.5 ± 14.3 to 66.4 ± 21.7 six months after the procedure ($p < 0.001$). Pain also significantly decreased from 37.5 ± 25.1 to 12.9 ± 20.9 ($p < 0.001$). No difference was observed on MRI parameters. Conclusion: A single injection of large volume of very pure PRP is associated with significant functional improvement and pain relief, allowing initiation of daily PRP injection within our hospital.

Keywords: PRP; knee arthrosis; growth factors

---

1. Introduction

Osteoarthritis (OA) of the knee is a progressive joint disease involving the intra-articular (IA) tibiofemoral and patellofemoral cartilage and all surrounding IA and periarticular structures [1]. In the United States, symptomatic OA affects more than 50 million adults, resulting in annual costs exceeding

$ 100 billion due to medical expenses and lost wages [2]. Non pharmacological approaches such as exercise and lifestyle modifications are often associated with poor compliance [3] and pharmacological therapies (including analgesics, non-steroid anti-inflammatory drugs and corticosteroid injections) are not curative and induce side effects in the long term [4,5]. Hyaluronic acid (HA) injections were described as more effective in the long term compared to corticosteroids injection [6] with highly variable association with pain [7]. However, the American Academy of Orthopaedic Surgeons (AAOS) clinical practice guidelines provide evidence against HA viscosupplementation injections in patients with symptomatic knee OA [8]. This situation has led to the emergence of cell-based therapy options also called orthobiologics. Among them, platelet-rich plasma (PRP) is defined as an autologous plasma suspension of platelets, characterized by a platelet concentration higher than in physiological blood [9] and able to release growth factors (GFs) involved in reparative and regenerative processes. PRP has been the subject of increased clinical interest in the orthopaedic field and a recent meta analysis indicates that, compared with HA and saline, an intra-articular PRP injection may have more benefits in pain relief and functional improvement in patients with symptomatic knee OA at one year post-injection [10], providing orthopaedic surgeons and rheumatologists a new validated non-invasive option to improve knee OA related symptoms [11]. However, there is significant variation in the production of autologous PRP, including heterogeneity in the harvesting method, the type of anticoagulant used and the production method. Substantial differences in the content of platelets concentrates produced by the various automated and manual protocols have been described [12,13] and their consequences on clinical results in PRP therapy is currently being investigated [14,15]. Thus, the initiation of PRP injection activity within a hospital necessitates the selection of dedicated material and the establishment of a precise patient care procedure which should take into account recent recommendations from the AAOS regarding minimum reporting standards for clinical studies evaluating PRP [16].

In this context, the aim of this study was to document the efficacy of a single PRP injection to treat knee OA in routine care procedure. We assumed that PRP would allow to recover 50% of responders three months after treatment, using OMERACT-OARSI criteria. We also analyzed the relationship between clinical results and PRP composition through a precise biological characterization of the injected PRP, including platelets, leukocytes and red blood cells (RBCs) counts.

2. Results

2.1. Characteristics of Patients

Out of 61 screened patients, 60 were injected and 57 were finally analyzed. One patient was originally included in the study population but finally excluded before the injection. Three patients were injected but could not be included in the analysis (one patient with lost follow up after one month and two patients with misunderstanding in inclusion criteria) (Figure 1). Patients were aged 63.3 ± 9.6 years old and presented grade 2 (40.3%) and grade 3 (59.7%) knee OA according to the Kellgren-Laurence scale (Table 1). 42 (73.7%) and 6 (10.5%) patients had previously had IA injection of HA or corticosteroids, respectively.

Table 1. Baseline characteristics of patients included (n = 57) in statistical analysis.

Sex, male:female, n	24:33
Age, year, mean ± SD	63.3 ± 9.6
BMI, kg/m^2, mean ± SD	25.4 ± 3.9
Symptom duration, mo, mean ± SD	8.4 ± 9.9
Kellgren Laurence Grade of knee OA grade 2: grade 3, n	23:34
Previous corticosteroids injection: HA injection, n	6:42
Flexion, °, mean ± SD	124.1 ± 10.3

Table 1. *Cont.*

Extension, °, mean ± SD	15.0 ± 4.6
KOOS total score, mean ± SD	43.9 ± 14.6
KOOS other symptoms score, mean ± SD	56.0 ± 20.9
KOOS pain score, mean ± SD	51.3 ± 13.3
KOOS function in daily living score, mean ± SD	54.5 ± 17.1
KOOS sport and recreation score, mean ± SD	27.5 ± 19.0
KOOS quality of life, mean ± SD	30.3 ± 18.0
Observed Pain on 50-foot walk test (0–100), mean ± SD	38.6 ± 25.3
Previous week VAS arthrosis activity (0–100)	57.9 ± 18.4
Previous week VAS damages caused by arthrosis (0–100)	63.0 ± 19.3
Previous week VAS global health (0–100)	72.6 ± 16.2
SF-36 PCS (0–100)	37.1 ± 9.3
SF-36 MCS (0–100)	40.4 ± 8.9

SD, standard deviation; BMI, body mass index; mo, months; OA, osteoarthritis; HA, hyaluronic acid; KOOS, Knee Injury and Osteoarthritis Score; VAS, visual analog scale; SF-36, Short Form Health Survey; PCS, Physical Component Summary; MCS, Mental Component Summary.

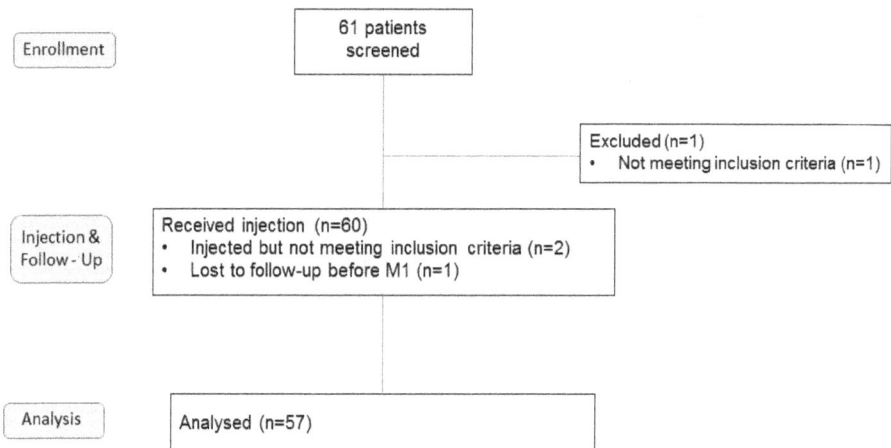

Figure 1. Flow diagram of the clinical trial. M1, month 1.

2.2. Biological Characteristics of PRP

Table 2 summarizes the biological characteristics of injected PRP. The final injected volume was 8.8 ± 1.1 mL. The mean recovery rate in platelets was 68.3 ± 16.5%. The mean increases in platelets and leukocytes compared with blood were 1.4 ± 0.4 and 0.1 ± 0.1, respectively. The percentage of platelets was 96.2 ± 2.5% with low contamination from RBCs (3.7 ± 2.4%) and leukocytes (0.1 ± 0.1%). The mean number of injected platelets was 2.5 ± 0.5 billion resulting in very pure PRP and a CCA rate according to DEPA (Dose, Efficiency, Purity, Activation) classification [17].

Table 2. Biological characteristics of platelet-rich plasma (PRP) (*n* = 57).

	Mean ± Standard Deviation
Blood	
Volume of whole blood collected, mL	18.0 ± 0.0
Red Blood Cells concentration, T/L	4.22 ± 0.65
Platelets concentration, G/L	197 ± 37
Leukocytes concentration, G/L	5.71 ± 1.22
PRP	
Volume of PRP injected, mL	8.8 ± 1.1
Red Blood Cells concentration, T/L	0.01 ± 0.01
Platelets concentration, G/L	288 ± 95
Leukocytes concentration, G/L	0.22 ± 0.27
Quantity of injected Red Blood Cells, millions	92 ± 53
Quantity of injected Red Blood Cells (%)	3.7 ± 2.4
Quantity of injected Platelets, millions	2517 ± 812
Quantity of injected Platelets (%)	96.2 ± 2.5
Quantity of injected Leukocytes, millions	2 ± 2
Quantity of injected Leukocytes (%)	0.1 ± 0.1
Recovery rate in platelets (%)	68.3 ± 16.5
Increase factor in platelets	1.4 ± 0.4
Increase factor in leukocytes	0.1 ± 0.1
DEPA Classification	CDA

2.3. Effect of Single Autologous PRP Injection in Knee OA

The main objective of the study was reached with 84.2% of OMERACT-OARSI responders at three months. This result was stable with 82.5% and 80.7% of responders one and six months after the injection, respectively. Single injection of PRP was effective in improving knee functional status with a significant increase in KOOS total score from 43.5 ± 14.3 to 66.4 ± 21.7, six months after the procedure ($p < 0.001$, Figure 2). Interestingly, this significant difference was observed already after one month after the treatment and was reflected on all KOOS subscores (Figure 2 and Supplemental Table S1). Assessment of pain through a 50-foot walk test also resulted in significant decrease of pain from the baseline (37.5 ± 25.1) as of one month after the injection (20.2 ± 23.3; $p < 0.001$, Supplemental Table S1) with a continuous effect until six months (12.9 ± 20.9; $p < 0.001$, Supplemental Table S1). Assessment of damages caused by the arthrosis were also reduced from 62.3 ± 19.6 at baseline to 42.1 ± 42.5 at six months with significant reduction at all follow-up ($p < 0.001$; Supplemental Table S1). Physical component score from the SF-36 significantly improved at all follow-up ($p < 0.001$, Supplemental Table S1). However, mental component score from the SF-36 did not change, which is consistent with the lack of improvement relative to patients' global health that was relatively good at the beginning of the study (72.1 ± 16.0) (Supplemental Table S1). 78.9% of the patients and 80.7% of the rheumatologists were either satisfied or very satisfied regarding the procedure six months after the injection. Evolution of MRI parameters are presented in Table 3 without significant change six months after injection. Regarding safety, four adverse events (AE) were reported in four patients. AE were shoulder pain in two cases, acute pulmonary edema and peripheral arterial obstructive disease. None were considered related to the study treatment.

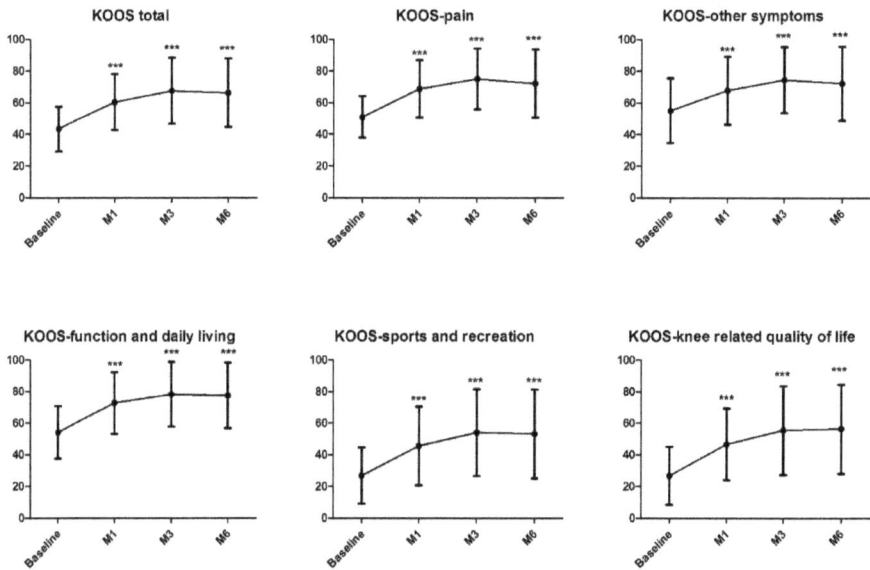

Figure 2. Evolution of KOOS total score and subscales. All follow-ups were statistically significant in comparison to baseline (***: $p < 0.001$; see Supplemental Table S1). KOOS, Knee Injury and Osteoarthritis Score. M1, month 1; M3, month 3; M6, month 6.

Table 3. MRI assessment pre-injection and six months post-injection of PRP ($n = 49$).

	Pre-Operative	6 Months Post Injection	p
Presence of edema (number of patients)			
Grade 0	23	26	
Grade 1	18	13	$p = 1$
Grade 2	6	10	
Grade 3	2	8	
Presence of joint effusion (number of patients)			
Grade 0	14	14	
Grade 1	17	16	$p = 1$
Grade 2	14	13	
Grade 3	4	6	
Articular thickness (mm, mean $\pm$ SD)			
IFT-F compartment	1.16 ± 0.72	1.14 ± 0.77	$p = 0.72$
IFT-T compartment	1.67 ± 0.85	1.64 ± 0.89	$p = 0.82$
LFT-F compartment	1.60 ± 0.60	1.62 ± 0.60	$p = 0.75$
LFT-T compartment	2.08 ± 0.91	2.14 ± 1.01	$p = 0.26$
IFP compartment	2.27 ± 0.75	2.33 ± 0.77	$p = 0.22$
LFP compartment	2.61 ± 1.03	2.68 ± 1.06	$p = 0.22$

KOOS, Knee Injury and Osteoarthritis Score; I, internal; L, Lateral; FT, femorotibial; FP, femoropatellar; F, femur; T, tibia.

3. Discussion

Single administration of high volume of autologous pure PRP provided significant clinical benefit to more than 80% of responders at three months according to OMERACT-OARSI definition, in patients presenting knee OA in stage 2 or 3 according Kellgren–Laurence scale. These results are consistent with meta-analysis results from Dai et al. indicating functional improvement and pain relief one year after PRP injection [8]. Our study targeted patients similar to Dai et al. meta-analysis i.e., over 50 years old, presenting stage 2 or 3 on the Kellgren–Laurence scale. However, the therapeutic schema was different as the 10 randomized clinical trial (RCT) selected in that meta-analysis included multiple PRP injections whereas one of the originality of our study was to perform a single large volume PRP injection. Interestingly, only 3/10 of these RCT injected 8 mL whereas other studies injected 3 to 5.5 mL. From our point of view, PRP preparation for OA knee injection should take into account the articular capacity of the knee in order to favor a better distribution of PRP throughout the joint. It was recently recommended that the volume for knee-specific injection should be at 9 mL [18]. Thus, the medical device used in this study was validated in order to reach this condition. It was also selected to provide a pure PRP with limited contamination in RBCs and leukocytes and a platelets dose of around 2.5 billion in accordance with the results of Louis et al. [19]. Indeed, this study demonstrates that a single injection of very pure PRP (mean platelets dose $\pm$ SD of 2.4 $\pm$ 0.8 billion and platelets purity of 91.4 $\pm$ 4.1%) offers a significant clinical improvement equivalent to a single HA injection. This RCT also identified that higher platelets doses were correlated to higher levels of Transforming Growth Factor-β1 and Platelets Derived Growth Factor-AB as well as with knee function impairment, hence supporting limiting the injected dose of platelets. In our study, comparison between biological characteristics of PRP injected between OMERACT-OARSI responders (n = 48) and non-responders (n = 9) patients was performed without noticeable difference. This could be explained by (i) the small number of non-responder patients, (ii) the high reproducibility of the PRP produced in this study and (iii) the absence of GF quantification. This also suggests that this kind of correlation should be performed in RCT to limit the impact of placebo effect in the interpretation of biological data. Despite the excellent results of our study on pain and knee function, no statistical difference was observed compared to baseline in the parameters assessed by MRI. These results are consistent with the study of Buendia-Lopez et al. [20] who also assessed the articular thickness in all knee articular compartments and reached a similar conclusion. However, Lisi et al. [21] used a different methodology where they compared the number of patients with at least one grade improvement using MRI, according the Shahriaree classification system [22], six months after PRP or HA injections. They describe a significant difference with 16/31 patients reaching this improvement in PRP group and 8/31 in HA group, suggesting that guidelines for MRI interpretation in the context of regenerative medicine are needed.

The major limitation of our study is the absence of a control group which is an important weakness knowing the important placebo effect on arthrosis care. Indeed, it is important to recall that placebo can relieve pain in OA patients (effect size of 0.51) or improve function and stiffness (effect size of 0.49 and 0.43), particularly when administered through injections [23]. The absence of a placebo group was a conscious decision as many patients are discouraged to participate to a RCT involving PRP whereas it is daily and routinely injected in several rheumatology and orthopedic departments. Also, an adequately resourced RCT would require a higher number of patients and entail higher costs. Finally, it would have been interesting to document efficacy and MRI parameters one year after the injection, and extend the characterization of PRP to GF contents.

To conclude, our study indicates that a single injection of a large volume of very pure PRP is associated with a responders' rate of around 80%, up to six months after the injection, supporting the initiation of daily PRP injection in OA patients in Saint Joseph hospital.

In light of the growing evidence of its benefit and taking into account the current complex and heterogeneous context, a feasibility study according to AAOS guidelines would be desirable or even mandatory, prior to initiating regular PRP injection in OA.

4. Materials and Methods

4.1. Patients

To obtain a homogeneous study population, the patient suitability for inclusion was assessed (after a first screening by a physician), according to the following inclusion criteria: Age between 20 and 80 years old, symptomatic knee osteoarthritis grade 2 or 3 in Kellgren–Lawrence scale and according to the criteria of the American College of Rheumatology, axial deformity of the lower limb equal to or lower than 5°, at least moderate pain and difficulty to walk on a plain surface, ability to perform rehabilitation exercises, articular pain > 6 months, Hemoglobin (Hb) >10 g/dL, negative pregnancy test and written informed consent. The exclusion criteria were: Axial deformity of the lower limb over 5°, knee instability, important knee injuries or knee surgery less than 52 weeks before inclusion, Body Mass Index >35, thrombocytopenia <150 G/L or >450 G/L, thrombopathy, Hb <10 g/dL, infectious disease or positive serology to HIV, HCV, HBV and syphilis, actual chronic treatment by oral corticosteroid (or last dose taken less than two weeks before), intra articular knee injection of corticosteroid less than eight weeks before inclusion, intra articular knee injection of hyaluronic acid less than 24 weeks before inclusion, NSAID or anti platelets treatment completed less than two weeks before inclusion, fever or recent disease, auto immune disease, inflammatory arthritis, immune deficit, pregnancy and patient under guardianship or involved in another clinical trial.

4.2. Study Design and Intervention

This monocentric prospective routine care trial was performed in the rheumatology department of Saint Joseph Hospital between March 2016 and August 2018. Patients received a single injection of PRP. After the injection, patients returned home with instructions to restrict movement of the leg for at least 48 hours and to use paracetamol or ice on the injected area to relieve pain if necessary. Non-steroidal anti-inflammatory drugs were prohibited during seven days following the injection. During the follow-up, no treatment restriction was applied and subsequently a gradual resumption of normal sport or recreational activities was tolerated.

The protocol was approved by the ethics committee and national health regulatory authority (CPP Ile de France 1 authorization #14243ND, 15th November 2016). The study was carried out in accordance with the Declaration of Helsinki and the principles of Good Clinical Practice. All patients gave written informed consent before their participation. The study was registered at clinicaltrials.gov (NCT 03082430).

4.3. Autologous PRP Preparation Method

After a four-fold skin decontamination (antiseptic foaming solution, rinsing with sterile water, drying, and alcoholic dermal antiseptic), a nurse collected 18 mL of blood by venipunture using a 21-gauge needle filling one 20 mL syringe containing 2 mL of ACD-A (Fidia, Abano Terme, Itlay). The blood was transferred into the Hy-tissue 20 PRP device (Fidia, Abano Terme, Itlay) before centrifugation using the Omnigrafter 3.0 (Fidia, Abano Terme, Itlay) and PRP Large Volume Cycle (3200 rpm during 10 minutes). All plasma was recovered using a 10 mL syringe through the Push-out system. 300 μL of whole blood and each autologous PRP preparation were sampled to determine platelets, leukocytes and RBCs concentrations using automated haematology blood cell analyzers Beckman Coulter DxH 801 (Beckman Coulter, Miami, FL, USA) according to recent guidelines [24].

4.4. Injection

The intra articular knee injection was performed with a 21 Gauge needle after conventional skin aseptic decontamination and under echographic control (HITACHI Aloka F37 Hitachi Aloka Medical Systems, Tokyo, Japan).

4.5. Evaluation Tools and Follow-Up

Patients were prospectively assessed at baseline and one, three, and six months after injection. Evaluation included the Knee Injury and Osteoarthritis Score (KOOS), Observed Pain on 50-foot walk test, Visual Analog Scale (VAS) assessments (0–100 mm scale) during the previous week regarding arthrosis activity, damages related to arthrosis and global health. Quality-of-life was evaluated using the 36-Item Short Form Health Survey (SF-36) which was divided into two summary measures: The Physical (PCS) and Mental (MCS) Component Summary scores. Magnetic Resonance Imaging (MRI) analysis was performed at baseline and six months after the procedure using 1.5T MAGNETOM Aera and Avanto^{fit} (Siemens Healthcare, Erlangen, Germany). The presence of edema and joint effusion was graded as follows: 0 (absence), 1 (low), 2 (moderate), 3 (severe). The highest articular thickness was evaluated on same sequences for six compartments: Internal and lateral femoro-tibial compartments on femur and tibial parts respectively and internal and lateral femoro-patellar compartments.

Patients and rheumatologists satisfaction were rated at six months on a 5-level scale: Not satisfied, Few Satisfied, Moderately Satisfied, Satisfied and Very satisfied. Adverse events were recorded. Primary endpoint measure was defined as the percentage of OMERACT-OARSI responders at three months. OMERACT-OARSI criteria define responders patients if they satisfy either of the following criteria: (i) High improvement ($\geq$50% and absolute change ≥ 10) in pain domain (pain observed on 50-foot walk test) or function (KOOS function in daily living subscore) or (ii) improvement ($\geq$20% and absolute change ≥ 10) in at least 2/3 of the following domains: Pain, function or patient's global assessment (VAS assessment on arthrosis activity previous week).

4.6. Statistical Analysis

Data were analyzed according to the intention-to-treat principle. The continuous variables were described by their mean and standard deviation. The categorical variables were described by their size and percentage. Comparisons over time, between two or more time points, were done using statistical test for repeated measurements. For situations involving two time points, we used Chi-square test, or Fisher's exact test if the expected count in any cell was <5 for categorical data and Wilcoxon's for continuous data. Correlation between covariates were quantified and tested using Pearson coefficient correlation. Friedman's test was used to consider trend over times. The tests were performed bilaterally and were considered statistically significant when *p*-values $\leq$ 0.05. To deal with multiple testing in trend analysis, we used Holm's method to produce *p*-values adjusted. The statistical analysis was performed with R software (version 3.1.0).

Supplementary Materials: Supplementary materials can be found at http://www.mdpi.com/1422-0067/20/6/1327/s1.

Author Contributions: For research articles with several authors, a short paragraph specifying their individual contributions must be provided. The following statements should be used "conceptualization, C.G., C.C., M.R., J.M., and D.A.; methodology, A.B., R.G., J.M., and D.A.; validation, C.G., C.C., G.E.L.G., and J.M.; formal analysis, A.B., and R.G.; investigation, C.G., C.C., F.X.D., G.E.L.G.; writing—original draft preparation, C.G. and J.M.; writing—review and editing, C.G., C.C., M.R., A.B., F.X.D., G.E.L.G., R.G., J.M. and D.A.; supervision, C.G., C.C., G.E.L.G., and J.M.

Funding: This research received no external funding.

Conflicts of Interest: The authors declare no conflict of interest.

References

1. Lane, N.E.; Brandt, K.; Hawker, G.; Peeva, E.; Schreyer, E.; Tsuji, W.; Hochberg, M.C. OARSI-FDA initiative: Defining the disease state of osteoarthritis. *Osteoarthr. Cartil.* **2011**, *19*, 478–482. [CrossRef]
2. Barbour, K.E.; Helmick, C.G.; Boring, M.; Zhang, X.; Lu, H.; Holt, J.B. Prevalence of Doctor-Diagnosed Arthritis at State and County Levels—United States, 2014. *MMWR Morb. Mortal. Wkly. Rep.* **2016**, *65*, 489–494. [CrossRef] [PubMed]

3. Felson, D.T.; Zhang, Y.; Anthony, J.M.; Naimark, A.; Anderson, J.J. Weight loss reduces the risk for symptomatic knee osteoarthritis in woman. The Framingham Study. *Ann. Intern. Med.* **1992**, *116*, 535–539. [CrossRef] [PubMed]

4. Bellamy, N.; Campbell, J.; Welch, V.; Gee, T.L.; Bourne, R.; Wells, G.A. Intraarticular corticosteroid for treatment of osteoarthritis of the knee. *Cochrane Database Syst. Rev.* **2006**, *19*, CD005328.

5. Hepper, C.T.; Halvorson, J.J.; Duncan, S.T.; Gregory, A.J.; Dunn, W.R.; Spindler, K.P. The efficacy and duration of intra-articular corticosteroid injection for knee osteoarthritis: A systematic review of level I studies. *J. Am. Acad. Orthop. Surg.* **2009**, *17*, 638–646. [CrossRef] [PubMed]

6. Bannuru, R.R.; Natov, N.S.; Obadan, I.E.; Price, L.L.; Schmid, C.H.; McAlindon, T.E. Therapeutic trajectory of hyaluronic acid versus corticosteroids in the treatment of knee osteoarthritis: A systematic review and meta-analysis. *Arthritis Rheum.* **2009**, *61*, 1704–1711. [CrossRef] [PubMed]

7. Gregori, D.; Giacovelli, G.; Minto, C.; Barbetta, B.; Gualtieri, F.; Azzolina, D.; Vaghi, P.; Rovati, L.C. Association of Pharmacological Treatments with Long-term Pain Control in Patients With Knee Osteoarthritis: A Systematic Review and Meta-analysis. *JAMA* **2018**, *320*, 2564–2579. [CrossRef] [PubMed]

8. Brown, G.A. AAOS clinical practice guidelines. Treatment of osteoarthritis of the knee: Evidence-based guideline, 2ded. *J. Am. Acad. Orthop. Surg.* **2013**, *21*, 577–579. [PubMed]

9. Marx, R.E. Platelet-rich plasma (PRP): What is PRP and what is not PRP? *Implant Dent.* **2001**, *10*, 225–228. [CrossRef] [PubMed]

10. Dai, W.L.; Zhou, A.G.; Zhang, H.; Zhang, J. Efficacy of Platelet-Rich Plasma in the Treatment of Knee Osteoarthritis: A Meta-analysis of Randomized Controlled Trials. *Arthroscopy* **2017**, *33*, 659–670. [CrossRef] [PubMed]

11. Hunt, T.J. Editorial Commentary: The Time Has Come to Try Intra-articular Platelet-Rich Plasma Injections for Your Patients with Symptomatic Knee Osteoarthritis. *Arthroscopy* **2017**, *33*, 671–672. [CrossRef]

12. Magalon, J.; Bausset, O.; Serratrice, N.; Giraudo, L.; Aboudou, H.; Veran, J.; Magalon, G.; Dignat-Georges, F.; Sabatier, F. Characterization and comparison of 5 Platelet-Rich Plasma preparations in a single donor model. *Arthroscopy* **2014**, *30*, 629–638. [CrossRef] [PubMed]

13. Castillo, T.N.; Pouliot, M.A.; Kim, H.J.; Dragoo, J.L. Comparison of growth factor and platelet concentration from commercial platelet-rich plasma separation systems. *Am. J. Sports Med.* **2011**, *39*, 266–271. [CrossRef]

14. Riboh, J.C.; Saltzman, B.M.; Yanke, A.B.; Fortier, L.; Cole, B.J. Effect of leukocyte concentration on the efficacy of Platelet rich Plasma in the treatment of knee osteoarthritis. *Am. J. Sports Med.* **2016**, *44*, 792–800. [CrossRef] [PubMed]

15. Simental-Mendía, M.; Vílchez-Cavazos, J.F.; Peña-Martínez, V.M.; Said-Fernández, S.; Lara-Arias, J.; Martínez-Rodríguez, H.G. Leukocyte-poor platelet-rich plasma is more effective than the conventional therapy with acetaminophen for the treatment of early knee osteoarthritis. *Arch. Orthop. Trauma Surg.* **2016**, *136*, 1723–1732. [CrossRef] [PubMed]

16. Chu, C.R.; Rodeo, S.; Bhutani, N.; Goodrich, L.R.; Huard, J.; Irrgang, J.; LaPrade, R.F.; Lattermann, C.; Lu, Y.; Mandelbaum, B.; et al. Optimizing Clinical Use of Biologics in Orthopaedic Surgery: Consensus Recommendations from the 2018 AAOS/NIH U-13 Conference. *J. Am. Acad. Orthop. Surg.* **2019**, *27*, e50–e63. [CrossRef] [PubMed]

17. Magalon, J.; Chateau, A.L.; Bertrand, B.; Louis, M.L.; Silvestre, A.; Giraudo, L.; Veran, J.; Sabatier, F. DEPA classification: A proposal for standardising PRP use and a retrospective application of available devices. *BMJ Open Sport Exerc. Med.* **2016**, *2*, e000060. [CrossRef] [PubMed]

18. Rastogi, A.K.; Davis, K.W.; Ross, A.; Rosas, H.G. Fundamentals of Joint Injection. *Am. J. Roentgenol.* **2016**, *207*, 484–494. [CrossRef] [PubMed]

19. Louis, M.L.; Magalon, J.; Jouve, E.; Bornet, C.E.; Mattei, J.C.; Chagnaud, C.; Rochwerger, A.; Veran, J.; Sabatier, F. Growth Factors Levels Determine Efficacy of Platelets Rich Plasma Injection in Knee Osteoarthritis: A Randomized Double Blind Noninferiority Trial Compared with Viscosupplementation. *Arthroscopy* **2018**, *34*, 1530–1540. [CrossRef]

20. Buendía-López, D.; Medina-Quirós, M.; Marín, M.Á. Clinical and radiographic comparison of a single LP-PRP injection, a single hyaluronic acid injection and daily NSAID administration with a 52-week follow-up: A randomized controlled trial. *J. Orthop. Traumatol.* **2018**, *19*, 3. [CrossRef] [PubMed]

21. Lisi, C.; Perotti, C.; Scudeller, L.; Sammarchi, L.; Dametti, F.; Musella, V.; Di Natali, G. Treatment of knee osteoarthritis: Platelet-derived growth factors vs. hyaluronic acid. A randomized controlled trial. *Clin. Rehabil.* **2018**, *32*, 330–339. [CrossRef] [PubMed]
22. Woertler, K.; Buerger, H.; Moeller, J.; Rummeny, E.J. Patellar articular cartilage lesions: in vitro MR imaging evaluation after placement in gadopentetate dimeglumine solution. *Radiology* **2004**, *230*, 768–773. [CrossRef] [PubMed]
23. Zhang, W.; Robertson, J.; Jones, A.C.; Dieppe, P.A.; Doherty, M. The placebo effect and its determinants in osteoarthritis: Meta-analysis of randomised controlled trials. *Ann. Rheum Dis.* **2008**, *67*, 1716–1723. [CrossRef] [PubMed]
24. Graiet, H.; Lokchine, A.; Francois, P.; Velier, M.; Grimaud, F.; Loyens, M.; Berda-Haddad, Y.; Veran, J.; Dignat-George, F.; Sabatier, F.; et al. Use of platelet-rich plasma in regenerative medicine: Technical tools for correct quality control. *BMJ Open Sport Exerc. Med.* **2018**, *13*, e000442. [CrossRef]

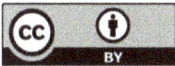

International Journal of
Molecular Sciences

MDPI

Article

Development of Autologous Platelet-Rich Plasma Mixed-Microfat as an Advanced Therapy Medicinal Product for Intra-Articular Injection of Radio-Carpal Osteoarthritis: From Validation Data to Preliminary Clinical Results

Alice Mayoly [1], Aurélie Iniesta [1], Caroline Curvale [1], Najib Kachouh [1], Charlotte Jaloux [2], Julia Eraud [2], Marie Vogtensperger [3], Julie Veran [3], Fanny Grimaud [3], Elisabeth Jouve [4], Dominique Casanova [2], Florence Sabatier [3,5], Régis Legré [1] and Jérémy Magalon [3,5,*]

[1] Department of Hand and Limb Reconstructive Surgery, Assistance Publique–Hôpitaux de Marseille, La Timone University Hospital, 13005 Marseille, France; alice.mayoly@ap-hm.fr (A.M.); aurelie.iniesta@gmail.com (A.I.); caroline.curvale@ap-hm.fr (C.C.); najib.kachouh@ap-hm.fr (N.K.); regis.legre@ap-hm.fr (R.L.)
[2] Department of Plastic and Reconstructive Surgery, Assistance Publique–Hôpitaux de Marseille, La Conception University Hospital, 13005 Marseille, France; charlotte.jaloux@ap-hm.fr (C.J.); julia.eraud@ap-hm.fr (J.E.); dominique.casanova@ap-hm.fr (D.C.)
[3] Cell therapy department, Assistance Publique–Hôpitaux de Marseille, INSERM, CBT-1409, La Conception University Hospital, Marseille 13005, France; marie.vogtensperger@ap-hm.fr (M.V.); julie.veran@ap-hm.fr (J.V.); fanny.grimaud@ap-hm.fr (F.G.); florence.sabatier@ap-hm.fr (F.S.)
[4] Aix-Marseille University, Assistance Publique–Hôpitaux de Marseille, INSERM, Inst Neurosci Syst, Service de Pharmacologie Clinique et Pharmacovigilance, CIC-CPCET, 13005 Marseille, France; elisabeth.jouve@ap-hm.fr
[5] Aix-Marseille University, INSERM, INRA, C2VN, 13005 Marseille, France
[*] Correspondence: jeremy.magalon@ap-hm.fr; Tel.: +33-491-38-1486; Fax: +33-491-38-3685

Received: 15 February 2019; Accepted: 28 February 2019; Published: 5 March 2019

check for updates

Abstract: Wrist osteoarthritis (OA) is one of the most common conditions encountered by hand surgeons with limited efficacy of non-surgical treatments. The purpose of this study is to describe the Platelet-Rich Plasma (PRP) mixed-microfat biological characteristics of an experimental Advanced Therapy Medicinal Product (ATMP) needed for clinical trial authorization and describe the clinical results obtained from our first three patients 12 months after treatment (NCT03164122). Biological characterization of microfat, PRP and mixture were analysed in vitro according to validated methods. Patients with stage four OA according to the Kellgren Lawrence classification, with failure to conservative treatment and a persistent daily painful condition >40 mm according to the visual analog scale (VAS) were treated. Microfat-PRP ATMP is a product with high platelet purity, conserved viability of stromal vascular fraction cells, chondrogenic differentiation capacity in vitro and high secretion of IL-1Ra anti-inflammatory cytokine. For patients, the only side effect was pain at the adipose tissue harvesting sites. Potential efficacy was observed with a pain decrease of over 50% (per VAS score) and the achievement of minimal clinically important differences for DASH and PRWE functional scores at one year in all three patients. Microfat-PRP ATMP presented a good safety profile after an injection in wrist OA. Efficacy trials are necessary to assess whether this innovative strategy could delay the necessity to perform non-conservative surgery.

Keywords: wrist osteoarthritis; microfat; platelet-rich plasma; cell therapy; adipose tissue

1. Introduction

Osteoarthritis (OA) of the wrist is one of the most common conditions encountered by hand surgeons. It is a chronic non-inflammatory joint disease characterised by degenerative lesions of the cartilage, which can result in major functional impairment including painful condition, and a loss of strength and motion [1]. Its incidence is constantly increasing due to the ageing population and sport-related traumatic injuries. Most of OA cases are post-traumatic and may be secondary to scapholunate ligament tears leading to carpal disorganization (named scapholunate advanced collapse or SLAC) or bone injury (sequelae of intra-articular distal radius fracture or scaphoid non-union named scaphoid nonunion advanced collapse also known as SNAC). Idiopathic causes such as idiopathic carpal avascular necrosis (Kienböck's or Preiser's disease) or congenital wrist abnormalities (Madelung's deformity) are rare, but can also lead to wrist OA [2,3].

The first line therapeutic measures are currently limited to symptomatic treatment: contention by splints, analgesics and anti-inflammatory drugs [3,4] whereas, intra-articular injections of corticosteroids or hyaluronic acid are used in common practice [3] without high levels of evidence. Whereas, their use in other hand joints is still debated [5]. Surgery is indicated after conservative treatment failure. The main objective is to ensure pain relief, while restoring strength and preserving as much wrist motion as possible. Palliative wrist denervation is usually the first step of treatment due to its lesser consequences on wrist mobility. However, it is inefficient in a quarter to more than a third of cases [6,7]. The other surgical alternatives are: first row carpectomy, total or partial wrist arthrodesis and sometimes prosthesis wrist arthroplasty. These palliative procedures require wrist immobilization, intensive post-operative rehabilitation and can only preserve partial function of the wrist [8–13].

Thus, minimally invasive therapeutic alternative that could delay the use of these heavy and non-conservative surgeries represent a medico-surgical challenge in management of wrist OA after failure of well-conducted medical treatment. Recently, the emergence of biological therapies has led to the evaluation of intra-articular injections of autologous Platelet-Rich Plasma (PRP) in treatment of chondral degenerative diseases with satisfactory results [14–18]. Briefly, activated platelets release growth factors (GF) with beneficial impacts on regenerative and reparative processes. In addition, autologous adipose tissue has gained great interest because it represents a rich and convenient source of cells for regenerative medicine. The stromal vascular fraction (SVF) cells constitute a heterogeneous cell population, including a large proportion of mesenchymal multipotent stem cells (Adipose-derived stem cells, ADSCs), which are located in the adipose tissue vasculature. Thus, the high abundance of adipose tissue within the body, its high surgical accessibility, and the demonstrated multipotency of ADSCs, especially towards the chondrogenic lineage [19–23], highlighted the potential of adipose tissue-derived products for cartilage repair. Among them, microfat is simply obtained through dedicated fat harvesting that uses a multi perforated cannula with holes of 1 mm allowing to harvest smaller lobules of fat (around 600 μm) [24].

We previously described the safety profile of combining autologous microfat and PRP as a mixed regenerative product injected in the carpus or the fetlock joint of sport horses presenting with degenerative joint disease [25]. A significant lameness reduction, together with an early return to compete were also indicative of potential efficacy. However, from a regulatory point of view, the intra-articular use of PRP mixed-microfat was considered by the French National Agency for Medicines and Health Products Safety (Agence Nationale de Sécurité du Médicament (ANSM)) as an Advanced Therapy Medicinal Product (ATMP) according to the directive No. 1394/2007 from the European Parliament and the European Council [26]. This classification is based on the non-homologous use of microfat in the wrist joint. The consequences are that the preparation of the product should comply with Good Manufacturing Practice (GMP), meaning it is relocated in a cell therapy facility, including the achievement of process validation batches with outstanding characterization of the final product, and definition of biological acceptance criteria. For safety concerns, ANSM also imposes a one-month delay between the treatment of each of the three first patients for safety concerns.

Here, we aimed to outline the phases of biological validation of a GMP-compliant PRP mixed-microfat. ATMP performed prior to approval by the French Agency. We also report the preliminary clinical results at 12 months with the follow-up obtained from the first three patients enrolled in a clinical trial evaluating PRP mixed-microfat in wrist OA.

2. Results

2.1. Process Validation Batches

In the biological data characterising the experimental PRP, microfat and the mixed ATMP are obtained from the process validation batches. As summarised in Table 1A–C, the PRP obtained was a very pure PRP according to the DEPA (Dose Efficiency Purity Activation) classification [27] with a mean ± SD of 97.4 ± 0.2 % platelets purity at the end of the preparation. Increase factor in platelet concentration compared to whole blood was 2.0 ± 0.4. Platelet aggregation in response to different inductors was considered effective for all conditions tested. All PRP preparations were free of microorganisms, and presented stable biological characteristics at 3 h after the end of the preparation. Production of microfat resulted in a macroscopically pure product with less than 10% of oily or bloody phase with stable results at 3 h after the end of the production.

Table 1. Biological characteristics of PRP (A), microfat (B), and PRP mixed-microfat (C) obtained from the analysis of GMP compliant process validation batches.

(A)	T0	T + 3 h
Platelets Purity (%)	97.4 ± 0.2	97.4 ± 0.1
RBCs Contamination (%)	2.5 ± 0.1	2.5 ± 0.1
Leukocytes Contamination (%)	0.04 ± 0.04	0.03 ± 0.03
Potential Dose of Injected Platelets (10^6/ 2 mL)	775.3 ± 35.8	766.7 ± 25.8
Increase Factor in Platelets	2.0 ± 0.4	2.0 ± 0.4
Platelets Aggregation Response (%)		
ADP 5 µM	74.2 ± 9.8	69.0 ± 2.6
ADP 2.5 µM	55.5 ± 7.5	47.8 ± 1.9
Arachidonic Acid 0.5 mg/ mL	91.6 ± 3.5	87.5 ± 1.6
Collagen 3.3 µg/mL	90.1 ± 2.9	91.1 ± 2.4
Ristocetin 1.25 mg/mL	97.7 ± 2.5	96.9 ± 4.0
Microbiological Assay	Free of germ (3/3)	Free of germ (3/3)
(B)	T0	T + 3 h
Macroscopical Aspect	Absence of blood and oily phase (3/3)	Absence of blood and oily phase (3/3)
Microbiological Assay	Free of germ (3/3)	Free of germ (3/3)
(C)	T0	-
SVF Viability (%)	75.7 ± 1.3	-
SVF Viable Nucleated Cells (x10^6 / 4 mL)	1.3 ± 0.6	-
Chondrocytes Differentiation * (Micromass Formed/Control Group)	17/1 10/0	-
GF Release (pg/mL)		
VEGF	22.0 ± 30.1	-
PDGF	394.0 ± 128.1	-
FGF2	171.8 ± 83.1	-
TGF-β1	ND	-
IL1-β	0.2 ± 0.1	-
IL-1RA	82.0 ± 73.3	-
IL-1RA/IL1-β ratio	443.3 ± 348.0	-

Results are expressed in mean ± SD except for microbiological assay, macroscopical aspect, and chondrocytes differentiation. Red Blood Cells, (RBCs); Growth Factors, (GF); Stromal Vascular Fraction (SVF) * performed only on two samples.

PRP mixed-microfat manufacturing lead to a product containing 1.3 ± 0.6 million viable nucleated Stromal Vascular Fraction (SVF) cells with a mean $\pm$ SD viability of 75.7 ± 1.3 %. ADSCs obtained from the mixture were able to differentiate in chondrocytes under specific culture conditions compared to control (Figure 1). Results of stability assays conducted at 3 h on PRP and microfat were similar to t0 data. Finally, PRP mixed-microfat release detectable quantity of regenerative growth factors (VEGF, PDGF, FGF2) whereas, only TGF-β1 was not. Interestingly, IL-1Ra/IL1-β ratio presented a mean $\pm$ SD of 443.3 ± 348.0 suggesting a potential anti-inflammatory effect.

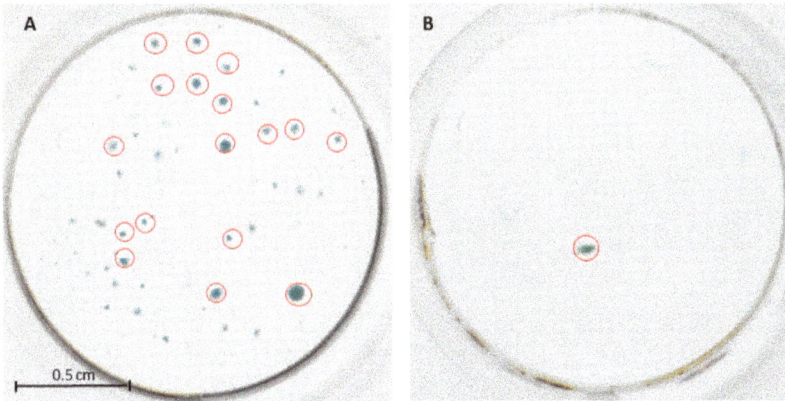

Figure 1. Macroscopic aspect of chondrocytes micromass obtained from adipose-derived stem cells (ADSCs) derived microfat-PRP in the presence of chondrogenic differentiation media (**A**) or control media (**B**). Red circles represent micromass with area > 0.05 mm^2.

The final investigational product used for the clinical trial was then defined as two interconnected 5 mL syringes containing 2 mL of microfat and 2 mL of PRP that had to be injected within 3 h after the end of manufacturing. Aspect of the final product delivered to the operating room and release criteria from microfat and PRP were defined and validated by ANSM according to the results of process validation batches and are listed in Figure 2.

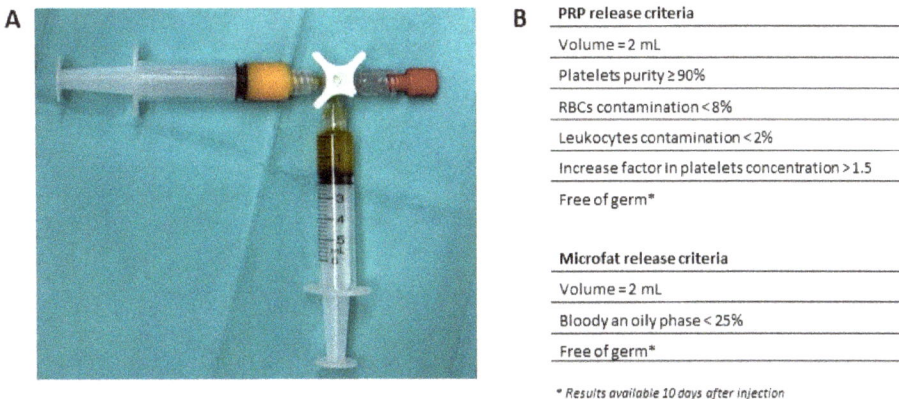

B PRP release criteria
Volume = 2 mL
Platelets purity ≥ 90%
RBCs contamination < 8%
Leukocytes contamination < 2%
Increase factor in platelets concentration > 1.5
Free of germ*

Microfat release criteria
Volume = 2 mL
Bloody an oily phase < 25%
Free of germ*

* Results available 10 days after injection

Figure 2. (**A**) Microfat-PRP investigational Advanced Therapy Medicinal Product (ATMP) delivered to the operating room for intra articular injection in radio-carpal joint (without labelling). (**B**) Release criteria from PRP and microfat checked by the responsible pharmacist from the ATMP manufacturing Department before delivery to the operating room.

2.2. Preliminary Data from Clinical Trials

The first three patients were treated between June and August 2017 respecting a one-month delay between each patient, as required by ANSM. Characteristics of patients and injected products are described in Table 2.

Table 2. Patients and injected products characteristics obtained from the first three patients treated with microfat-PRP ATMP.

	Patient 1	Patient 2	Patient 3
Gender	Female	Female	Male
Age, years	65	62	59
Dominant hand	Right	Right	Right
Injured wrist	Left	Left	Left
Etiology	Radius fracture	SLAC	SLAC
Kellgren Lawrence grade	4	4	4
Seat(s) of osteoarthritis	RC	RC and IC	RC
Volume of microfat PRP injected (mL)	2.7	4.0	3.8
Dose of injected platelets (10^6)	720.9	674.0	708.7
Platelets purity (%)	96.0	94.2	97.4
PRP microbiological assay	Free of germ	Free of germ	Free of germ
Microfat microbiological assay	Free of germ	Free of germ	Free of germ

R, Radiocarpal; IC, Intracarpal; SLAC, scapholunate advanced collapse.

There was 2.7 to 4 mL of mixture injected with a platelet dose around 700 million and a platelet purity over 95%. Absence of pain was observed during injection (Visual Analog Scale: 0). All patients were able to get back to their regular activities one week after injection. No serious adverse event was recorded in these three patients. In addition, there was no infectious complication observed. The only reported side effect was pain at the sites of the adipose tissue harvesting, which was systematically reported at day seven in a postoperative visit and was relieved by grade 1 analgesics and completely disappeared after one month. All three patients presented with at least a 50% decrease in pain compared to baseline at three months. This effect was maintained until one year after the injection, except for patient three. Disabilities of the Arm and Shoulder (DASH) improvement reached 11 points, corresponding to the minimal clinically important difference (MCID) [28] for patient two and patient three at three months and for all patients at six months. Patient-Rated Wrist Evaluation (PRWE) improvement reached 14 points corresponding to MCID [29] since the third month after treatment for all patients. These observations were stable until the last visit at one year. No significant improvement was observed in grip strength and wrist range of motion during the follow-up. All three patients were either satisfied or very satisfied after the procedure at all follow-up. Figure 3 summarises the results of the pain Visual Analog Scale (VAS), DASH and PRWE scores up to one year.

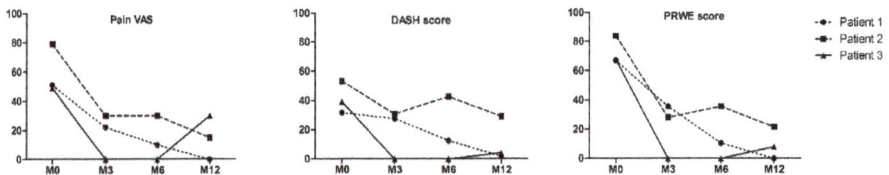

Figure 3. Evolution of pain according to Visual Analog Scale (VAS), Disabilities of the Arm and Shoulder (DASH) and Patient-Rated Wrist Evaluation (PRWE) scores at baseline, and months 3, 6 and 12 for patients 1, 2 and 3.

3. Discussion

To our knowledge, this study is the first to report the use of a combined microfat-PRP product as ATMP for joint injection in humans. Indeed, an introduction of adipose tissue in the joint was considered as an ATMP, according to European regulation No. 1394/2007 due to the non-homologous use of adipose tissue in the wrist joint. Thus, a set of accurate biological and pharmaceutical characterisations of the final injected product was conducted, as requested by the regulatory French Agency ANSM prior to any clinical trial authorization. Testing of the process validation batches attested that the PRP mixed-microfat is a sterile product with limited contamination in Red Blood Cells (RBCs) and leukocytes, preserved viability of SVF cells, chondrogenic differentiation ability in vitro and high secretion of IL1Ra anti-inflammatory cytokine. Characteristics of the product were stable upon 3 h after the end of the manufacturing.

These data allowed to obtain a clinical trial authorization for a phase I study with the constraint to wait one month during the treatments of each of the three first patients for safety reason. The only reported side effect was pain at the site of adipose tissue harvesting. Clinical results achieved MCID for DASH and PRWE scores in all patients one year after injection. MCID is not clearly defined in the literature for VAS scale, which measures pain for wrist OA. That said, VAS scale MCID for surgical treatment of shoulder diseases is between 14 and 30 mm [30,31]. Interestingly, the three patients reached a final improvement at one year of 51, 64 and 19 mm, respectively. The profile of patient three is a matter of discussion, as he presented with an impressive improvement in pain and function up until six months with a slight impairment in pain at one year. In contrast, patient 1 and 2 showed progressive improvement up until one year after treatment. This was explained by a pain wrist crisis in the weeks before the one-year evaluation. However, these subjective assessments were not supported by the objective improvement in measures of strength or range of motion, and should therefore be interpreted carefully.

Absence of adverse event is consistent with other published studies in the literature. Indeed, no infectious or neoplasic complications related to the intra-articular injection of cell-based products (including PRP, cultured ADSCs and/or minimally processed adipose tissue), has been reported to date [15,32,33]. However, very few studies have been designed to address the upper limb, and mainly concern the thumb carpometacarpal joint. Autologous intra-articular fat injection has been studied for the treatment of the thumb carpometacarpal joint OA in two studies. Herold et al. assessed the efficacy of the intra-articular injection of centrifuged adipose tissue in the treatment of rhizarthrosis. They had significantly less pain and a better DASH score at all postoperative time points up until the 12-month follow-up, when they analysed all of the patients together. However, severe patients (grade 4) only presented a slight improvement in DASH score from 57 ± 23 to 51 ± 31 at 12 months with a near return to preoperative value for VAS pain [34]. Kemper et al. [35] assessed the efficacy of surgical arthroscopic debridement combined with autologous fat injections in the treatment of early stages of thumb carpometacarpal osteoarthritis. They showed pain relief at rest, and under stress and an improvement of the QuickDASH score after three to six months, which kept improving over two years. These approaches differ from our procedure, as we used a dedicated harvesting device to obtain small lobules of adipose tissue, also called "microfat" and presenting greater trophic and regenerative qualities than adipose tissue harvested according to "standard" technique [36]. Furthermore, none of these studies have associated PRP to improve the outcomes.

From a regulatory point of view, the preparation and injection of adipose tissue within these two studies were performed in the same surgical procedure, which is simpler and faster than our ATMP procedure. However, the strict application of European Regulation No. 1394/2007 [26] or from the corresponding Food and Drug Administration guidance [37] considered that "regenerating or promoting the regeneration of cartilage or tendon is not a basic function of adipose tissue which is generally not considered a homologous use". This question is still under debate, as some countries believe the entire procedure can be performed routinely in the operating room and more precision and harmonisation from national and international governing bodies are urgently needed. Nevertheless, the manufacturing of our innovative therapy remains simple, conservative, and minimally invasive and can be performed in a one-day surgery including two consecutive surgeries under local anesthesia. As ATMP production must occur in accordance with the pharmaceutical industry GMP, production costs have increased. However, we were aware that the microfat-PRP ATMP had to be manufactured within a few hours, to anticipate potential sustainability for public institutions in the future. This point should be considered from a cost-effectiveness perspective.

Regarding the mechanism of action, the association of microfat and PRP could be interesting in order to potentiate trophic and regenerative effects on damaged cartilage sites. From a theoretical point of view, the combination of these two products, which are respectively rich in autologous multipotent stem cells and growth factors, aims to create an optimal environment for cartilage cells regeneration. Furthermore, microfat could play the role of scaffold limiting PRP resorption [38,39]. However, this regenerative potential could only be confirmed by the use of appropriate magnetic resonance imaging of the wrist.

The major limitation of this study is the absence of a control group, which is an important weakness knowing the substantial placebo effect in arthrosis care [40]. Furthermore, due to the low number of patients assessed (only three patients), no statistical analysis was conducted.

4. Material and Methods

4.1. Obtention of Human Tissues and Regulatory Approval

For the process of validation batches, human peripheral blood and abdominal adipose tissue were harvested from three healthy volunteers (42, 33 and 31-year-old females who were not taking any drugs) during esthetic liposuction and after the collection of written informed consent collection.

The clinical trial was approved by the ethics committee (authorization for AMIPREP trial #16-65 from Comité de Protection des Personnes Sud Méditerranée #1 received 22nd of August 2016) and the ANSM (authorization for AMIPREP trial #160879A-12 received 28th of April 2017) and registered in Clinicaltrials.gov website (NCT03164122 and EudraCT #2016-002648-18). All experiments were conducted in the Cell Therapy facility (authorization #ETI/14/O/005) of our university hospital in compliance with Good Manufacturing Practice.

4.2. PRP Preparation

After seven steps of skin decontamination (antiseptic foaming solution, rinsing with sterile water, drying, antiseptic foaming solution, rinsing with sterile water, drying and alcoholic dermal antiseptic), 18 mL of blood was collected by venipuncture using a 21-gauge needle filling one 20 mL syringe containing 2 mL of ACD-A (Proteal, Barcelona, Spain). The blood was transferred into the Orthopras 20+ ® device (Proteal, Barcelona, Spain) before centrifugation using the Omnigrafter III ® (Proteal, Barcelona, Spain) at 3200 rpm over 10 min. The PRP was recovered using the Push Out system and 2 mL of PRP was sampled in a 5 mL syringe.

For process validation batches, the following analyses were performed on the PRP: cell counting, platelet aggregation test and microbiological assay at t = 0 (immediately after manufacturing) and t = 3 h (claimed shelf life with storage at 18–24°C).

Cell counting and microbiological assay were performed on clinical trial PRP batches.

4.2.1. Blood and PRP Cell Counting

300 μL from whole blood and each PRP preparation were sampled to determine platelets, leukocytes and red blood cells counts using automated haematology blood cell analyzers Sysmex XN-10 (Sysmex, Kobe, Japan) in accordance with recently published guidelines [41].

4.2.2. Platelets Aggregation Test

Platelets aggregation was assessed by light transmittance aggregometry (LTA) on a four-channel APACT 4004 aggregometer (Elitech, France). To obtain homologous Platelet-Poor Plasma (PPP) as negative control, 1.8 mL of PRP was centrifuged at $2500 \times g$ during 10 min. Maximal (peak) platelet aggregation (%) induced by ADP 5 µM, ADP 2.5 µM, collagen 3.3 µg/mL, ristocetin 1.25 mg/mL, arachidonic acid 0.5 mg/mL was measured in PRP.

4.3. Microfat Preparation

After seven steps of skin decontamination, harvesting the adipose tissue was performed either in the abdominal area (process validation batches) or in the subcutaneous adipose area of the inner side of the knees (clinical trial batches) after local anesthesia. The microfat harvesting technique was performed using a Hapifat® kit (Benew Medical, Melesse, France). Briefly, a St'rim cannula was both connected to a 10 mL syringe and a purification Puregraft 50® bag through a Fat Lock System®. Adipose tissue was then purified two times using 1:1 rinsing with saline solution [42] allowing for the elimination of fluid excess, lipid phase, blood cells, and fragments through filtration by the Puregraft bag membrane. Finally, 2 mL of microfat was sampled in a 5 mL syringe.

For process validation batches, following analyses were performed on microfat: assessment of macroscopic aspect and microbiological assay at t = 0 and t = 3 h.

For clinical trial batches, following analyses were performed: assessment of macroscopic aspect and microbiological assay.

4.3.1. Macroscopic Assessment of Microfat

The 5 mL syringe containing 2 mL of microfat was placed vertically allowing sedimentation of oily and bloody phases, considered as contaminants. Quantification was performed visually using syringe graduations by an experimented technician. Contamination lower than 25% of the final volume (0.5 mL) in oil and/or blood was expected.

4.3.2. Microbiological Assay

250 µL of PRP or microfat were sampled in Bactec culture bottles (Peds Plus Aerobic/F and Plus Anaerobic/F culture vials, containing each 40 mL of medium). The Bactec method (Becton Dickinson, Sparks, MD, USA) uses a computer-controlled incubation/detection system. The media used contained proprietary factors designed to inactivate a wide variety of antibacterial and antifungal agents [43]. Bactec culture bottles were incubated at 37 °C for a total of 10 days, and automated readings were taken every 10 min. Detection of organisms resulted in an audible alarm and automatic recording of time to detection.

4.4. Microfat-PRP Mixture

The two 5 mL syringes were connected and mixed by gently shaking the two syringes back and forth ten times to obtain a final product of 4 mL of a homogeneous mixed product.

For process validation batches, following the analyses performed on Microfat-PRP: SVF viability and cell content, ability to differentiate in chondrocytes, GF release.

For clinical trial batches, following analyses were performed: GF release.

4.4.1. Stromal Vascular Fraction (SVF) Extraction

From 2 to 4 mL of mixture were sampled for SVF extraction. SVF was purified from the Microfat-PRP mixture by collagenase digestion (0.25 U/mL, NB5, Heideberg, Germany) at 37 °C with 5% CO_2 for 45 min. Total viable nucleated cell recovery and cell viability were determined using the Nucleocounter NC100 instrument (ChemoMetec, Denmark).

4.4.2. Chondrocytes Differentiation

ADSCs were isolated following SVF cells plating in a 25 cm^2 flask in the following proliferation media (45% DMEM / 45% HAMS-F12/ 10% fetal bovine serum (Gibco, Thermo Fisher Scientific, Waltham, MA, USA)), GlutaMAX® (100×, Gibco) gentamicin (Panpharma Luitré, France) penicillin G (Panpharma Luitré, France), fungizone (Bristol-Myers Squibb, New York, NY, USA) for ADSCs proliferation. At 80% confluence, ADSCs were trypsined and plated in 24 well-plate in either a chondrocyte differentiation media (StemPro®, Thermo Fisher Scientific, Waltham, MA, USA) or proliferation media (considered as control media) at the concentration of 80,000 cells/5 µL. At 10 days, cells were washed using DPBS Ca++/Mg++-free medium (Life Technologies, Carlsbad, California, USA), coloured with 0.015% Alcian Blue 8GX (Sigma-Aldrich, Saint-Quentin-Fallavier, France) to stain glycosaminoglycan cartilage and fixed in 60% ethanol/40% acetic acid to observe chondrocytes micromass. Standardized photographs were taken using a Canon Eos 50D (Canon, Tokyo, Japan) with a 100 mm F2.8 Macro lens. All micromass area $\geq$0.05 mm^2 were quantified using NIH ImageJ software and compared with the control group.

4.4.3. Microfat-PRP Growth Factors Release Measurement

The microfat-PRP mixture (500 µL) was placed in a 48-well collagen coated plate (CellAffix, APSciences, Columbia, MD, USA) and incubated for 30 min at 37°C with 5% CO_2 to allow contact with collagen. After this incubation, 500 µL of non supplemented DMEM (Gibco, Thermo Fisher Scientific, Waltham, MA, USA) was added to the mixture and incubated for 24 h at 37 °C with 5% CO_2. After 24 h the samples were centrifuged (Multifuge Heraus 3 S-R centrifuge, Thermo Scientific, Indianapolis, IN) at 1500 rpm for 5 min to remove microfat, and samples were stored at −80 °C until used for analysis. A combination of 6 cytokines and growth factors (Vascular Endothelial Growth Factor, Interleukin-1 Receptor antagonist, Fibroblast Growth Factor 2, Interleukin-1β, Transforming Growth Factor β1, Platelet Derived Growth Factor AA-BB or AB-BB) were measured using a Magpix instrument (Luminex xMAP Technology, Luminex Inc., Austin, TX, USA) allowing simultaneous measurement of the different analytes in small sample volume.

4.5. Patients

According to the Kellgren and Lawrence classification [44] and with the informed written patient consent, males and females between 18 to 75 years of age who suffered from radio-carpal OA stage four were enrolled. OA resulted from post-traumatic malunion of an articular distal radius fracture or SLAC or SNAC. Only patients that failed conservative treatments (analgesics, anti-inflammatory drugs, splinting, and physiotherapy), defined as having a persistent daily painful condition > 40 mm according to VAS, and that would have otherwise been a candidate to surgery were included.

4.5.1. Surgical Procedure and Injection

Operative procedure included two consecutive surgical steps performed under local anesthesia in the same day. The first step consisted of lipoaspiration for microfat and harvesting the blood sample. Lipoaspirate and the blood sample were transported in sterile bags to the authorized ATMP manufacturing Unit. Microfat and PRP were prepared as described above and two interconnected syringes were sent back to the operating room within 2 h after harvesting. The second step consisted of the injection of PRP mixed-microfat. Before the intra-articular injection, microfat and PRP were pooled together by making ten transfers between the two connected syringes. After local anesthesia subcutaneously on the dorsal side of the wrist with xylocaine (10 mg/mL) without adrenaline, 4 mL of microfat and PRP was injected using a 16 gauge needle into the radio-carpal joint under X-ray guidance (Ziehm Solo FD, Ziehm Imaging GmbH, Nürnberg, Deutschland). An analgesic immobilization by a specific cast involving compression, contention and cryotherapy (IGLOO®) was immediately put in place for seven days.

4.5.2. Clinical Assessment

The primary endpoint was the safety of the treatment evaluated by the occurrence of adverse events up to one month after the injection (visits at Day 7 and Month 1). Secondary endpoints were the following criteria at 3, 6 and 12 months: subjective pain rating according to VAS (0–100 mm), functional evaluation according to the DASH and the PRWE scores, objective wrist strength measured by dynamometry, and the objective wrist range of motion measured using a goniometer. Patient's satisfaction was rated on a 5-level scale: Not satisfied, Few Satisfied, Moderately Satisfied, Satisfied, and Very satisfied.

4.6. Statistical Analysis

Data are presented as mean ± standard deviation except for microbiological assay (presence/free of germ), chondrocytes differentiation (number of micromass formed compared to control), macroscopic aspect of the microfat (presence/absence of contaminants > 25%). The increase factor in platelets was obtained by dividing the concentration of platelets in PRP by the concentration in whole blood. Doses of platelets in PRP were obtained by multiplying the volume of PRP injected by the corresponding concentration. Platelets purity was obtained by dividing the quantity of platelets in the PRP by the sum of platelets, red blood cells and leukocytes. No statistical analysis was performed due to the low number of samples or patients described in the study.

5. Conclusion

The present report demonstrates the feasibility to manufacture, control, and inject a PRP mixed-microfat investigational ATMP and its short-term good tolerance for wrist OA. However, only a greater number of patients documented will improve the safety of the procedure. If this endpoint is met, efficacy trials could then be implemented to define whether this non-invasive strategy can be proposed in selected patients with a history of wrist OA with drug-refractory failure, and be advantageous compared to invasive and non-conservative surgical wrist procedures.

Author Contributions: Conceptualization: A.M., J.V., F.G., F.S., R.L., J.M.; Methodology: J.V., F.G., E.J., J.M.; Validation: D.C., F.S., R.L.; Formal Analysis: M.V., E.J., J.M.; Investigation: A.M., A.I., C.C., N.K., C.J., J.E., D.C., R.L.; Original Draft Preparation: A.M., M.V., J.M.; Writing-Review and Editing: A.M., A.I., C.C., N.K., C.J., J.E., M.V., J.V., F.G., E.J., D.C., F.S., R.L., J.M.; Supervision: D.C., F.S., R.L., J.M.

Funding: This research received no external funding

Acknowledgments: Medical devices Orthopras 20+® device (Proteal, Barcelona, Spain) and Hapi® fat (Benew Medical, Melesse, France) kit were provided for free by companies.

Conflicts of Interest: The authors declare no conflict of interest

References

1. Laulan, J.; Marteau, E.; Bacle, G. Wrist osteoarthritis. *Orthop. Traumatol. Surg. Res. OTSR* **2015**, *101* (Suppl. 1), S1–S9. [CrossRef] [PubMed]
2. Watson, H.K.; Ballet, F.L. The SLAC wrist: Scapholunate advanced collapse pattern of degenerative arthritis. *J. Hand Surg.* **1984**, *9*, 358–365. [CrossRef]
3. Weiss, K.E.; Rodner, C.M. Osteoarthritis of the wrist. *J. Hand Surg.* **2007**, *32*, 725–746. [CrossRef] [PubMed]
4. Lane, N.E.; Shidara, K.; Wise, B.L. Osteoarthritis year in review 2016: Clinical. *Osteoarthr. Cartil.* **2017**, *25*, 209–215. [CrossRef] [PubMed]
5. Lue, S.; Koppikar, S.; Shaikh, K.; Mahendira, D.; Towheed, T.E. Systematic review of non-surgical therapies for osteoarthritis of the hand: An update. *Osteoarthr. Cartil.* **2017**, *25*, 1379–1389. [CrossRef] [PubMed]
6. Fuchsberger, T.; Boesch, C.E.; Tonagel, F.; Fischborn, T.; Schaller, H.E.; Gonser, P. Patient Rated Long-Term Results after Complete Denervation of the Wrist. *J. Plast. Reconstr. Aesthet. Surg.* **2018**, *71*, 57–61. [CrossRef] [PubMed]

7. Rothe, M.; Rudolf, K.-D.; Partecke, B.-D. Long-term results following denervation of the wrist in patients with stages II and III SLAC-/SNAC-wrist. *Handchir. Mikrochir. Plast. Chir. Organ.* **2006**, *38*, 261–266. [CrossRef] [PubMed]

8. Sauerbier, M.; Kluge, S.; Bickert, B.; Germann, G. Subjective and objective outcomes after total wrist arthrodesis in patients with radiocarpal arthrosis or Kienböck's disease. *Chir. Main* **2000**, *19*, 223–231. [CrossRef]

9. Aita, M.A.; Nakano, E.K.; de Schaffhausser, H.L.; Fukushima, W.Y.; Fujiki, E.N. Randomized clinical trial between proximal row carpectomy and the four-corner fusion for patients with stage II SNAC. *Rev. Bras. Ortop.* **2016**, *51*, 574–582. [CrossRef] [PubMed]

10. Dacho, A.K.; Baumeister, S.; Germann, G.; Sauerbier, M. Comparison of proximal row carpectomy and midcarpal arthrodesis for the treatment of scaphoid nonunion advanced collapse (SNAC-wrist) and scapholunate advanced collapse (SLAC-wrist) in stage II. *J. Plast. Reconstr. Aesthet. Surg.* **2008**, *61*, 1210–1218. [CrossRef] [PubMed]

11. Garcia-Elias, M.; Lluch, A.; Ferreres, A.; Papini-Zorli, I.; Rahimtoola, Z.O. Treatment of radiocarpal degenerative osteoarthritis by radioscapholunate arthrodesis and distal scaphoidectomy. *J. Hand Surg.* **2005**, *30*, 8–15. [CrossRef] [PubMed]

12. Le Nen, D.; Richou, J.; Simon, E.; Le Bourg, M.; Nabil, N.; de Bodman, C.; Bacle, G.; Saint-Cast, Y.; Obert, L.; Saraux, A.; et al. The arthritic wrist. I–The degenerative wrist: Surgical treatment approaches. *Orthop. Traumatol. Surg. Res.* **2011**, *97*, S31–S36. [CrossRef] [PubMed]

13. Cavaliere, C.M.; Chung, K.C. A Systematic Review of Total Wrist Arthroplasty Compared with Total Wrist Arthrodesis for Rheumatoid Arthritis. *Plast. Reconstr. Surg.* **2008**, *122*, 813–825. [CrossRef] [PubMed]

14. Xie, X.; Zhang, C.; Tuan, R.S. Biology of platelet-rich plasma and its clinical application in cartilage repair. *Arthritis Res. Ther.* **2014**, *16*, 204. [CrossRef] [PubMed]

15. Dai, W.-L.; Zhou, A.-G.; Zhang, H.; Zhang, J. Efficacy of Platelet-Rich Plasma in the Treatment of Knee Osteoarthritis: A Meta-analysis of Randomized Controlled Trials. *Arthrosc. J. Arthrosc. Relat. Surg.* **2017**, *33*, 659–670. [CrossRef] [PubMed]

16. Meheux, C.J.; McCulloch, P.C.; Lintner, D.M.; Varner, K.E.; Harris, J.D. Efficacy of Intra-articular Platelet-Rich Plasma Injections in Knee Osteoarthritis: A Systematic Review. *Arthrosc. J. Arthrosc. Relat. Surg.* **2016**, *32*, 495–505. [CrossRef] [PubMed]

17. Khoshbin, A.; Leroux, T.; Wasserstein, D.; Marks, P.; Theodoropoulos, J.; Ogilvie-Harris, D.; Gandhi, R.; Takhar, K.; Lum, G.; Chahal, J. The Efficacy of Platelet-Rich Plasma in the Treatment of Symptomatic Knee Osteoarthritis: A Systematic Review with Quantitative Synthesis. *Arthrosc. J. Arthrosc. Relat. Surg.* **2013**, *29*, 2037–2048. [CrossRef] [PubMed]

18. Laudy, A.B.M.; Bakker, E.W.P.; Rekers, M.; Moen, M.H. Efficacy of platelet-rich plasma injections in osteoarthritis of the knee: A systematic review and meta-analysis. *Br. J. Sports Med.* **2015**, *49*, 657–672. [CrossRef] [PubMed]

19. English, A.; Jones, E.A.; Corscadden, D.; Henshaw, K.; Chapman, T.; Emery, P.; McGonagle, D. A comparative assessment of cartilage and joint fat pad as a potential source of cells for autologous therapy development in knee osteoarthritis. *Rheumatology* **2007**, *46*, 1676–1683. [CrossRef] [PubMed]

20. Maumus, M.; Manferdini, C.; Toupet, K.; Peyrafitte, J.-A.; Ferreira, R.; Facchini, A.; Gabusi, E.; Bourin, P.; Jorgensen, C.; Lisignoli, G.; et al. Adipose mesenchymal stem cells protect chondrocytes from degeneration associated with osteoarthritis. *Stem Cell Res.* **2013**, *11*, 834–844. [CrossRef] [PubMed]

21. Erickson, G.R.; Gimble, J.M.; Franklin, D.M.; Rice, H.E.; Awad, H.; Guilak, F. Chondrogenic Potential of Adipose Tissue-Derived Stromal Cells in Vitro and in Vivo. *Biochem. Biophys. Res. Commun.* **2002**, *290*, 763–769. [CrossRef] [PubMed]

22. Huang, J.I.; Zuk, P.A.; Jones, N.F.; Zhu, M.; Lorenz, H.P.; Hedrick, M.H.; Benhaim, P. Chondrogenic Potential of Multipotential Cells from Human Adipose Tissue. *Plast. Reconstr. Surg.* **2004**, *113*, 585–594. [CrossRef] [PubMed]

23. Zuk, P.A.; Zhu, M.; Ashjian, P.; De Ugarte, D.A.; Huang, J.I.; Mizuno, H.; Alfonso, Z.C.; Fraser, J.K.; Benhaim, P.; Hedrick, M.H. Human adipose tissue is a source of multipotent stem cells. *Mol. Biol. Cell* **2002**, *13*, 4279–4295. [CrossRef] [PubMed]

24. Nguyen, P.S.; Desouches, C.; Gay, A.M.; Hautier, A.; Magalon, G. Development of micro-injection as an innovative autologous fat graft technique: The use of adipose tissue as dermal filler. *J. Plast. Reconstr. Aesthet. Surg.* **2012**, *65*, 1692–1699. [CrossRef] [PubMed]

25. Bembo, F.; Eraud, J.; Philandrianos, C.; Bertrand, B.; Silvestre, A.; Veran, J.; Sabatier, F.; Magalon, G.; Magalon, J. Combined use of platelet rich plasma & micro-fat in sport and race horses with degenerative joint disease: Preliminary clinical study in eight horses. *Muscles Ligaments Tendons J.* **2016**, *6*, 198–204. [PubMed]

26. The European Parliament and the Council of the European Union. Regulation (EC) No 1394/2007 of the European Parliament and of the Council of 13 November 2007 on advanced therapy medicinal products and amending Directive 2001/83/EC and Regulation (EC) No 726/2004. *Off. J. Eur. Union* **2007**, *L 324*, 121–137.

27. Magalon, J.; Chateau, A.L.; Bertrand, B.; Louis, M.L.; Silvestre, A.; Giraudo, L.; Veran, J.; Sabatier, F. DEPA classification: A proposal for standardising PRP use and a retrospective application of available devices. *BMJ Open Sport Exerc. Med.* **2016**, *2*, e000060. [CrossRef] [PubMed]

28. Franchignoni, F.; Vercelli, S.; Giordano, A.; Sartorio, F.; Bravini, E.; Ferriero, G. Minimal Clinically Important Difference of the Disabilities of the Arm, Shoulder and Hand Outcome Measure (DASH) and Its Shortened Version (QuickDASH). *J. Orthop. Sports Phys. Ther.* **2014**, *44*, 30–39. [CrossRef] [PubMed]

29. Walenkamp, M.M.J.; de Muinck Keizer, R.-J.; Goslings, J.C.; Vos, L.M.; Rosenwasser, M.P.; Schep, N.W.L. The Minimum Clinically Important Difference of the Patient-rated Wrist Evaluation Score for Patients with Distal Radius Fractures. *Clin. Orthop. Relat. Res.* **2015**, *473*, 3235–3241. [CrossRef] [PubMed]

30. Tashjian, R.Z.; Deloach, J.; Porucznik, C.A.; Powell, A.P. Minimal clinically important differences (MCID) and patient acceptable symptomatic state (PASS) for visual analog scales (VAS) measuring pain in patients treated for rotator cuff disease. *J. Shoulder Elbow Surg.* **2009**, *18*, 927–932. [CrossRef] [PubMed]

31. Tashjian, R.Z.; Hung, M.; Keener, J.D.; Bowen, R.C.; McAllister, J.; Chen, W.; Ebersole, G.; Granger, E.K.; Chamberlain, A.M. Determining the minimal clinically important difference for the American Shoulder and Elbow Surgeons score, Simple Shoulder Test, and visual analog scale (VAS) measuring pain after shoulder arthroplasty. *J. Shoulder Elbow Surg.* **2017**, *26*, 144–148. [CrossRef] [PubMed]

32. Pak, J.; Chang, J.-J.; Lee, J.H.; Lee, S.H. Safety reporting on implantation of autologous adipose tissue-derived stem cells with platelet-rich plasma into human articular joints. *BMC Musculoskelet. Disord.* **2013**, *14*, 337. [CrossRef] [PubMed]

33. Centeno, C.; Pitts, J.; Al-Sayegh, H.; Freeman, M. Efficacy of autologous bone marrow concentrate for knee osteoarthritis with and without adipose graft. *Biomed. Res. Int.* **2014**, *2014*, 370621. [CrossRef] [PubMed]

34. Herold, C.; Rennekampff, H.O.; Groddeck, R.; Allert, S. Autologous Fat Transfer for Thumb Carpometacarpal Joint Osteoarthritis: A Prospective Study. *Plast. Reconstr. Surg.* **2017**, *140*, 327–335. [CrossRef] [PubMed]

35. Kemper, R.; Wirth, J.; Baur, E.-M. Arthroscopic Synovectomy Combined with Autologous Fat Grafting in Early Stages of CMC Osteoarthritis of the Thumb. *J. Wrist Surg.* **2018**, *7*, 165–171. [CrossRef] [PubMed]

36. Alharbi, Z.; Opländer, C.; Almakadi, S.; Fritz, A.; Vogt, M.; Pallua, N. Conventional vs. micro-fat harvesting: How fat harvesting technique affects tissue-engineering approaches using adipose tissue-derived stem/stromal cells. *J. Plast. Reconstr. Aesthet. Surg.* **2013**, *66*, 1271–1278. [CrossRef] [PubMed]

37. Food and Drug Administration. *Regulatory Considerations for Human Cells, Tissues, and Cellular and Tissue-Based Products: Minimal Manipulation and Homologous Use*; Guidance for Industry and Food and Drug Administration Staff; Availability, Federal Register, 82 (221/Friday, November 17); Food and Drug Administration: Silver Spring, MD, USA, 2017; pp. 54290–54292.

38. Mojallal, A.; Lequeux, C.; Shipkov, C.; Rifkin, L.; Rohrich, R.; Duclos, A.; Brown, S.; Damour, O. Stem cells, mature adipocytes, and extracellular scaffold: What does each contribute to fat graft survival? *Aesthet. Plast. Surg.* **2011**, *35*, 1061–1072. [CrossRef] [PubMed]

39. Bosetti, M.; Borrone, A.; Follenzi, A.; Messaggio, F.; Tremolada, C.; Cannas, M. Human Lipoaspirate as Autologous Injectable Active Scaffold for One-Step Repair of Cartilage Defects. *Cell Transplant.* **2016**, *25*, 1043–1056. [CrossRef] [PubMed]

40. Zhang, W.; Robertson, J.; Jones, A.C.; Dieppe, P.A.; Doherty, M. The placebo effect and its determinants in osteoarthritis: Meta-analysis of randomised controlled trials. *Ann. Rheum. Dis.* **2008**, *67*, 1716–1723. [CrossRef] [PubMed]

41. Graiet, H.; Lokchine, A.; Francois, P.; Velier, M.; Grimaud, F.; Loyens, M.; Berda-Haddad, Y.; Veran, J.; Dignat-George, F.; Sabatier, F.; et al. Use of platelet-rich plasma in regenerative medicine: Technical tools for correct quality control. *BMJ Open Sport Exerc. Med.* **2018**, *4*, e000442. [CrossRef] [PubMed]

42. Sautereau, N.; Daumas, A.; Truillet, R.; Jouve, E.; Magalon, J.; Veran, J.; Casanova, D.; Frances, Y.; Magalon, G.; Granel, B. Efficacy of Autologous Microfat Graft on Facial Handicap in Systemic Sclerosis Patients. *Plast. Reconstr. Surg. Glob. Open* **2016**, *4*, e660. [CrossRef] [PubMed]

43. Khuu, H.M.; Stock, F.; McGann, M.; Carter, C.S.; Atkins, J.W.; Murray, P.R.; Read, E.J. Comparison of automated culture systems with a CFR/USP-compliant method for sterility testing of cell-therapy products. *Cytotherapy.* **2004**, *6*, 183–195. [CrossRef] [PubMed]

44. Kellgren, J.H.; Lawrence, J.S. Radiological assessment of osteo-arthrosis. *Ann. Rheum. Dis.* **1957**, *16*, 494–502. [CrossRef] [PubMed]

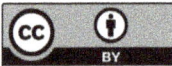

International Journal of
Molecular Sciences

MDPI

Article

Redifferentiation of Articular Chondrocytes by Hyperacute Serum and Platelet Rich Plasma in Collagen Type I Hydrogels

Vivek Jeyakumar [1],*[ORCID], Eugenia Niculescu-Morzsa [1], Christoph Bauer [1], Zsombor Lacza [2] and Stefan Nehrer [1]

[1] Center for Regenerative Medicine, Danube University Krems, 3500 Krems, Austria;
eugenia.niculescu-morzsa@donau-uni.ac.at (E.N.-M.); christoph.bauer@donau-uni.ac.at (C.B.);
stefan.nehrer@donau-uni.ac.at (S.N.)
[2] OrthoSera GmbH, 3500 Krems, Austria; zsombor.lacza@orthosera.com
* Correspondence: vivek.jeyakumar@donau-uni.ac.at

Received: 4 December 2018; Accepted: 10 January 2019; Published: 14 January 2019

✔ check for updates

Abstract: Matrix-assisted autologous chondrocyte transplantation (MACT) for focal articular cartilage defects often fails to produce adequate cartilage-specific extracellular matrix in vitro and upon transplantation results in fibrocartilage due to dedifferentiation during cell expansion. This study aimed to redifferentiate the chondrocytes through supplementation of blood-products, such as hyperacute serum (HAS) and platelet-rich plasma (PRP) in vitro. Dedifferentiated monolayer chondrocytes embedded onto collagen type I hydrogels were redifferentiated through supplementation of 10% HAS or 10% PRP for 14 days in vitro under normoxia (20% O_2) and hypoxia (4% O_2). Cell proliferation was increased by supplementing HAS for 14 days ($p < 0.05$) or by interchanging from HAS to PRP during Days 7–14 ($p < 0.05$). Sulfated glycosaminoglycan (sGAG) content was deposited under both HAS, and PRP for 14 days and an interchange during Days 7–14 depleted the sGAG content to a certain extent. PRP enhanced the gene expression of anabolic markers COL2A1 and SOX9 ($p < 0.05$), whereas HAS enhanced COL1A1 production. An interchange led to reduction of COL1A1 and COL2A1 expression marked by increased MMP13 expression ($p < 0.05$). Chondrocytes secreted less IL-6 and more PDGF-BB under PRP for 14 days ($p < 0.05$). Hypoxia enhanced TGF-β1 and BMP-2 release in both HAS and PRP. Our study demonstrates a new approach for chondrocyte redifferentiation.

Keywords: articular cartilage; cartilage repair; redifferentiation; collagen hydrogels; biologics; hyperacute serum; platelet-rich plasma

1. Introduction

The articular cartilage of the synovial joints, being avascular and limited for endogenous repair capacity, consists of sparsely distributed specialized cells called chondrocytes embedded within its extracellular matrix (ECM), which provide the cartilage with remarkable mechanical and low friction properties. A traumatic injury or anomalous loading to the joint results in a cartilage defect in the short-term. For full articular cartilage defects, cell-scaffold-based tissue engineering approaches, such as the matrix-assisted autologous chondrocyte transplantation (MACT), are some of the standardized treatment methods among many others. MACT involves a two-step surgical intervention by isolating a cartilage biopsy from the non-load bearing site for obtaining and expanding autologous chondrocytes in vitro onto 2D substrates in order to attain sufficient cell populations and then further embedding it onto biological scaffolds and transplantation [1]. The autologous chondrocytes are expanded both under 2D and 3D conditions in the presence of autologous human serum (HS) supplemented along the growth medium [2]. Chondrocyte dedifferentiation is a well-known phenomenon that occurs during 2D expansion, and redifferentiation occurs when cultured on a 3D scaffold [3]. Most often, studies indicating redifferentiation potential on scaffolds utilize fetal calf serum (FCS) and not autologous HS. MACT involves a clinical approach and thereby the use of autologous HS for culturing cell-scaffold constructs. However, supplementing HS does not necessarily redifferentiate in many settings and instead leads to a fibrocartilaginous phenotype usually marked by an increased type I collagen expression with no or less type II collagen expression [4]. Various cell sources other than autologous chondrocytes are investigated for cartilage repair, including bone marrow mesenchymal stem cells, adipose tissue derived mesenchymal stem cells, synovium-derived mesenchymal stem cells and infrapatellar fat pad stem cells. These sources of cells are advantageous for the low donor site morbidity and in obtaining higher cell yield.

HS and platelet-rich plasma (PRP) are blood products. The latter has gained attention over the last two decades for use in cell-culture supplements to expand bone marrow or adipose-derived mesenchymal stem cells (MSCs) [5] and for its advantage over the autologous source. Both autologous and allogeneic pooled PRP have been shown to maintain the stemness and concomitantly support differentiation of MSCs into the osteogenic, chondrogenic and adipogenic lineages. PRP constitutes a milieu of growth factors, chemokines/cytokines, proteases/antiproteases, adhesive proteins, trophic factors, small molecules, and catabolic/anti-catabolic factors [6]. In the clinical context, leukocyte-free PRP is used as intra-articular injections in patients with knee joint degeneration enrolled for randomized controlled trials (RCTs). It provides symptomatic pain relief for up to 12 months, noticed through local adverse inflammation reactions initially after multiple PRP injections, which diminishes over time [7–9]. Ex vivo expansion of bone marrow MSCs using autologous PRP has been proposed as and treatment option for articular cartilage defects in a case study with repair, less pain, and mobility but no RCTs have further progressed in this regard [10]. Several in vitro studies investigating the biological effects of leukocyte-free PRP on porcine and human articular chondrocytes observe an increase in both proliferation and differentiation [11–13]. Discrepancies among PRP preparations and the mode of activation remains a concern owing to the uncertainty of biological effects and clinical outcomes. A recent alternative derivative of platelet-rich fibrin (PRF) is hyperacute serum (HAS) and HAS which has been consistently reported for its regenerative capacity by increasing the cell proliferation capacity, as reported for chondrocytes [14], bone-marrow mesenchymal stem cells [15], and in an ex vivo model of bone ischemia recently [16]. HAS involves the activation of the natural coagulation cascade by a single-step centrifugation process, and its chemical composition comprises serum proteins, albumin, growth factor, and cytokines. Advantages of HAS over PRP include: there is no cellular reminiscence, it is free from fibrinogen and there is no over-concentration of the plasma content.

An important consideration when using biological scaffolds to regenerate the articular cartilage extracellular matrix is the interaction between chondrocyte and its surrounding niche. In this study, we aimed to test PRP and HAS as an alternative to replace HS for in vitro supplementation in the culture of MACT constructs, namely the collagen type I hydrogel used herein under normoxic/hypoxic conditions. We evaluated the effect of supplementing chondrocytes with HAS and PRP and observed the changes to chondrogenic markers encoding the synthesis of ECM and proteoglycan content. Subsequently as the next approach, we cultured chondrocytes with HAS for seven days and interchanged to PRP during Days 7–14. This way we hypothesized to achieve cell proliferation with HAS and an interchange to PRP would enhance the ECM synthesis. Dedifferentiated chondrocytes were obtained by expansion on 2D substrates for 14 days and subsequently cultured onto collagen hydrogels for another 14 days. Redifferentiation was assessed by analyzing anabolic cartilage matrix gene expression and glycosaminoglycan production as the critical evaluation criteria. Furthermore, the secreted anabolic growth factors and catabolic inflammatory cytokines responsible for modulation of the dedifferentiated or redifferentiation fate were measured in the cell-construct culture supernatant using ELISA.

2. Results

2.1. HAS Increases Chondrocyte Proliferation and Accumulates sGAG Content but PRP Enhances Anabolic Markers of the Cartilage Extracellular Matrix

The rate of proliferation over the course of chondrocyte redifferentiation analyzed on Days 7 and 14 revealed that PRP inhibited the proliferation over Days 0–14 with no change in cell numbers from the initial seeding density. HAS increased the cell number by three-fold on Day 7 ($p < 0.0019$) and by eight-fold as compared to PRP ($p < 0.0001$) (Figure 1A). DMMB assay quantification of the sulfated glycosaminoglycan (sGAG) illustrated that the total amount of sGAG per construct was enhanced under both HAS and PRP (Figure 1B). The total sGAG content normalized to total dsDNA content denotes an increase in HAS on Day 7 as compared to in PRP ($p < 0.0121$) (Figure 1C).

The redifferentiation potential of the monolayer dedifferentiated chondrocytes embedded in collagen type I hydrogels was assessed for the anabolic/catabolic chondrocyte markers of gene expression. Chondrocytes cultured for 14 days with PRP showed higher expression of COL2A1 on Days 7 ($p < 0.05$) and 14 ($p < 0.0.5$) (Figure 1E) and of SOX9 on Days 7 ($p = 0.0428$) and 14 ($p = 0.0396$) (Figure 1F) than in HAS. Concomitantly, the expression of COL1A1 had a seven-fold increase in HAS during Days 7–14 ($p < 0.0404$), whereas no COL1A1 expression was observed in PRP at both time points (Figure 1D). MMP3 was downregulated as compared to Day 0 in both groups (Figure 1G). MMP13 and VCAN were upregulated in PRP during Days 7–14, whereas, in HAS, MMP13 and VCAN were downregulated during Days 7–14 (Figure 1H,I).

2.2. An Interchange in Supplementation from HAS to PRP Enhances Proliferation but Depletes Anabolic Markers of the Cartilage Extracellular Matrix Marked by High Upregulation of MMP13

To achieve both proliferation and redifferentiation of the chondrocytes, an interchange from HAS to PRP during Days 7–14 was performed. The interchange did not arrest cell proliferation (Figure 2A), and the total sGAG content was significantly higher over 14 days ($p < 0.0238$) (Figure 2B). The total sGAG content normalized to total dsDNA content over 7–14 days was decreased by one-fold, denoting a depletion of the sGAG content (Figure 2C).

The anabolic/catabolic chondrocyte markers of gene expression indicated a seven-fold decrease in COL1A1 expression ($p < 0.05$) over 14 days indicating dedifferentiation (Figure 2D). Interchange during Days 7–14 did not enhance the COL2A1 expression (Figure 2E), but SOX9 increased by two-fold ($p = 0.0952$) (Figure 2F). MMP3 was significantly downregulated on Day 14 ($p < 0.0476$) and VCAN was downregulated by three-fold. MMP13 was significantly upregulated by 20-fold ($p < 0.0238$), suggesting that MMP13 upregulation could result in depletion of the extracellular matrix markers and the sGAG content.

2.3. Chondrocytes Secrete More Anabolic Growth Factors and Less Catabolic Inflammatory Cytokines When Supplemented by PRP under Normoxia

ELISA quantification of inflammatory cytokine secretion levels under normoxic conditions (20% O_2) revealed that the chondrocytes secreted higher levels of IL-6 under HAS as compared to the controls; however, in the PRP group, IL-6 secretion was significantly reduced by 10-fold during Days 7–14 ($p < 0.0446$) (Figure 3A). IL-1β levels under PRP were less in the chondrocytes when compared to HAS at 14 days, but no significant difference was observed (Figure 3B). Quantification of anabolic growth factors revealed that PDGF-BB levels secreted by chondrocytes had a two-fold increase in the PRP group during Days 7–14 ($p < 0.0312$) as compared to HAS (Figure 3C). Lower IGF-1 levels were secreted by the chondrocytes than observed in the controls (Figure 3D). BMP-2 was present in a higher amount in both the HAS and PRP controls but the chondrocytes did not secrete BMP-2 under HAS supplementation. Under PRP supplementation, chondrocytes secreted high BMP-2 levels on Day 7, which decreased significantly by Day 14 ($p < 0.0496$) (Figure 3E). No significant differences were observed in the TGF-β1 levels among all groups (Figure 3F).

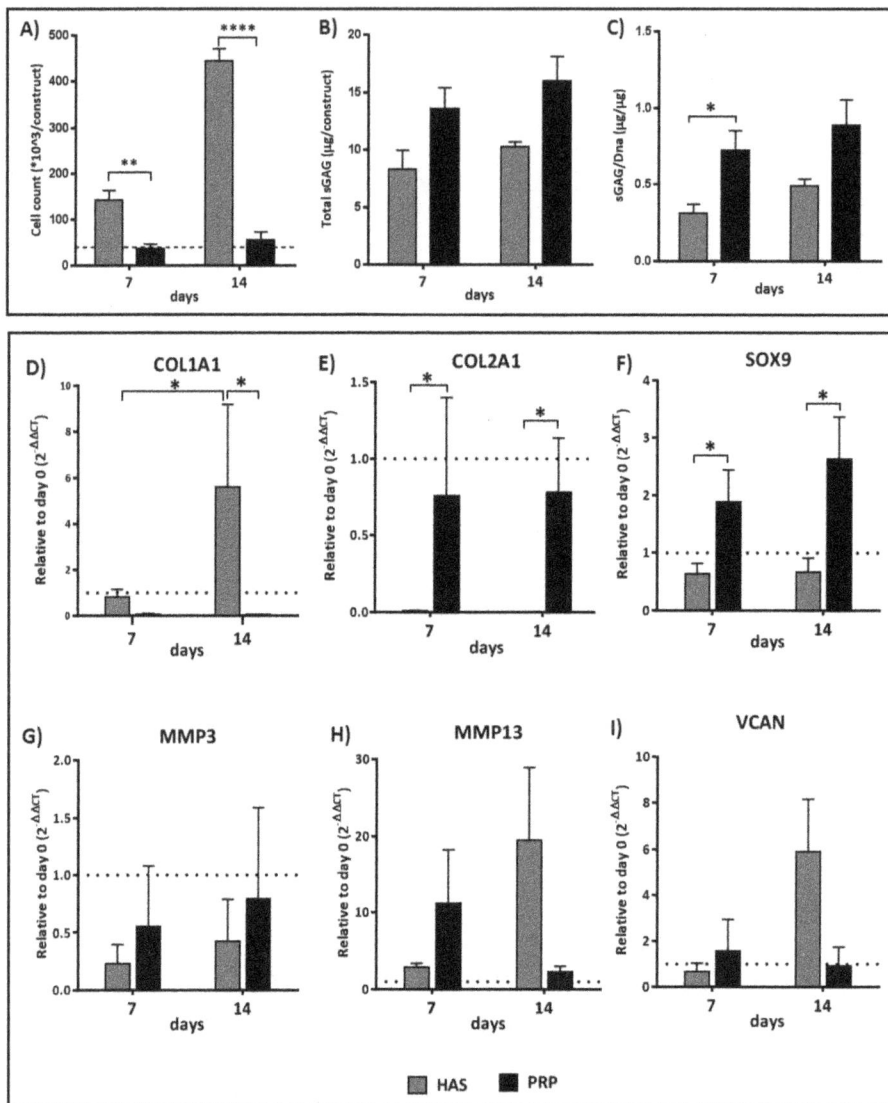

Figure 1. Analysis of: cell proliferation (**A**); total sGAG quantification (**B**); and sGAG/DNA quantification (**C**). Differences in relative expression of chondrogenic markers for COL1A1, COL2A1, SOX9, MMP3, MMP13, and VCAN (**D–I**) as determined by reverse transcriptase quantitative real-time PCR of chondrocytes cultured in hyperacute serum (HAS) and platelet-rich plasma (PRP) under normoxia (20% O_2). Significant difference at * $p < 0.05$, ** $p < 0.01$, **** $p < 0.0001$; $n = 6$ biological replicates.

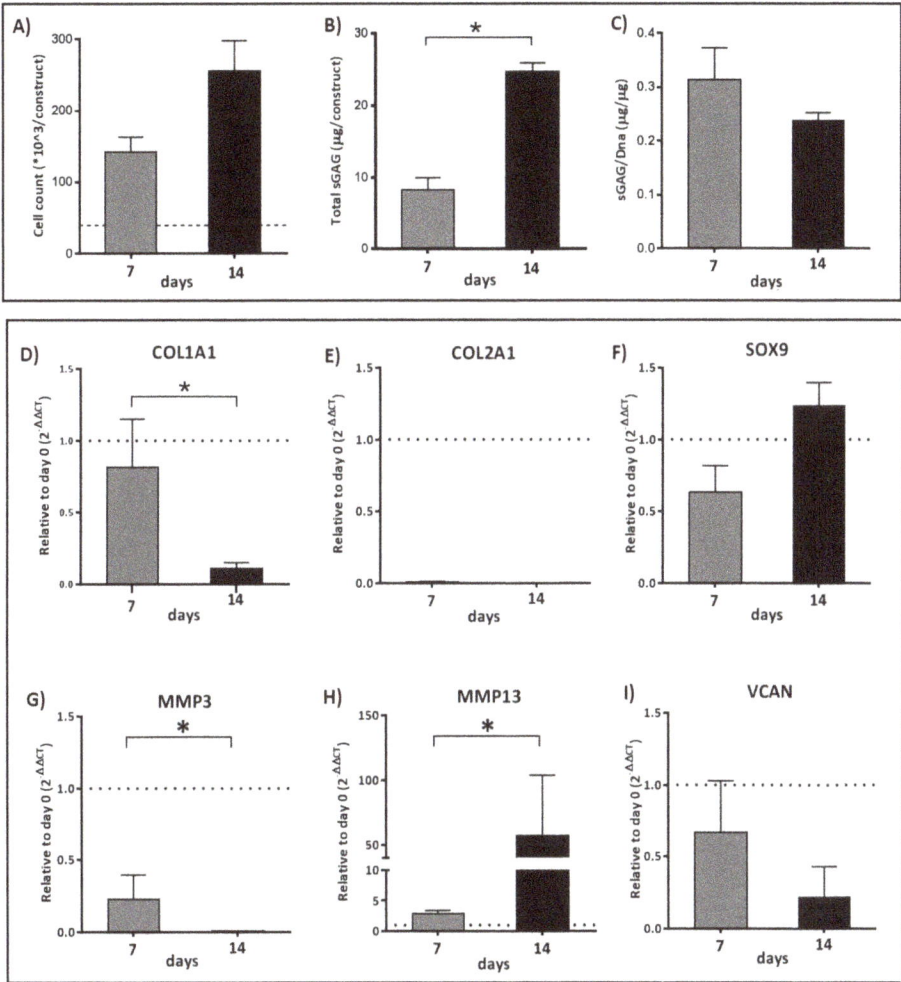

Figure 2. Analysis of: cell proliferation (**A**); total sGAG quantification (**B**); and sGAG/DNA quantification (**C**). Differences in relative expression of chondrogenic markers for COL1A1, COL2A1, SOX9, MMP3, MMP13, and VCAN (**D–I**) as determined by reverse transcriptase quantitative real-time PCR of chondrocytes cultured in hyperacute serum (HAS) for seven days and interchanged to platelet-rich plasma (PRP) during Days 7–14 under normoxia (20% O_2). Significant difference at * $p < 0.05$; $n = 6$ biological replicates.

2.4. Secretion of BMP and TGF-β1 by Chondrocytes Is Enhanced by Both HAS and PRP Supplementation under Hypoxia

ELISA quantification of inflammatory cytokine secretion levels under hypoxic conditions (4% O_2) revealed that the chondrocytes secreted higher levels of IL-6 under HAS as compared to the controls but in the PRP group IL-6 secretion was significantly reduced by seven-fold during Days 7–14 ($p < 0.0348$) (Figure 4A). Lower IL-1β levels under PRP were less secreted by the chondrocytes as compared to HAS at 14 days, but no significant difference was observed (Figure 4B). Quantification of anabolic growth factors revealed that PDGF-BB levels secreted by chondrocytes increased two-fold in the PRP group during Days 7–14 ($p < 0.0496$) as compared to HAS (Figure 4C). Lower IGF-1 levels were secreted by the chondrocytes than observed in the controls (Figure 4D). The above factors were secreted similarly as seen under normoxic conditions. Differences from normoxia were observed in BMP-2 and TGF-β1, where BMP-2 was consistently secreted over 14 days in both PRP and HAS (Figure 4E). Similarly, TGF-β1 was secreted consistently under PRP but decreased over 14 days under HAS. No significant differences were observed between the groups (Figure 4F).

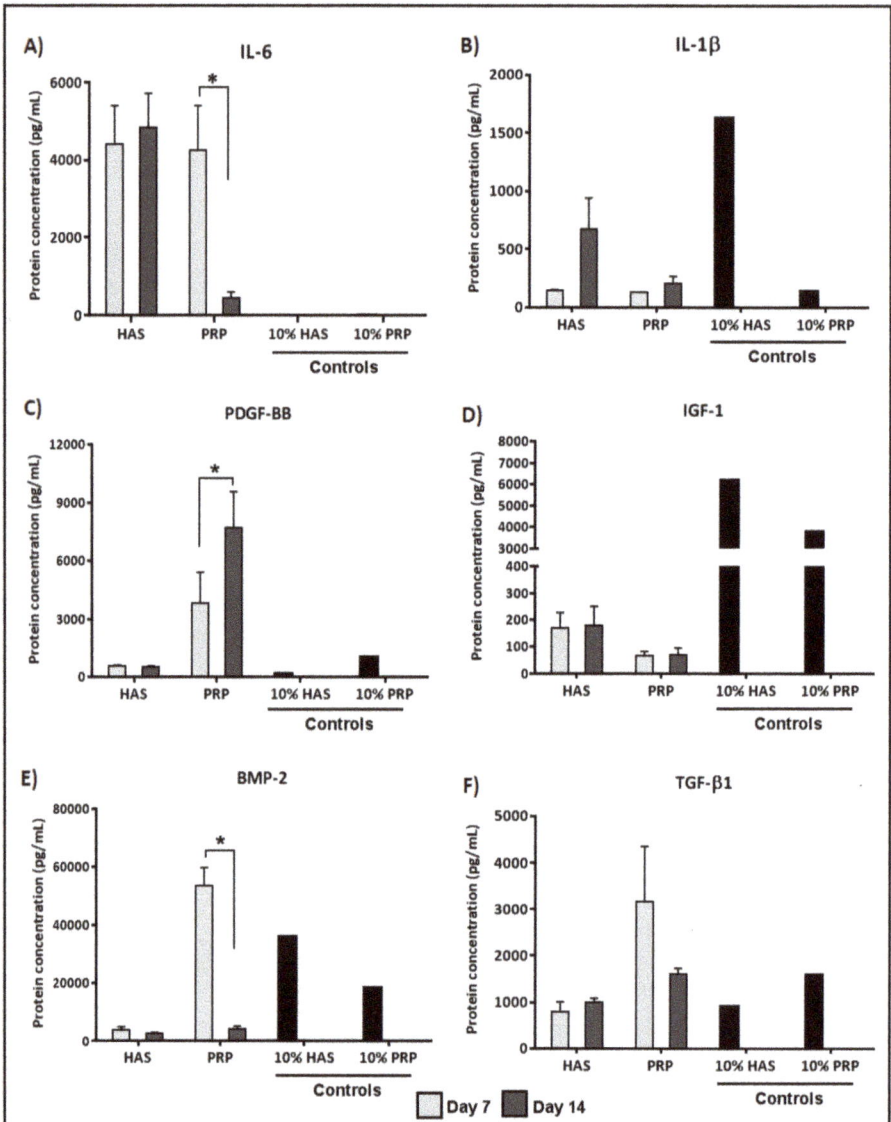

Figure 3. Analysis of determined catabolic inflammatory cytokines (IL-6 (**A**); and IL-1β (**B**)) and anabolic growth factors (PDGF-BB (**C**); IGF-1 (**D**); BMP-2 (**E**); and TGF-β1 (**F**)) secreted by the chondrocytes during the culture period of 7 and 14 days under normoxic conditions (20% O_2). Significant difference at * $p < 0.05$; $n = 6$ biological replicates.

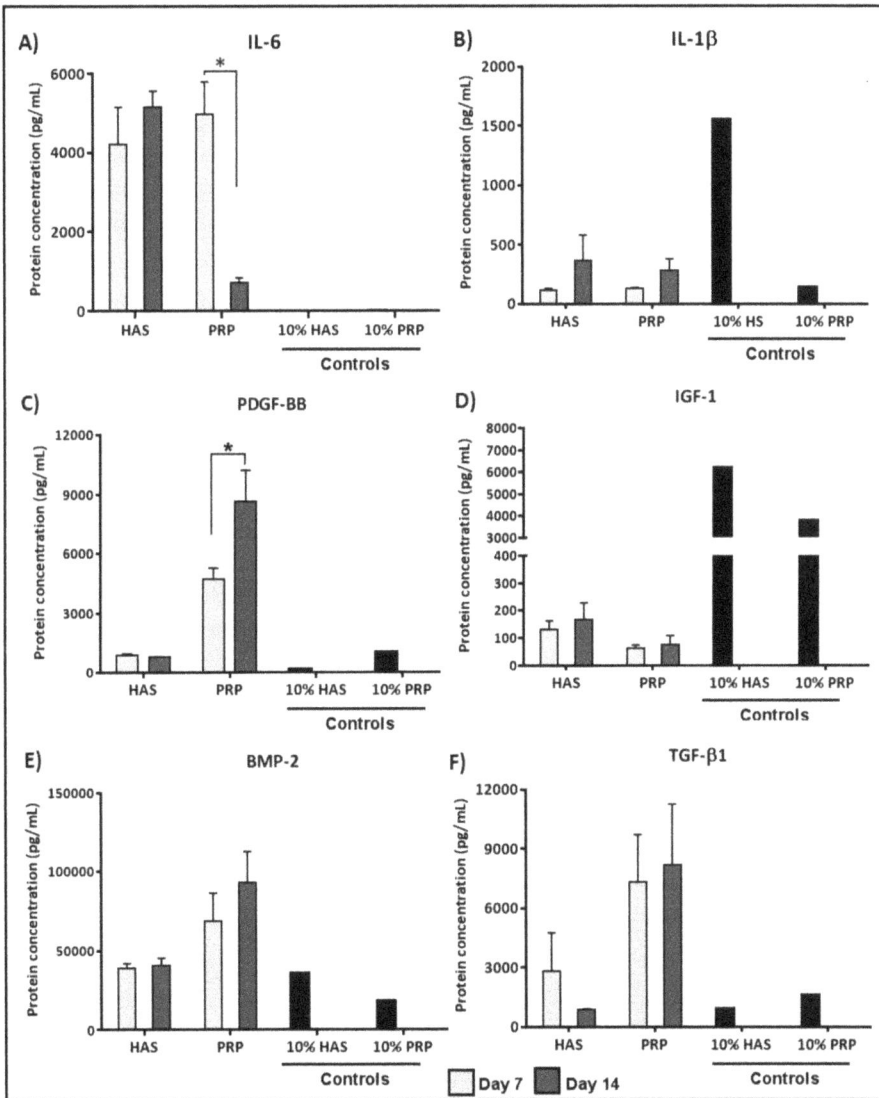

Figure 4. Analysis of determined catabolic inflammatory cytokines (IL-6 (**A**); and IL-1 β (**B**)) and anabolic growth factors (PDGF-BB (**C**); IGF-1 (**D**); BMP-2 (**E**); and TGF- β1 (**F**)) secreted by the chondrocytes during the culture period of 7 and 14 days under hypoxic conditions (4% O_2). Significant difference at * $p < 0.05$; $n = 6$ biological replicates.

3. Discussion

MACT in specific systems utilizes in vitro expansion for engineered cartilage constructs for cartilage repair. We investigated blood products as a natural mixture of bioactive molecules on the chondrocyte microenvironment. Our objective was to assess the redifferentiation potential of dedifferentiated chondrocytes cultured in collagen type I hydrogels for 14 days under supplementation of HAS and PRP in the culture media under normoxia/hypoxia and an interchange from HAS to PRP during Days 7–14. Cell growth was enhanced only by supplementing HAS, and an interchange from HAS to PRP led to enhancement of cell growth. However, the redifferentiation of chondrocytes was achieved only by supplementing PRP for the entire 14-day culture. Proteoglycan accumulation was observed under all conditions, but an interchange led to a decrease in the content at 14 days. Chondrocytes secreted higher pro-inflammatory cytokine IL-6 at seven days under all conditions but reduced at 14 days under PRP. The IL-1β secretion was comparatively lower than IL-6 secretion. The anabolic growth factor secretion of PDGF-BB was higher in PRP at both 7 and 14 days, while IGF-1 remained at same levels under all conditions. Under hypoxia, TGF-β1 and BMP-2 were higher in PRP than in normoxia and vice versa in HAS. The highest magnitude of gene expression encoding cartilage matrix synthesis, namely COL2A1 and SOX9, occurred when supplementing PRP for 14 days, but an interchange from HAS to PRP did not support the synthesis.

MACT involving culture of autologous chondrocytes is often cultured under cell culture medium supplementation of autologous human serum (HS) as a gold standard, but there is not much clarity on the subsequent redifferentiation of monolayer expanded dedifferentiated chondrocytes to MACT constructs for transplantation. Autologous human serum in cell culture supplementation for MACT is known for its progressive proliferation capacity [2], but the MACT constructs very often result in a fibrocartilage tissue formation upon implantation, rather than a hyaline cartilage tissue formation. Discrepancies in analogy with regard to different serum preparations have not been investigated in many of the previous studies articulating MACT constructs. In recent years, several in vitro studies have demonstrated the redifferentiation potential of chondrocytes by platelet derivatives [14,17]. We found different effects on chondrogenesis with different formulations of platelet and serum derivatives wherein our study, PRP inhibited the cellular growth in specific to collagen hydrogels, but matrix turnover markers were enhanced. This mimics the natural environment of chondrocytes as articular cartilage under normal conditions maintains a low matrix turnover and is resilient to proliferation and end-stage differentiation [18]. This result is coherent with several reports that indicate that chondrocytes are involved in the process of proliferation during cell cycle phase or committed to the differentiated state [19–21]. Liou et al [22] recently reported that PRP promotes proliferation of mesenchymal stem cells from bone marrow and infrapatellar fat pad in hydrogel encapsulated cultures. This effect could be specific to mesenchymal stem cells and inapplicable to chondrocytes in hydrogels.

Low oxygen tension between 1% and 5% O_2 is reported to maintain the chondrogenic phenotype during cell expansion and maintain the matrix metabolism in 3D constructs [23–25]. However, not all commercially available MACT systems utilize hypoxic conditions for MACT procedures. A few systems, e.g., NeoCart®, apply 2% hypoxia in a bioreactor together with hydrostatic pressure stimulation. On the one hand, obtaining clinically sufficient cell numbers without monolayer expansion continues to be a challenge. On the other hand, restoring the functional properties of articular cartilage is insubordinate in tissue-engineered cartilage. To tackle the limitation in increasing cell number while simultaneously enhancing the chondrocytes to resuscitate its matrix synthesis activity in a short culture period within the MACT constructs, an interchange of supplementation of HAS for the proliferation of cells switched to PRP for matrix synthesis was tested in our study. The interchanging of culture conditions, however, did not favor the hypothesis, as proliferation achieving matrix synthesis did not occur, which was indicative of higher MMP13 upregulation after the interchange. The fact that MMP13 is temporarily and not permanently active in articular cartilage as well as its higher activity, based on the congregation of several factors such as insulin-like growth factor (IGF-1), which subsequently results in abnormal homeostasis and breakdown of the proteoglycans [26,27].

Chondrocyte dedifferentiation results from the failure of metabolic imbalance to sustain the anabolic/catabolic equilibrium during synthesis of the ECM involving a multitude of anabolic and catabolic cytokines/growth factors [28]. PRP constitutes a natural milieu of growth factors/cytokines and embodies as an alternative cell culture supplementation to avoid chondrocyte dedifferentiation for MACT procedures. Our study is consistent with other studies where PRP concentrated platelets release the cytokines/growth factors from their α-granules [29,30]. Sundman et al [31] compared the concentrations of anabolic and catabolic growth factors/cytokines in the cellular composition of leukocyte-rich and leukocyte free PRP, and determined that leukocyte-rich PRP (Lr-PRP) released higher levels of catabolic cytokines such as IL-1β, and a higher concentration of platelet content in Lr-PRP released more anabolic growth factors such as TGF-β1 and PDGF-AB. Contrary to the above-mentioned statement, our study involving leukocyte-poor PRP (Lp-PRP) released less IL-1β associated with less TGF-β1 and PDGF-BB. Remarkably, the chondrocytes secreted higher levels of TGF-β1 and PDGF-BB with no increase in IL-1β when supplemented with Lp-PRP. We found an increased secretion of BMP2 by the chondrocytes during the culture period under hypoxic conditions in HAS, which was more in PRP supplementation, as well as the stable release of TFG-β1 throughout the culture time. BMP2 was observed to disappear during monolayer expansion, and the addition of BMP2 was superior to TGF-β1 in preventing chondrocyte dedifferentiation [27]. BMP-2 has been strongly correlated with hypoxia on expression of the matrix gene COL2A1, which is tightly controlled through the p38MAK pathway [32]. However, we did not observe differences in matrix gene expression and the sulfated glycosaminoglycan content between normoxic and hypoxic conditions. This could be attributed to the fact that there might be a prevalence of hypoxia gradients inside the collagen hydrogel. Future investigations should decipher the hypoxia levels and make them more precisely controllable.

This limitation to our current study includes the lack of histological characterization for additional confirmation of the matrix synthesis and remodeling. Deciphering the underlying signaling mechanism between secreted growth factor and cytokines on the ECM turnover would have provided more insights on the effect of PRP and HAS. Taken together, these factors have been considered for future investigations. The current state of the art for cartilage repair envisions on a broad range of tissue engineering strategies and towards this direction a compliant GMP structure can expedite the production of tissue engineered implants and biologics at the premises of the surgical facility. Towards this context additive manufacturing technologies such as 3D bioprinting are advantageous as biomaterials for MACT procedures can be controlled for a high degree of porosity with hierarchical anisotropic architecture for cells to produce collagen fibers vertically, which subsequently helps during the phase of matrix remodeling.

4. Materials and Methods

4.1. Ethics

The local ethical committee of Lower Austria approved the study protocol on 1st January 2013 (approval No. GS4-EK-4/249-2013). All subjects gave written informed consent in accordance with the Declaration of Helsinki.

4.2. Isolation and Culture of OA Chondrocytes

Human osteoarthritic cartilage was obtained from the surgical wastes of 12 donors undergoing total knee arthroplasty (60 ± 3 years old) after written informed consent was given. The cartilage pieces from the superficial zone areas where no cartilage loss occurred were determined then rinsed in phosphate buffered saline (PBS) and minced into fine pieces. Chondrocytes from the articular surface of the cartilage were isolated by enzymatic digestion, as previously reported [4]. Chondrocytes were seeded at a density of 10,000 cells/cm^2 and expanded in a growth medium (GIBCO® DMEM/F12 GlutaMAX™-I, Invitrogen, Vienna, Austria) containing 2.5 µg/mL Amphotericin B and 0.1 mg/mL streptomycin (Sigma, Steinheim, Germany) with 10% FCS (PAA Laboratories GmbH, Linz, Austria). All further experiments were performed on passage 1 chondrocytes to reduce the point of dedifferentiation over passaging.

4.3. Preparation of Hyperacute Serum and Platelet-Rich Plasma

Whole blood was collected from 15 individual healthy male and female blood donors (36 ± 10 years old) after written informed consent was given. HAS was prepared by centrifuging whole blood onto 9 mL silicon coated blood collection tubes (VACUETTE® z serum clot activator, Greiner bio-one, Kremsmünster, Austria) at 1770 g for 10 min. The top layer containing the supernatant was removed and the resulting fibrin clot (middle layer) was separated from the tube by discarding the bottom part containing red blood cells. The fibrin clot was gently squeezed with a non-absorbable sterile material in a petri dish to extrude HAS. HAS was pooled from the individual 15 blood donors and stored at −80 °C. Leukocyte poor PRP (lpPRP) was prepared by transferring whole blood from the same donors onto 9 mL EDTA coated blood collection tubes (VACUETTE® K3EDTA, Greiner bio-one, Kremsmünster, Austria) and centrifuged at 440 g for 10 min. The platelet enriched plasma (middle layer) along the poor platelet plasma (top layer) was further transferred to 15 mL falcon tubes leaving the leukocytes and RBC region and secondary centrifugation at 1770 g for 10 min was performed. The resulting lpPRP was pooled from individual donors and stored at −80 °C. Pooled lpPRP enclosed on average 1×10^6 platelets/mL.

4.4. Re-Differentiation of OA Chondrocytes by Supplementing Hyper Acute Serum and Platelet-Rich Plasma

Ten milligrams of collagen type I solution (BD Biosciences) were diluted to a final concentration of 2.5 mg/mL in a neutral buffer containing $10\times$ PBS, ultra-pure distilled water, and 1 N NaOH with a final pH of 7.4. Passage 1 dedifferentiated chondrocyte were encapsulated onto collagen type I hydrogels at a density of 40,000 cells/cm^2 at 4 °C and left to polymerize at 37 °C/5% in a CO$_2$ incubator for 30 min. Post-polymerization constructs were re-differentiated in growth medium supplemented with either 10% HAS or 10% PRP for 7 and 14 days under normoxia (20% O$_2$) or hypoxia (4% O$_2$). Another set of experiments were performed where constructs were redifferentiated in a growth medium supplemented with 10% HAS until 7 days and switched to medium supplementation with 10% PRP post for Days 7–14 under normoxia (20% O$_2$) or hypoxia (4% O$_2$).

4.5. Real-Time Quantitative PCR

Collagen gel-chondrocyte constructs were collected and digested with 120 units/mL collagenase in a serum-free medium for 30 min to release the cells. The RNA was isolated using the High Pure RNA Isolation kit (Roche Diagnostics GmbH, Mannheim, Germany) in accordance with the manufacturer's instructions. The mRNA was reverse transcripted with a First Strand cDNA Synthesis Kit (Roche Diagnostics GmbH, Mannheim, Germany), and cDNA samples were amplified with RT-qPCR in a cycler. GAPDH was used as an endogenous external reference gene, and the ΔΔCt method was used to evaluate the relative expression level of mRNA for each target gene. The values are depicted with the Day 0 monolayer dedifferentiated chondrocyte as a control. The following human primers were used in this study: *GAPDH* (forward (F) 5′-CTCTGCTCCTCCTGTTCGAC-3′; reverse (R) 5′-ACGACCAAATCCGTTGACTC-3′), *COL2A1* (F, 5′-GTGTCAGGGCCAGGATGT-3; R, 5′-TCCCAGTGTCACAGACACAGAT-3′), *COL1A1* (F, 5′-GGGATTCCCTGGACCTAAAG-3′; R, 5′-GGAACACCTCGCTCTCCAG-3′), *SOX9* (F, 5′-TACCCGCACTTGCACAAC-3′; R, 5′-TCTCGCTCTCGTTCAGAAGTC-3′), *VCAN* (F, 5′-GCACCTGTGTGCCAGGATA-3′; R, 5′-CAGGGATTAGAGTGACATTCATCA-3′), *MMP3* (F, 5′-CAAAACATATTTCTTTGTAGAGGACAA-3′; R, 5′-TTCAGETATTCGCTTGGGAAA-3′), *MMP13* (F, 5′-TTTCCTCCTGGGCCAAAT-3′; R, 5′-GCAACAAGAAACAAGTTGTAGCC-3′).

4.6. Sulfated Glycosaminoglycan (sGAG) and DNA Quantification

Constructs were collected on Days 7 and 14, frozen at −80 °C and lyophilized at 20 °C to evaporate the water content and measure the produced matrix content. sGAG quantification was achieved by treating constructs overnight with 25 U/mL proteinase K enzyme at 56 °C. Enzyme inactivation was then performed at 90 °C for 10 min. One hundred microliters of the supernatant were frozen at −80 °C for DNA quantification and the resultant solution was transferred to ultra-free filter reaction tubes of 0.1 μm pore size (Millipore, Billerica, MA, USA) and centrifuged at 12,000 g for min. sGAG was measured through complexation and decomplexation with a 1.9 dimethyl methylene blue solution (DMMB). The absorbance was measured at 656 nm in a plate reader. The DNA content was measured fluorometrically using the Quant-iT™ PicoGreen® assay (Molecular Probes, Vienna, Austria) in accordance with the manufacturer's instructions (excitation wavelength 480 nm; emission wavelength 528 nm).

4.7. Growth Factor and Cytokine Quantification

The above supernatant constructs were collected every 2 days during total media exchange and pooled until Day 7 or Day 14 of incubation as experimental end time points for an enzyme-linked immunosorbent assay (ELISA). The 10% HAS and 10% PRP served as internal controls to the constructs supplemented with 10% HAS and 10% PRP. ELISA kits were used to measure the production of human IGF-I (Quantikine®, R&D Systems, Abingdon, UK), PDGF-BB, TGF-β1, BMP-2, FGF-18, IL-1β, and IL-6, and quantified according to the manufacturer's instructions and measured for absorbance at 450 nm in a microplate reader.

4.8. Statistical Analysis

Non-parametric Mann–Whitney two-tailed U-test was performed for comparisons between two datasets at a time. Multiple comparisons were performed using non-parametric Kruskal–Wallis test followed by Dunn's multiple comparisons test. All data are presented as the mean $\pm$ SEM. Significance level was set at $p < 0.05$. All statistical analyses were performed using the GraphPad Prism software (Graphpad Prism Software Inc., San Diego, CA, USA).

5. Conclusions

The current study showed that; (i) PRP supplementation over 14 days to collagen-gel chondrocyte constructs enhances the anabolic gene expression markers of cartilage regeneration; (ii) an interchange from HAS to PRP achieves proliferation of chondrocytes but impairs matrix anabolic metabolism; and (iii) hypoxic conditions favor increased secretion of TGF-β1 and BMP-2 by chondrocytes compared to normoxia under both HAS and PRP. Our study proposes a step towards the continual improvement of the existing MACT procedure based on in vitro culture conditions specific to collagen type I hydrogels by instructing the embedded chondrocytes to produce hyaline-like cartilage upon transplantation. Further strategies should be developed for embedding autologous chondrocytes with rapid eTnzymatic digestion post arthroscopy in a PRP-augmented collagen hydrogel, aimed at a one-step cartilage repair procedure.

Author Contributions: Conceptualization, V.J., Z.L. and S.N.; Data curation, V.J., E.N.-M. and C.B.; Funding acquisition, S.N.; Investigation, V.J.; Methodology, V.J., E.N.-M. and C.B.; Project administration, V.J.; Visualization, V.J. and Z.L.; Writing—original draft, V.J.; and Writing—review and editing, Z.L. and S.N.

Acknowledgments: The authors gratefully acknowledge the financial support of Life science calls (Project Id: LSC12-001) from NÖ Forschungs- und Bildungsges.m.b.H (NFB) and the provincial government of Lower Austria.

Conflicts of Interest: Z Lacza owns stock in a start-up company OrthoSera GmbH that holds patents on HAS. All other authors declare no competing interests.

References

1. Dehne, T.; Karlsson, C.; Ringe, J.; Sittinger, M.; Lindahl, A. Chondrogenic differentiation potential of osteoarthritic chondrocytes and their possible use in matrix-associated autologous chondrocyte transplantation. *Arthritis Res. Ther.* **2009**, *11*, 1–14. [CrossRef] [PubMed]
2. Tallheden, T.; Van Der Lee, J.; Brantsing, C.; Månsson, J.E.; Sjögren-Jansson, E.; Lindahl, A. Human serum for culture of articular chondrocytes. *Cell Transplant.* **2005**, *14*, 469–479. [CrossRef] [PubMed]
3. Caron, M.M.J.; Emans, P.J.; Coolsen, M.M.E.; Voss, L.; Surtel, D.A.M.; Cremers, A.; van Rhijn, L.W.; Welting, T.J.M. Redifferentiation of dedifferentiated human articular chondrocytes: Comparison of 2D and 3D cultures. *Osteoarthr. Cartil.* **2012**, *20*, 1170–1178. [CrossRef] [PubMed]

4. Jeyakumar, V.; Halbwirth, F.; Niculescu-Morzsa, E.; Bauer, C.; Zwickl, H.; Kern, D.; Nehrer, S. Chondrogenic Gene Expression Differences between Chondrocytes from Osteoarthritic and Non-OA Trauma Joints in a 3D Collagen Type I Hydrogel. *Cartilage* **2017**, *8*, 191–198. [CrossRef] [PubMed]

5. Lohmann, M.; Walenda, G.; Hemeda, H.; Joussen, S.; Drescher, W.; Jockenhoevel, S.; Hutschenreuter, G.; Zenke, M.; Wagner, W. Donor age of human platelet lysate affects proliferation and differentiation of mesenchymal stem cells. *PLoS ONE* **2012**, *7*, e37839. [CrossRef] [PubMed]

6. Andia, I.; Maffulli, N. Platelet-rich plasma for managing pain and inflammation in osteoarthritis. *Nat. Rev. Rheumatol.* **2013**, *9*, 721–730. [CrossRef] [PubMed]

7. Sánchez, M.; Fiz, N.; Azofra, J.; Usabiaga, J.; Aduriz Recalde, E.; Garcia Gutierrez, A.; Albillos, J.; Gárate, R.; Aguirre, J.J.; Padilla, S.; et al. A randomized clinical trial evaluating plasma rich in growth factors (PRGF-Endoret) versus hyaluronic acid in the short-term treatment of symptomatic knee osteoarthritis. *Arthrosc. J. Arthrosc. Relat. Surg.* **2012**, *28*, 1070–1078. [CrossRef]

8. Smith, P.A. Intra-articular Autologous Conditioned Plasma Injections Provide Safe and Efficacious Treatment for Knee Osteoarthritis: An FDA-Sanctioned, Randomized, Double-blind, Placebo-controlled Clinical Trial. *Am. J. Sports Med.* **2016**, *44*, 884–891. [CrossRef]

9. Filardo, G.; Kon, E.; Di Martino, A.; Di Matteo, B.; Merli, M.L.; Cenacchi, A.; Fornasari, P.M.; Marcacci, M. Platelet-rich plasma vs hyaluronic acid to treat knee degenerative pathology: Study design and preliminary results of a randomized controlled trial. *BMC Musculoskelet. Disord.* **2012**, *13*, 229. [CrossRef]

10. Centeno, C.J.; Busse, D.; Kisiday, J.; Keohan, C.; Freeman, M.; Karli, D. Increased Knee Cartilage Volume in Degenerative Joint Disease using Percutaneously Implanted, Autologous Mesenchymal Stem Cells. *Pain Phys.* **2008**, *11*, 343–353.

11. Akeda, K.; An, H.S.; Okuma, M.; Attawia, M.; Miyamoto, K.; Thonar, E.J.-M.A.; Lenz, M.E.; Sah, R.L.; Masuda, K. Platelet-rich plasma stimulates porcine articular chondrocyte proliferation and matrix biosynthesis. *Osteoarthr. Cartil.* **2006**, *14*, 1272–1280. [CrossRef] [PubMed]

12. Drengk, A.; Zapf, A.; Stürmer, E.K.; Stürmer, K.M.; Frosch, K.H. Influence of platelet-rich plasma on chondrogenic differentiation and proliferation of chondrocytes and mesenchymal stem cells. *Cells Tissues Organs* **2009**, *189*, 317–326. [CrossRef] [PubMed]

13. Spreafico, A.; Chellini, F.; Frediani, B.; Bernardini, G.; Niccolini, S.; Serchi, T.; Collodel, G.; Paffetti, A.; Fossombroni, V.; Galeazzi, M.; et al. Biochemical investigation of the effects of human platelet releasates on human articular chondrocytes. *J. Cell. Biochem.* **2009**, *108*, 1153–1165. [CrossRef] [PubMed]

14. Jeyakumar, V.; Niculescu-Morzsa, E.; Bauer, C.; Lacza, Z.; Nehrer, S. Platelet-Rich Plasma Supports Proliferation and Redifferentiation of Chondrocytes during In Vitro Expansion. *Front. Bioeng. Biotechnol.* **2017**, *5*, 1–8. [CrossRef]

15. Kuten, O.; Simon, M.; Hornyák, I.; De Luna-Preitschopf, A.; Nehrer, S.; Lacza, Z. The Effects of Hyperacute Serum on Adipogenesis and Cell Proliferation of Mesenchymal Stromal Cells. *Tissue Eng. Part A* **2018**, *24*, 1011–1021. [CrossRef]

16. Vácz, G.; Major, B.; Gaál, D.; Petrik, L.; Horváthy, D.B.; Han, W.; Holczer, T.; Simon, M.; Muir, J.M.; Hornyák, I.; et al. Hyperacute serum has markedly better regenerative efficacy than platelet-rich plasma in a human bone oxygen-glucose deprivation model. *Regen. Med.* **2018**, *13*, 531–543. [CrossRef] [PubMed]

17. Muraglia, A.; Nguyen, V.T.; Nardini, M.; Mogni, M.; Coviello, D.; Dozin, B.; Strada, P.; Baldelli, I.; Formica, M.; Cancedda, R.; et al. Culture Medium Supplements Derived from Human Platelet and Plasma: Cell Commitment and Proliferation Support. *Front. Bioeng. Biotechnol.* **2017**, *5*, 66. [CrossRef]

18. Dreier, R. Hypertrophic differentiation of chondrocytes in osteoarthritis: The developmental aspect of degenerative joint disorders. *Arthritis Res. Ther.* **2010**, *12*, 216. [CrossRef]

19. Tallheden, T.; Bengtsson, C.; Brantsing, C.; Sjögren-Jansson, E.; Carlsson, L.; Peterson, L.; Brittberg, M.; Lindahl, A. Proliferation and differentiation potential of chondrocytes from osteoarthritic patients. *Arthritis Res. Ther.* **2005**, *7*, 560–568. [CrossRef]

20. Takahashi, T.; Ogasawara, T.; Asawa, Y.; Mori, Y.; Uchinuma, E.; Takato, T.; Hoshi, K. Three-dimensional microenvironments retain chondrocyte phenotypes during proliferation culture. *Tissue Eng.* **2007**, *13*, 1583–1592. [CrossRef]

21. Elder, S.; Thomason, J. Effect of platelet-rich plasma on chondrogenic differentiation in three-dimensional culture. *Open Orthop. J.* **2014**, *8*, 78–84. [CrossRef] [PubMed]

22. Liou, J.-J.; Rothrauff, B.B.; Alexander, P.G.; Tuan, R.S. Effect of Platelet-Rich Plasma on Chondrogenic Differentiation of Adipose- and Bone Marrow-Derived Mesenchymal Stem Cells. *Tissue Eng. Part A* **2018**, *24*, 1432–1443. [CrossRef] [PubMed]

23. Markway, B.D.; Cho, H.; Johnstone, B. Hypoxia promotes redifferentiation and suppresses markers of hypertrophy and degeneration in both healthy and osteoarthritic chondrocytes. *Arthritis Res. Ther.* **2013**, *15*, R92. [CrossRef] [PubMed]

24. Heywood, H.K.; Lee, D.A. Low oxygen reduces the modulation to an oxidative phenotype in monolayer-expanded chondrocytes. *J. Cell. Physiol.* **2010**, *222*, 248–253. [CrossRef] [PubMed]

25. Henderson, J.H.; Ginley, N.M.; Caplan, A.I.; Niyibizi, C.; Dennis, J.E. Low oxygen tension during incubation periods of chondrocyte expansion is sufficient to enhance postexpansion chondrogenesis. *Tissue Eng. Part A* **2010**, *16*, 1585–1593. [CrossRef] [PubMed]

26. Borzı, R.M.; Olivotto, E.; Pagani, S.; Vitellozzi, R.; Neri, S.; Battistelli, M.; Falcieri, E.; Facchini, A.; Flamigni, F.; Penzo, M.; et al. Matrix Metalloproteinase 13 Loss Associated With Impaired Extracellular Matrix Remodeling Disrupts Chondrocyte Differentiation by Concerted Effects on Multiple Regulatory Factors. *Arthritis Rheum.* **2010**, *62*, 2370–2381. [CrossRef] [PubMed]

27. Schmidt, M.B.; Chen, E.H.; Lynch, S.E. A review of the effects of insulin-like growth factor and platelet derived growth factor on in vivo cartilage healing and repair. *Osteoarthr. Cartil.* **2006**, *14*, 403–412. [CrossRef]

28. Duan, L.; Ma, B.; Liang, Y.; Chen, J.; Zhu, W.; Li, M.; Wang, D. Cytokine networking of chondrocyte dedifferentiation in vitro and its implications for cell-based cartilage therapy. *Am. J. Transl. Res.* **2015**, *7*, 194–208.

29. McCarrel, T.; Fortier, L. Temporal growth factor release from platelet-rich plasma, trehalose lyophilized platelets, and bone marrow aspirate and their effect on tendon and ligament gene expression. *J. Orthop. Res.* **2009**, *27*, 1033–1042. [CrossRef]

30. Oh, J.H.; Kim, W.O.O.; Park, K.U.; Roh, Y.H. Comparison of the cellular composition and cytokine-release kinetics of various platelet-rich plasma preparations. *Am. J. Sports Med.* **2015**, *43*, 3062–3070. [CrossRef]

31. Sundman, E.A.; Cole, B.J.; Fortier, L.A. Growth Factor and Catabolic Cytokine Concentrations Are Influenced by the Cellular Composition of Platelet-Rich Plasma. *Am. J. Sports Med.* **2011**, *39*, 2135–2140. [CrossRef] [PubMed]

32. Lafont, J.E.; Poujade, F.A.; Pasdeloup, M.; Neyret, P.; Mallein-Gerin, F. Hypoxia potentiates the BMP-2 driven COL2A1 stimulation in human articular chondrocytes via p38 MAPK. *Osteoarthr. Cartil.* **2016**, *24*, 856–867. [CrossRef] [PubMed]

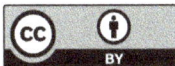

International Journal of
Molecular Sciences

MDPI

Article

The Composition of Hyperacute Serum and Platelet-Rich Plasma Is Markedly Different despite the Similar Production Method

Dorottya Kardos [1,*], Melinda Simon [1], Gabriella Vácz [1], Adél Hinsenkamp [1], Tünde Holczer [2], Domonkos Cseh [3], Adrienn Sárközi [3], Kálmán Szenthe [4], Ferenc Bánáti [4], Susan Szathmary [5], Stefan Nehrer [6], Olga Kuten [6,9], Mariana Masteling [1,7], Zsombor Lacza [1,8,9] and István Hornyák [1,9]

[1] Institute of Clinical Experimental Research, Semmelweis University, Budapest 1094, Hungary; melinda.simon@orthosera.com (M.S.); vaczgabi@gmail.com (G.V.); adel.hinsenkamp@orthosera.com (A.H.); mastelin@umich.edu (M.M.); zsombor.lacza@orthosera.com (Z.L.); istvan.hornyak@orthosera.com (I.H.)
[2] Department of Laboratory Medicine, Semmelweis University, Budapest 1089, Hungary; holczer.tunde@med.semmelweis-univ.hu
[3] Department of Physiology, Semmelweis University, Budapest, 1094 Hungary; cseh.domonkos@med.semmelweis-univ.hu (D.C.); sarkoziadrienn88@gmail.com (A.S.)
[4] RT-Europe Non-profit Research Center, Mosonmagyaróvár 9200, Hungary; kszenthe@rt-europe.org (K.S.); fbanati@rt-europe.org (F.B.)
[5] Galenbio Ltd., Mosonmagyaróvár 9200, Hungary; sszathmary@galenbio.com
[6] Danube University, Center for Regenerative Medicine, Krems an der Donau 3500, Austria; stefan.nehrer@donau-uni.ac.at (S.N.); olga.kuten@orthosera.com (O.K.)
[7] Faculdade de Engenharia da Universidade do Porto, Universidade do Porto, Porto 4200-465, Portugal
[8] University of Physical Education, Institution of Sport and Health Sciences, Budapest 1123, Hungary
[9] Orthosera GmbH, Krems an der Donau 3500, Austria
* Correspondence: dorottya.kardos@orthosera.com; Tel.: +36-70-426-9094

Received: 1 February 2019; Accepted: 5 February 2019; Published: 8 February 2019

check for updates

Abstract: Autologous blood derived products, such as platelet-rich plasma (PRP) and platelet-rich fibrin (PRF) are widely applied in regenerative therapies, in contrast to the drawbacks in their application, mainly deriving from the preparation methods used. Eliminating the disadvantages of both PRP and PRF, hyperacute serum (HAS) opens a new path in autologous serum therapy showing similar or even improved regenerative potential at the same time. Despite the frequent experimental and clinical use of PRP and HAS, their protein composition has not been examined thoroughly yet. Thus, we investigated and compared the composition of HAS, serum, PRP and plasma products using citrate and EDTA by simple laboratory tests, and we compared the composition of HAS, serum, EDTA PRP and plasma by Proteome Profiler and ELISA assays. According to our results the natural ionic balance was upset in both EDTA and citrate PRP as well as in plasma. EDTA PRP contained significantly higher level of growth factors and cytokines, especially platelet derived angiogenic and inflammatory proteins, that can be explained by the significantly higher number of platelets in EDTA PRP. The composition analysis of blood derivatives revealed that although the preparation method of PRP and HAS were similar, the ionic and protein composition of HAS could be advantageous for cell function.

Keywords: hyperacute serum; platelet-rich plasma; blood derived products; composition

1. Introduction

Autologous blood derived products, particularly platelet concentrates, are widely applied nowadays in different regenerative therapies which include wound healing, orthopedics, and dentistry [1–5]. Platelet derived growth factors are able to enhance soft and hard tissue regeneration by increasing cell migration and proliferation, and decreasing the rate of inflammation [6,7]. The most commonly used platelet concentrate products are PRP (platelet-rich plasma)—also known as first generation blood product—and PRF (platelet-rich fibrin), which is known as second generation blood product. PRP has a wide range of application in wound healing, cartilage, bone, musculoskeletal regeneration, oral surgery, dentistry, and cosmetics [8–13]. Moreover, PRP has been successfully applied in treating endometriosis, chronic skin ulcer and vitiligo in earlier studies [14,15]. Nevertheless, there are some drawbacks of using PRP [16]. For example, the lack of uniformity in PRP preparation methods [4,17] which is mainly caused by the treatment of blood with different anticoagulants like EDTA and citrate, which are the most preferred ones in PRP preparation. The information in the literature on the optimal anticoagulant for PRP preparation is contradictory. On the basis of previous studies, both EDTA and citrate (sodium citrate, acid citrate dextrose) have a negative effect on the balance of ionic content in the plasma fraction because of their chelating mechanism [18]. Higher platelet numbers can be obtained by using EDTA compared to citrate [19,20], however the mean platelet volume (MPV)—which is a marker of platelet function—can be higher than citrate using EDTA [20]. Other studies have claimed that platelet aggregation was inhibited more efficiently by using EDTA than acid citrate dextrose solution [19]. Using EDTA, spontaneous platelet activation can be avoided because EDTA has a stronger complex capacity with divalent cations than citrate. For the activation of citrate and EDTA, PRP thrombin and calcium–chloride or temperature activation can be used. [21] The addition of bovine thrombin during PRP preparation may lead to cross-reaction with human factor Va causing bleeding disorder, but it is more effective than activating PRP by repeated freezing and thawing [16].

With PRF the major disadvantages of PRP can be avoided. In addition, growth factors and cytokines are released from platelets over a longer period of time, whereas in PRP these factors are released immediately into the site of application [22,23]. Nevertheless, PRF is not capable of replacing PRP in all therapeutic areas because of its compact three-dimensional structure, which hinders its application as an injection [24–26]. Consequently, PRF is mainly used for replacing injured tissues in oral and dental surgery, orthopedics, and wound healing [27–31].

SPRF (serum from platelet-rich fibrin) or HAS (hyperacute serum) was developed to avoid the limitations of both PRF and PRP. The preparation method is the same as in the case of PRF, but the serum is squeezed out from the PRF clot at the end of the procedure [32]. Thus, it does not contain any anticoagulant or thrombin, and the final product is liquid. Based on our previous results, HAS has a better cell proliferative effect on mesenchymal stem cells, osteoblasts, and osteoarthritic chondrocytes compared to EDTA PRP [33]. Furthermore, HAS promotes MSCs lineage shift towards the osteoblastic line and results in a better preserved bone marrow structure in bone marrow explants compared to EDTA PRP treatments [32,34].

Despite the positive results of HAS in cell proliferation and migration, the composition of HAS has not been reported so far. However, angiogenic proteins were measured earlier both in HAS and PRP by Proteome Profiler, showing that EDTA PRP has more angiopoietic components, whereas HAS has more anti-angiopoietic components [35]. In the present study we investigated and compared the composition of HAS, PRP, blood serum, and plasma to understand the differences in the cell proliferative and regenerative effect of HAS and PRP. In the laboratory tests EDTA and citrate anticoagulated PRP were also compared. However, due to the more homogenous blood fraction separation that was achieved using EDTA, and based on the earlier cell culture experiments, the semi-quantitative and quantitative analysis was only done with PRP that was anticoagulated with EDTA in order to allow consequent results and interpretation.

2. Results

First, we measured the concentration of relevant metal ions, inorganic phosphate, the activity of ALP enzyme, and the quantity of cellular blood components in the serum and plasma samples by a general laboratory test. EDTA and citrate PRP were activated by thrombin and $CaCl_2$ with heparin together to prevent coagulation, thus the chelation capacity of both K_3EDTA and sodium citrate was reduced in PRP.

The concentration of calcium ions was significantly higher in EDTA and citrate PRP, and lower in EDTA and citrate plasma compared to the serum fractions. Both anticoagulants effectively chelate calcium and citrate is more effective in forming complexes with magnesium ions. The level of potassium ions was higher in EDTA plasma fractions due to the potassium content of K_3EDTA. The concentration of copper, zinc, and iron ions was also significantly lower in EDTA plasma and EDTA PRP due to the chelating ability of K_3EDTA. Sodium ion concentration was increased due to the sodium content of citrate while phosphate content was only significantly influenced using citrate PRP. The activity of ALP enzymes was also reduced significantly because EDTA naturally chelates Mg^{2+} and Zn^{2+} which have a crucial role in the structural stability of ALP enzyme (Figure 1A).

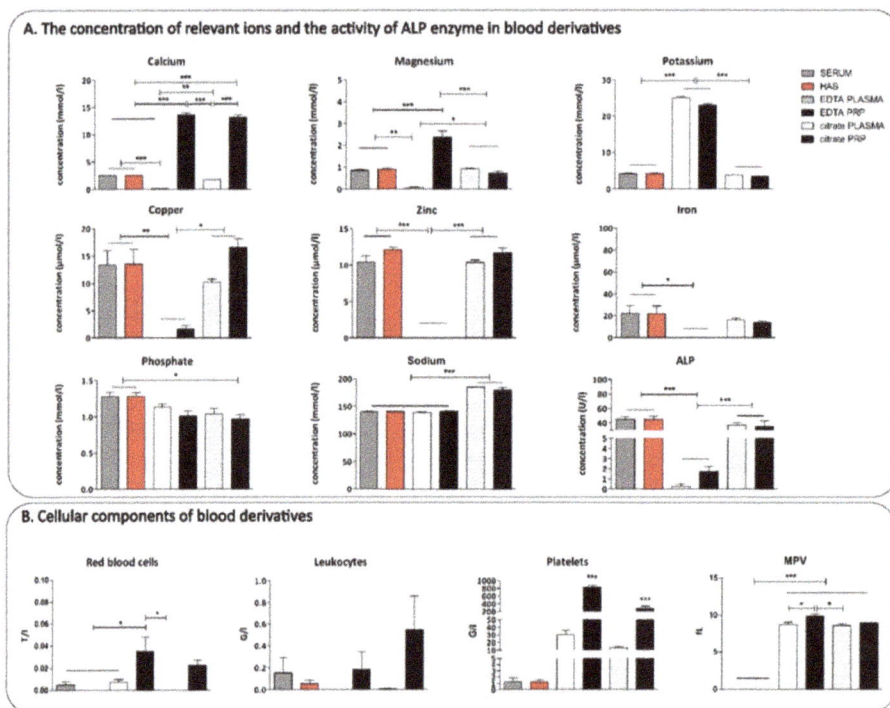

Figure 1. Quantitative determination of the concentration of relevant ions and the activity of alkaline phosphatase (ALP) enzyme (**A**) and the number of red blood cells, leukocytes and platelets in the serum and plasma fractions (**B**), $n = 4$. The significance level was $p > 0.05$, where * means that p is between 0.01 and 0.05, ** means that p is between 0.01 and 0.001, and *** means that p is lower than 0.001.

Sodium citrate has a weaker complex capacity with divalent cations than EDTA, thus the ion content of citrate plasma fractions was not influenced significantly except calcium ions, which were added both to citrate and EDTA PRP for activation. Cellular blood components were measured before activating PRP because activated platelets might have been disrupted. The number of leukocytes was the highest in citrate PRP and the standard error of mean was high in the case of EDTA and citrate

PRP as well. The number of platelets was higher in EDTA PRP compared to citrate PRP. The platelet number was extremely low in EDTA and citrate plasma, serum and HAS. Mean platelet volume (MPV), which is a marker of platelet function, was similar in EDTA and citrate PRP. (Figure 1B). For further examination EDTA plasma and PRP were used because a higher number of platelets could be isolated by EDTA than citrate with similar MPV values. Furthermore, EDTA enabled the most homogenous separation and therefore EDTA was used as an anticoagulant in our previous studies where the cell proliferation rate of different cell types was investigated.

For mapping the composition of serum, HAS, EDTA plasma, and PRP (Figure 2A), 138 different known cytokines and growth factors were screened using antibody-based dot-blot assays. The results were presented as relative values compared to the positive control for the secondary antibody. From the 138 cytokines and growth factors selected as known paracrine mediators of tissue regeneration, vascularization or inflammation, 82 proteins were neglected (AU < 2%) thus 56 proteins (AU > 2%) are presented in Figure 2A [35]. The whole data set containing the 138 cytokines and growth factors is shown in Table S1. We observed a general trend that the overall concentration of active molecules was the highest in PRP, followed by HAS, plasma, and serum, respectively (see in Figure 2A and Table S1). There were clear differences in the proteome profiler patterns of the blood derivatives, although the proteome profiler is not reliable enough for quantitative measurements and for the statistic comparison of the blood derivates. Thus, on the basis of these results and the literature [6,36–39] we set out to quantify the key inflammation related cytokines and proteins with ELISA or Luminex assays.

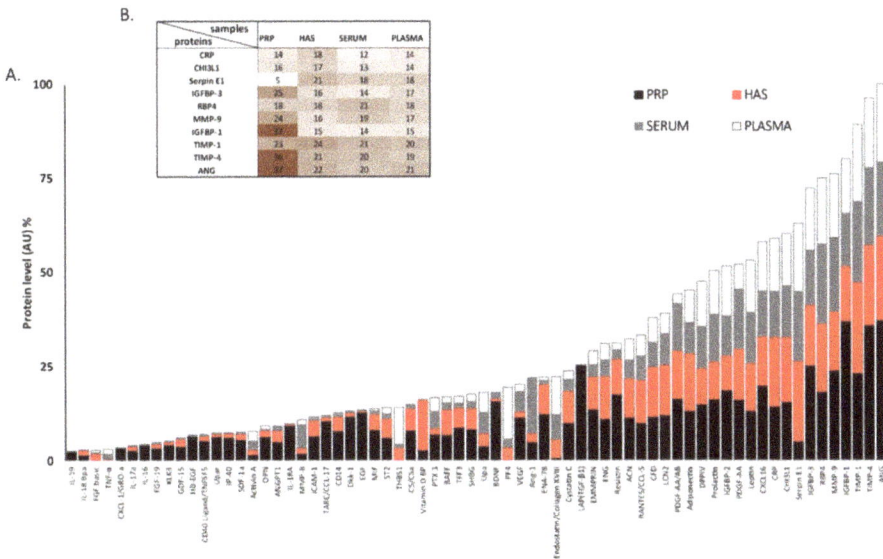

Figure 2. Semi-quantitative Proteome Profiler analysis of serum, hyperacute serum (HAS), plasma, and platelet-rich fibrin (PRP). On the bar chart proteins exceeding 2% (AU) of the total protein content (**A**) are presented. The level of the top 10 angiogenic proteins and cytokines are presented on a heat map. (**B**) The level of the proteins is expressed in % compared to the combined arbitrary unit of ANG that was considered to be 100%. *n* = 8.

For quantitative protein analysis, Luminex and ELISA assays were used where systemic pro-inflammatory molecules, complement system molecules, platelet-derived inflammation, angiogenesis related molecules, and anti-inflammatory molecules were investigated. Lipocalin-2, EMMPRIN (CD147), Osteopontin, IL-17A, and Chitinase-3-like protein 1 (CHI3L1) are similarly present in all blood derivates. While CD97 and Myeloperoxidase (MPO) were higher in serum derivates,

ALCAM was higher in plasma derivates. The concentration of CD40L was elevated in PRP compared to HAS, and CRP was significantly higher in plasma than in HAS and PRP (Figure 3A). From the complement system we measured C5a that showed the highest levels in plasma and C1qR1 which was highly elevated in all cases (Figure 3B).

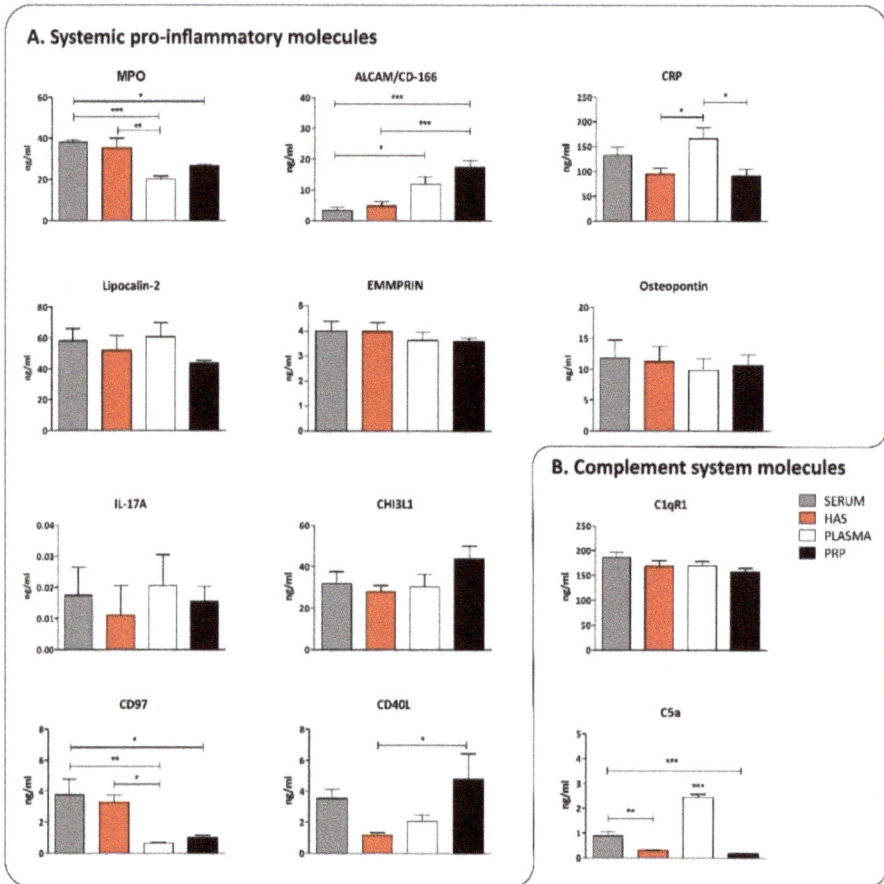

Figure 3. Concentration of systemic pro-inflammatory molecules (**A**) and complement system related molecules (**B**) in blood derivatives, *n* = 8. The significance level was *p* > 0.05, where * means that *p* is between 0.01 and 0.05, ** means that *p* is between 0.01 and 0.001, and *** means that *p* is lower than 0.001.

Platelet-derived pro-inflammatory cytokines and growth factors showed a very clear pattern: they were higher in PRP compared to other blood derivatives. In contrast, the fibrin/fibrinogen level was high both in plasma and PRP compared to serum and HAS, as the latter two were already coagulated and the clot was removed (Figure 4A). The anti-inflammatory cytokine IL-1RA was elevated in PRP and HAS. Angiopoietin-1 showed the highest level in serum but was present in all other blood derivatives in effective concentrations (Figure 4B).

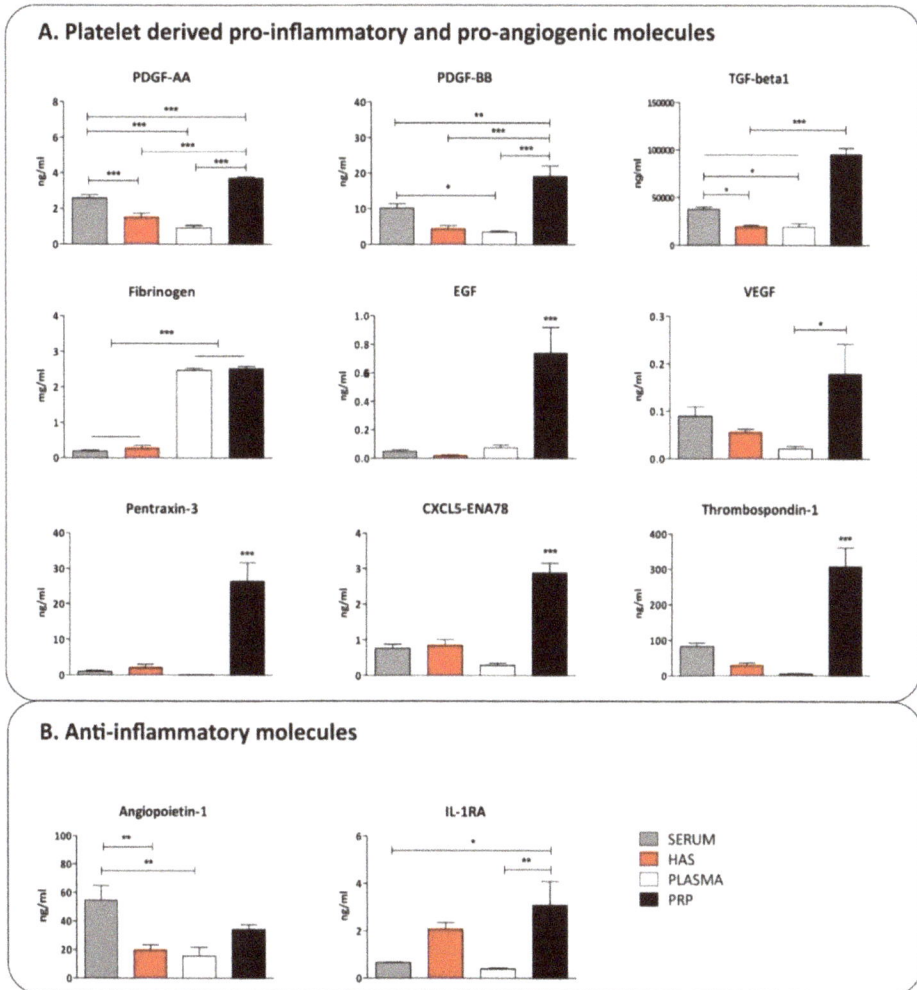

Figure 4. The concentration of platelet-derived inflammatory molecules (**A**) and anti-inflammatory molecules (**B**) in blood derivatives, $n = 8$. The significance level was $p > 0.05$, where * means that p is between 0.01 and 0.05, ** means that p is between 0.01 and 0.001, and *** means that p is lower than 0.001.

3. Discussion

In the present study we investigated and compared the composition of different blood derivatives, especially EDTA, citrate PRP and HAS. On the basis of the literature PRP has excellent regenerative effects in numerous clinical applications, such as bone and cartilage regeneration, in osteoarthritis, in dental and oral surgery, or in musculoskeletal regeneration [8,9,11,40]. However, there are numerous drawbacks in the application of PRP mainly caused by certain steps of the preparation methods which are not present in the preparation of HAS [19,20].

First, the blood derivatives were analyzed by laboratory tests, where the number of cellular blood components, the concentration of relevant ion contents and the activity of ALP enzymes were measured. The concentration of ions, such as iron, copper, and zinc which are all influenced by the chelating mechanism of EDTA, were significantly lower, whereas potassium was higher in PRP and plasma because K_3EDTA was used as an anticoagulant. The upset of the natural ionic balance due to EDTA PRP treatment may result in unexpected side effects when using it inside injured and/or inflamed tissue. As EDTA chelated both Zn^{2+} and Mg^{2+} the activity of ALP enzymes was reduced significantly. ALP has an important role in bone healing and regeneration, thus the reduced enzymatic activity has a negative effect in the case of injecting PRP into an osteoarthritic or injured joint [41]. The ionic balance of citrate PRP was much better, except for calcium ions which were added to PRP for platelet activation, and sodium because of the addition of sodium citrate. However, a significantly lower number of platelets could be isolated using citrate than EDTA, and the number of leukocytes was also much higher in citrate PRP.

The standard error of mean was high, indicating that the level of red blood cells and leukocytes in the samples depend mainly on the preparation method. During the preparation of HAS, the red blood cell containing fraction was cut away from the bottom of the PRF clot, while in case of PRP preparation, plasma fraction was removed by pipetting it carefully from the top of the red blood cell containing fraction. Using this isolation procedure, the PRP fraction contains some red blood cell fraction. The plasma isolation procedure is more complicated when citrate is used as an anticoagulant because the plasma and red blood cell fraction overlaps after centrifugation and the boundary could not be defined in a uniform manner. The mean platelet volume was similar in EDTA and citrate PRP, which indicates that platelet function was not influenced significantly by EDTA in our experiments. Using citrate, much better ionic composition can be achieved while the composition of blood shaped elements is much less favorable than EDTA PRP. On the basis of these results, and because only EDTA PRP was used in our previous studies for proteome profiler and luminex analysis, only EDTA PRP and plasma were used.

The level of angiogenic proteins [35] and cytokines was screened by semi-quantitative proteome profiler analysis. This method is not accurate enough for statistic comparison but was sufficient to determine that the overall concentration of proteins was the highest in EDTA PRP, followed by HAS, plasma, and the lowest was in serum. For quantitative protein measurement, inflammation-related molecules were chosen based on the proteome profiler results and relevant scientific literature [37–39].

The level of those molecules which are derived from systemic sources and are not affected by the preparation protocols, including MPO, ALCAM, CRP, Lipocalin-2, EMMPRIN, Osteopontin, IL-17A, CHI3L1, CD97, CD40L, was similar. From the elements of the complement system, C5a was present in the highest level in plasma, while C1qR1 was present in a similar concentration in all cases indicating that it was already activated after blood drawing regardless of the processing method. Platelet-derived pro-inflammatory cytokines and growth factors were all the highest in EDTA PRP compared to the other blood derivatives except for fibrinogen, which was high both in plasma and EDTA PRP compared to serum and HAS. This was due to the fibrin clot being separated from both HAS and serum after coagulation. Analyzing the concentration of anti-inflammatory cytokines in the samples, IL-1RA was elevated in EDTA PRP and HAS, and angiopoietin-1 was elevated in serum only. Interestingly the platelet-derived molecules were not increased in HAS or serum, although in both cases platelets are activated and release cytokines. This is probably due to the fact that serum is deprived of platelets and it contains only molecules which the platelets actively secrete. This is closer to the physiological conditions than disrupting all platelets and mixing their content into the plasma, as in the case of EDTA PRP activated by thrombin and calcium-chloride for example. The composition analysis of blood derivatives revealed that although the preparation method of EDTA PRP and HAS are similar, and they are typically considered interchangeable in clinical settings, there are marked differences. Most strikingly EDTA PRP contains excess EDTA, and as a consequence imbalanced ionic composition, higher growth factor content, and elevated pro-inflammatory cytokine content is present compared to HAS. According to previous results, EDTA PRP contains more angiogenic factors as well [31]. On the basis of our results so far, HAS eliminates the disadvantages of PRP preparation, such as the addition of EDTA, citrate, thrombin, or calcium chloride, which may cause side effects inside an injured tissue. HAS is free from activated platelets, which may be the reason why EDTA PRP is more pro-inflammatory than HAS. The presence of pro-inflammatory cytokines could further enhance inflammation in injured tissues. Further benefits of using HAS instead of EDTA PRP is the better cell proliferative effect on mesenchymal stem cells, osteoblasts, and osteoarthritic chondrocytes than EDTA PRP based on our previous results [32,34,35].

4. Materials and Methods

4.1. Isolation of Blood Derivates

Blood samples were obtained from healthy donors of both genders aged 24–45 years under IRB approval (IRB approval number 33106-1/2016/EKU, 12.07.2016.). The preparation method of serum, hyperacute serum, plasma and platelet-rich plasma is shown in Figures 5–8.

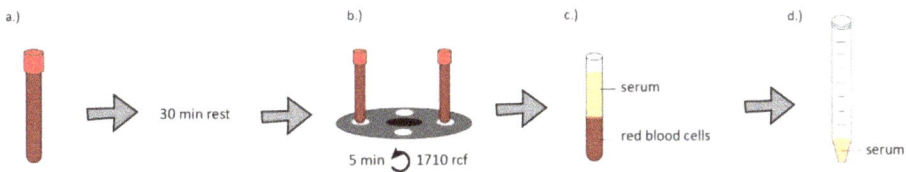

Figure 5. For serum isolation, whole blood was obtained from donors in VACUETTE® 9 mL Z Serum C/A tubes (Greiner Bio-One, Kremsmünster, Austria). Blood was allowed to clot for 30 min (**a**) and centrifuged at 1710× *g* for 5 min at room temperature (**b**). The supernatant formed after centrifugation is called serum (**c**,**d**).

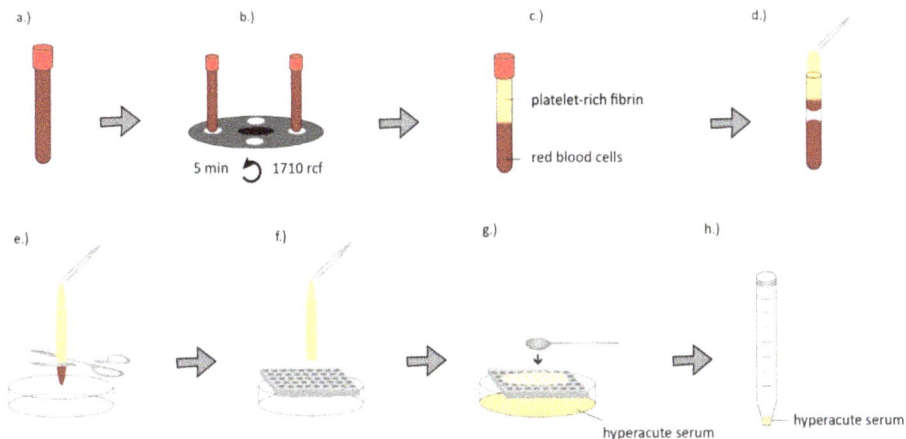

Figure 6. For hyperacute serum isolation, a whole blood sample was obtained from healthy donors (28–45 years) in VACUETTE® 9 mL Z Serum C/A tubes (Greiner Bio-One) (**a**) and it was immediately centrifuged at 1710× *g* for 5 min at room temperature (**b**). After centrifugation two layers were formed in the tubes. The top layer was the platelet-rich fibrin clot and the bottom layer contains red blood cells (**c**). PRF (platelet-rich fibrin) as removed using sterile forceps in a biosafety cabinet (**d**), red blood cells at the bottom of the fibrin clot were cut away (**e**) and the clot was placed onto a 110 mm long, 75 mm wide custom-made plastic grid with 5 mm diameter holes on it. It was sterilized in an autoclave before use (**f**). The hyperacute serum was squeezed out from the PRF clot using a sterile spatula (**g**,**h**) [24].

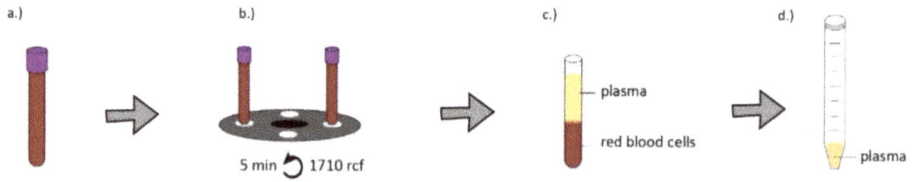

Figure 7. For PRP isolation, whole blood was obtained from donors in VACUETTE® 9 mL K3 EDTA blood collection tubes (Greiner Bio-One) and VACUTTE 3.5 mL sodium citrate 3.2% blood collection tubes (Greiner Bio-One) (**a**) then centrifuged at 1710× *g* for 5 min at room temperature (**b**). The supernatant formed after centrifugation is called plasma (**c,d**).

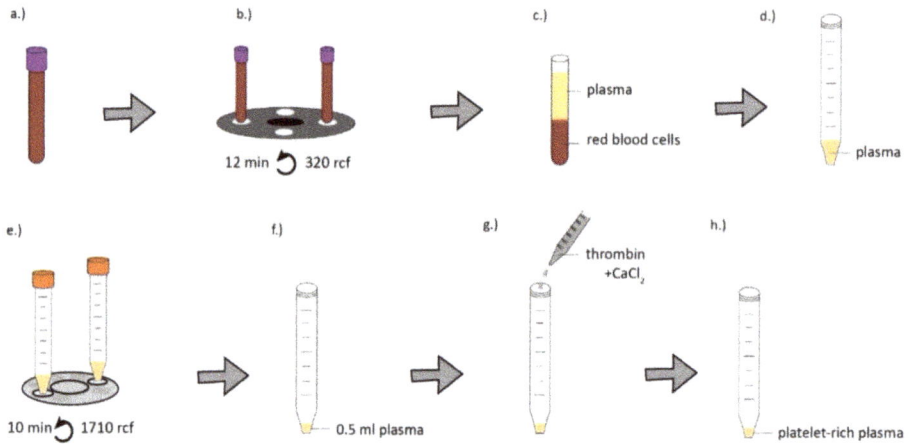

Figure 8. For PRP isolation, whole blood was obtained from donors in VACUETTE® 9 mL K3 EDTA blood collection tubes (Greiner Bio-One) and VACUTTE 3.5 mL sodium citrate 3.2% blood collection tubes (Greiner Bio-One) (**a**) then centrifuged at 320 *g* for 12 min at room temperature (**b**). The platelet-rich layer above the buffy coat was aspirated and transferred into a 15 mL tube (**c,d**) and centrifuged at 1710× *g* for 10 minutes (**e**). The resulting platelet pellet was resuspended in the same volume as the isolated hyperacute serum from the same donor (**f**). PRP was activated by 10 IU thrombin and 10 mg calcium-chloride (Sigma-Aldrich, St. Louis, MO, USA) in case of both EDTA and citrate tubes (**g,h**).

4.2. Laboratory Testing of Blood Derivates

A Sysmex XN-1000 Sa-01 cell counter was used for the quantitative determination of red blood cells, leukocytes and platelet number in the serum and plasma fractions. The concentration of ions, that may interfere with EDTA and sodium citrate (calcium, magnesium, copper, zinc, iron, sodium, phosphate, and potassium) and the activity of ALP enzymes were measured using a Beckman Coulter AU5800 automated laboratory machine (*n* = 4).

4.3. Comprehensive Protein Analysis

In order to quantify the cytokine and angiogenesis-related protein content of EDTA PRP and plasma serum a HAS Proteome Profiler Human Angiogenesis Array Kit (55 protein, R&D Systems, #ARY007) (R&D Systems Inc., Minneapolis, MN, USA) [35] and Proteome Profiler Human XL Cytokine Array Kit (102 protein R&D Systems, #ARY022) were used according to the manufacturer's instructions. Some cytokines were included in both the Proteome Profiler Human Angiogenesis Array Kit and Proteome Profiler Human XL Cytokine Array Kit, in these cases we used the mean of the results.

In total, 138 different cytokines were measured by the two different kits. Proteome Profiler individual protein levels were measured as spot intensities on the blots using Fiji Image J 1.47 (South Bend, IN, USA) and Adobe Photoshop CC 2015.5 software (San Jose, CA, USA). The results were expressed in % compared to the arbitrary unit of the highest AU value, which belonged to ANG. Thus, the combined protein level of ANG among the samples was considered to be 100% ($n = 8$).

4.4. Quantitative Protein Measurement by Multiplex Immunoassay and ELISA Assays

The key proteins, where clear differences were found during the proteome profiler measurements, were quantified using custom Human Magnetic Luminex Assay (CHI3L1, C5a, EGF, CD40L, VEGF, CRP, Il-17a, Osteopontin, Angiopoetin, IL-1RA, EMMPRIN, Lipocalin-2, Pentraxin-3, PDGF-AA, PDGF-BB) (R&D Systems Inc.) or ELISA assays (MPO, ALCAM, CD97, C1qR1, TGF-beta, Fibrinogen, Thrombospondin-1, CXCL-5) (Abcam, Cambridge, UK) ($n = 8$)

4.5. Statistical Analysis

One-way analysis of variance (ANOVA) was performed with a Tukey post hoc test to compare differences between the groups. The significance level was $p > 0.05$, where * means that p is between 0.01 and 0.05, ** means that p is between 0.01 and 0.001, and *** means that p is lower than 0.001. Prism 7 software (Irvine, CA, USA) was used for statistical analysis. Data are presented as mean $\pm$ SEM.

5. Conclusions

General trends can be observed in the composition changes of the blood products that were investigated. These trends are based on the characteristics of the additives and the steps of the production methods. For the preparation of PRPs calcium-chloride, thrombin, citrate or EDTA is added, which has a negative effect on the composition of these blood products. The exact mechanism of HAS on cells is not regenerative, only acts as a supplement but with the use of HAS the negative effects originating from the PRP's preparation methods can be circumvented, while maintaining the beneficial influence of PRP on cells and tissues in vitro. Our further aims include comparing the effect of HAS, EDTA and citrate PRP in clinical studies, whicht can be differ from the in vitro results.

Abbreviations

ALCAM	activated leukocyte cell adhesion molecule
ALP	alkaline phosphatase
CD40L	cluster of differentiation 40 ligand
CD97	cluster of differentiation 97
CHI3L1	chitinase 3-like protein 1
CRP	C-reactive protein
CXCL-5	chemokine (C-X-C motif) ligand 5
C1qR1	complement component 1 Q subcomponent receptor 1
C5a	complement component 5a
EDTA	ethylenediaminetetraacetic acid
EGF	epidermal growth factor
EMMPRIN	extracellular matrix metalloproteinase inducer
ELISA	enzyme-linked immunosorbent assay
HAS	hyperacute serum
IL-17	interleukin-17
IL-1RA	interleukin-1 receptor antagonist
MSC	mesenchymal stem cell
TGF-beta	transforming growth factor beta
PDGF-AA	platelet-derived growth factor AA
PDGF-BB	platelet-derived growth factor BB

PRF	platelet-rich fibrin
PRP	platelet-rich plasma
SPRF	serum from platelet-rich fibrin
VEGF	vascular endothelial growth factor

Supplementary Materials: Supplementary materials can be found at http://www.mdpi.com/1422-0067/20/3/721/s1.

Author Contributions: I.H., M.S., G.V., M.M., Z.L. and D.K. conceived and designed the experiments; I.H., M.S., G.V., A.S., D.C., T.H., K.S., F.B. and D.K. performed the experiments; I.H., M.S., M.M., Z.L., S.N., O.K. and D.K. analyzed the data; I.H., M.S., G.V., M.M., A.H., S.S., F.B., K.S. and D.K. contributed reagents/materials/analysis tools; D.K. and I.H. wrote the paper.

Funding: This research received no external funding.

Acknowledgments: The authors are thankful for OrthoSera GmbH for the research support to Semmelweis and Danube Universities. Disclaimer: authors Z.L., I.H. and S.N. are employees, stock holders, or advisory board members of OrthoSera GmbH, a startup company developing hyperacute serum technology towards clinical applications.

Conflicts of Interest: Z.L. owns stock in OrthoSera GmbH, a startup company developing the hyperacute serum technology towards clinical application.

References

1. Fotouhi, A.; Maleki, A.; Dolati, S.; Aghebati-Maleki, A.; Aghebati-Maleki, L. Platelet rich plasma, stromal vascular fraction and autologous conditioned serum in treatment of knee osteoarthritis. *Biomed. Pharmacother.* **2018**, *104*, 652–660. [CrossRef] [PubMed]

2. Le, A.D.K.; Enweze, L.; DeBaun, M.R.; Dragoo, J.L. Current Clinical Recommendations for Use of Platelet-Rich Plasma. *Curr. Rew. Musculoskelet. Med.* **2018**, *11*, 624–634. [CrossRef] [PubMed]

3. Amable, P.R.; Carias, R.B.V.; Teixeira, M.V.T.; da Cruz Pacheco, I.; Corrêa do Amaral, R.J.F.; Granjeiro, J.M.; Borojevic, R. Platelet-rich plasma preparation for regenerative medicine: Optimization and quantification of cytokines and growth factors. *Stem Cell Res. Ther.* **2013**, *4*, 67. [CrossRef] [PubMed]

4. Prakash, S.; Thakur, A. Platelet concentrates: Past, present and future. *J. Oral Maxillofac. Surg.* **2011**, *10*, 45–49. [CrossRef] [PubMed]

5. Andia, I.; Maffulli, N. Use of platelet-rich plasma for patellar tendon and medial collateral ligament injuries: Best current clinical practice. *J. KNEE Surg.* **2015**, *28*, 11–18. [CrossRef] [PubMed]

6. Masuki, H.; Okudera, T.; Watanebe, T.; Suzuki, M.; Nishiyama, K.; Okudera, H.; Nakata, K.; Uematsu, K.; Su, C.-Y.; Kawase, T. Growth factor and pro-inflammatory cytokine contents in platelet-rich plasma (PRP), plasma rich in growth factors (PRGF), advanced platelet-rich fibrin (A-PRF), and concentrated growth factors (CGF). *Int. J. Implant. Dent.* **2016**, *2*, 19. [CrossRef]

7. El-Sharkawy, H.; Kantarci, A.; Deady, J.; Hasturk, H.; Liu, H.; Alshahat, M.; Van Dyke, T.E. Platelet-rich plasma: Growth factors and pro- and anti-inflammatory properties. *J. Periodontol.* **2007**, *78*, 661–669. [CrossRef]

8. Badis, D.; Omar, B. The effectiveness of platelet-rich plasma on the skin wound healing process: A comparative experimental study in sheep. *Vet. World* **2018**, *11*, 800–808. [CrossRef]

9. Lee, K.S.; Wilson, J.J.; Rabago, D.P.; Baer, G.S.; Jacobson, J.A.; Borrero, C.G. Musculoskeletal applications of platelet-rich plasma: Fad or future? *AJR Am. J. Roentgenol.* **2011**, *196*, 628–636. [CrossRef]

10. Gentile, P.; Cole, J.P.; Cole, M.A.; Garcovich, S.; Bielli, A.; Scioli, M.G.; Orlandi, A.; Insalaco, C.; Cervelli, V. Evaluation of Not-Activated and Activated PRP in Hair Loss Treatment: Role of Growth Factor and Cytokine Concentrations Obtained by Different Collection Systems. *Int. J. Mol. Sci.* **2017**, *18*, 408. [CrossRef]

11. Montanez-Heredia, E.; Irizar, S.; Huertas, P.J.; Otero, E.; Del Valle, M.; Prat, I.; Diaz-Gallardo, M.S.; Peran, M.; Marchal, J.A.; Hernandez-Lamas, M.D.C. Intra-Articular Injections of Platelet-Rich Plasma versus Hyaluronic Acid in the Treatment of Osteoarthritic Knee Pain: A Randomized Clinical Trial in the Context of the Spanish National Health Care System. *Int. J. Mol. Sci* **2016**, *17*, 1064. [CrossRef]

12. Angelone, M.; Conti, V.; Biacca, C.; Battaglia, B.; Pecorari, L.; Piana, F.; Gnudi, G.; Leonardi, F.; Ramoni, R.; Basini, G.; et al. The Contribution of Adipose Tissue-Derived Mesenchymal Stem Cells and Platelet-Rich Plasma to the Treatment of Chronic Equine Laminitis: A Proof of Concept. *Int. J. Mol. Sci* **2017**, *18*, 2122. [CrossRef] [PubMed]

13. Andia, I.; Martin, J.I.; Maffulli, N. Advances with platelet rich plasma therapies for tendon regeneration. *Expert Opin. Biol. Ther.* **2018**, *18*, 389–398. [CrossRef] [PubMed]

14. Pinto, J.M.N.; Pizani, N.S.; Kang, H.C.; Silva, L.A.K. Application of platelet-rich plasma in the treatment of chronic skin ulcer - case report. *An. Brasileiros de Dermatologia* **2014**, *89*, 638–640. [CrossRef]

15. Shih, S. Platelet-rich plasma: Potential role in combined therapy for vitiligo. *Dermatol. Ther.* **2018**, e12773. [CrossRef] [PubMed]

16. Chu, C.R.; Rodeo, S.; Bhutani, N.; Goodrich, L.R.; Huard, J.; Irrgang, J.; LaPrade, R.F.; Lattermann, C.; Lu, Y.; Mandelbaum, B.; et al. Optimizing Clinical Use of Biologics in Orthopaedic Surgery: Consensus Recommendations From the 2018 AAOS/NIH U-13 Conference. *J. Am. Acad. Orthop. Surg.* **2018**, *27*, e50–e63. [CrossRef] [PubMed]

17. Andia, I.; Maffulli, N. A contemporary view of platelet-rich plasma therapies: Moving toward refined clinical protocols and precise indications. *Regenerative Med.* **2018**, *13*, 717–728. [CrossRef] [PubMed]

18. Giraldo, C.E.; Álvarez, M.E.; Carmona, J.U. Effects of sodium citrate and acid citrate dextrose solutions on cell counts and growth factor release from equine pure-platelet rich plasma and pure-platelet rich gel. *BMC Vet. Res.* **2015**, *11*, 60. [CrossRef]

19. Araki, J.; Jona, M.; Eto, H.; Aoi, N.; Kato, H.; Suga, H.; Doi, K.; Yatomi, Y.; Yoshimura, K. Optimized preparation method of platelet-concentrated plasma and noncoagulating platelet-derived factor concentrates: Maximization of platelet concentration and removal of fibrinogen. *Tissue Eng. C Methods* **2012**, *18*, 176–185. [CrossRef] [PubMed]

20. do Amaral, R.J.F.C.; da Silva, N.P.; Haddad, N.F.; Lopes, L.S.; Ferreira, F.D.; Filho, R.B.; Cappelletti, P.A.; de Mello, W.; Cordeiro-Spinetti, E.; Balduino, A. Platelet-Rich Plasma Obtained with Different Anticoagulants and Their Effect on Platelet Numbers and Mesenchymal Stromal Cells Behavior In Vitro. *Stem Cells Int.* **2016**, *2016*, 11. [CrossRef]

21. Schuff-Werner, P.; Steiner, M.; Fenger, S.; Gross, H.-J.; Bierlich, A.; Dreissiger, K.; Mannuß, S.; Siegert, G.; Bachem, M.; Kohlschein, P. Effective estimation of correct platelet counts in pseudothrombocytopenia using an alternative anticoagulant based on magnesium salt. *Br. J. Haematol.* **2013**, *162*, 684–692. [CrossRef] [PubMed]

22. Kumar, R.V.; Shubhashini, N. Platelet rich fibrin: A new paradigm in periodontal regeneration. *Cell Tissue Bank* **2013**, *14*, 453–463. [CrossRef]

23. Di Liddo, R.; Bertalot, T.; Borean, A.; Pirola, I.; Argentoni, A.; Schrenk, S.; Cenzi, C.; Capelli, S.; Conconi, M.T.; Parnigotto, P.P. Leucocyte and Platelet-rich Fibrin: A carrier of autologous multipotent cells for regenerative medicine. *J. Cell Mol. Med.* **2018**, *22*, 1840–1854. [CrossRef] [PubMed]

24. Kardos, D.; Hornyak, I.; Simon, M.; Hinsenkamp, A.; Marschall, B.; Vardai, R.; Kallay-Menyhard, A.; Pinke, B.; Meszaros, L.; Kuten, O.; et al. Biological and Mechanical Properties of Platelet-Rich Fibrin Membranes after Thermal Manipulation and Preparation in a Single-Syringe Closed System. *Int. J. Mol. Sci* **2018**, *19*, 3433. [CrossRef] [PubMed]

25. Jimenez-Aristizabal, R.F.; Lopez, C.; Alvarez, M.E.; Giraldo, C.; Prades, M.; Carmona, J.U. Long-term cytokine and growth factor release from equine platelet-rich fibrin clots obtained with two different centrifugation protocols. *Cytokine* **2017**, *97*, 149–155. [CrossRef]

26. Varela, H.A.; Souza, J.C.M.; Nascimento, R.M.; Araujo, R.F., Jr.; Vasconcelos, R.C.; Cavalcante, R.S.; Guedes, P.M.; Araujo, A.A. Injectable platelet rich fibrin: Cell content, morphological, and protein characterization. *Clin. Oral Investig.* **2018**. [CrossRef] [PubMed]

27. Kapse, S.; Surana, S.; Satish, M.; Hussain, S.E.; Vyas, S.; Thakur, D. Autologous platelet-rich fibrin: Can it secure a better healing? *Oral Surg. Oral Med. Oral Pathol. Oral Radiol. Endod.* **2018**. [CrossRef]

28. Wang, L.; Liu, G.; Li, Z.; Jia, B.C.; Wang, Y. Clinical application of platelet-rich fibrin in chronic wounds combined with subcutaneous stalking sinus. *Zhonghua Shao Shang Za Zhi* **2018**, *34*, 637–642.

29. Shah, R.; Gowda, T.M.; Thomas, R.; Kumar, T.; Mehta, D.S. Biological activation of bone grafts using injectable platelet-rich fibrin. *J. Prosthet. Dent.* **2018**. [CrossRef]

30. Wang, X.; Zhang, Y.; Choukroun, J.; Ghanaati, S.; Miron, R.J. Behavior of Gingival Fibroblasts on Titanium Implant Surfaces in Combination with either Injectable-PRF or PRP. *Int. J. Mol. Sci* **2017**, *18*, 331. [CrossRef]

31. Wong, C.C.; Kuo, T.-F.; Yang, T.-L.; Tsuang, Y.-H.; Lin, M.-F.; Chang, C.-H.; Lin, Y.-H.; Chan, W.P. Platelet-Rich Fibrin Facilitates Rabbit Meniscal Repair by Promoting Meniscocytes Proliferation, Migration, and Extracellular Matrix Synthesis. *Int. J. Mol. Sci* **2017**, *18*, 1722. [CrossRef] [PubMed]

32. Simon, M.; Major, B.; Vacz, G.; Kuten, O.; Hornyak, I.; Hinsenkamp, A.; Kardos, D.; Bago, M.; Cseh, D.; Sarkozi, A.; et al. The Effects of Hyperacute Serum on the Elements of the Human Subchondral Bone Marrow Niche. *Stem Cells Int.* **2018**, *2018*, 4854619. [CrossRef] [PubMed]

33. Jeyakumar, V.; Niculescu-Morzsa, E.; Bauer, C.; Lacza, Z.; Nehrer, S. Platelet-Rich Plasma Supports Proliferation and Redifferentiation of Chondrocytes during In Vitro Expansion. *Front. Bioeng. Biotechnol.* **2017**, *5*, 75. [CrossRef] [PubMed]

34. Kuten, O.; Simon, M.; Hornyak, I.; De Luna-Preitschopf, A.; Nehrer, S.; Lacza, Z. The Effects of Hyperacute Serum on Adipogenesis and Cell Proliferation of Mesenchymal Stromal Cells. *Tissue Eng. Part A* **2018**, *24*, 1011–1021. [CrossRef]

35. Vacz, G.; Major, B.; Gaal, D.; Petrik, L.; Horvathy, D.B.; Han, W.; Holczer, T.; Simon, M.; Muir, J.M.; Hornyak, I.; et al. Hyperacute serum has markedly better regenerative efficacy than platelet-rich plasma in a human bone oxygen-glucose deprivation model. *Regenerative Med.* **2018**, *13*, 531–543. [CrossRef] [PubMed]

36. Okuda, K.; Kawase, T.; Momose, M.; Murata, M.; Saito, Y.; Suzuki, H.; Wolff, L.F.; Yoshie, H. Platelet-rich plasma contains high levels of platelet-derived growth factor and transforming growth factor-beta and modulates the proliferation of periodontally related cells in vitro. *J. Periodontol.* **2003**, *74*, 849–857. [CrossRef] [PubMed]

37. Lubkowska, A.; Dolegowska, B.; Banfi, G. Growth factor content in PRP and their applicability in medicine. *J. Biol. Regul. Homeost. Agents* **2012**, *26*, 3s–22s. [PubMed]

38. Lee, J.W.; Kwon, O.H.; Kim, T.K.; Cho, Y.K.; Choi, K.Y.; Chung, H.Y.; Cho, B.C.; Yang, J.D.; Shin, J.H. Platelet-rich plasma: Quantitative assessment of growth factor levels and comparative analysis of activated and inactivated groups. *Arch. Plast. Surg.* **2013**, *40*, 530–535. [CrossRef]

39. Park, H.-B.; Yang, J.-H.; Chung, K.-H. Characterization of the cytokine profile of platelet rich plasma (PRP) and PRP-induced cell proliferation and migration: Upregulation of matrix metalloproteinase-1 and -9 in HaCaT cells. *Korean J. Hematol.* **2011**, *46*, 265–273. [CrossRef]

40. Andia, I.; Maffulli, N. Platelet-rich plasma for managing pain and inflammation in osteoarthritis. *Nat. Rev. Rheumatol.* **2013**, *9*, 721–730. [CrossRef]

41. Golub, E.E.; Harrison, G.; Taylor, A.G.; Camper, S.; Shapiro, I.M. The role of alkaline phosphatase in cartilage mineralization. *Bone Miner.* **1992**, *17*, 273–278. [CrossRef]

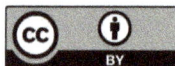

International Journal of
Molecular Sciences

MDPI

Communication

Growth Factor Quantification of Platelet-Rich Plasma in Burn Patients Compared to Matched Healthy Volunteers

Roos E. Marck [1,2,3] ⓘ, Kim L. M. Gardien [2,3], Marcel Vlig [4], Roelf S. Breederveld [2,5] and Esther Middelkoop [2,3,4,*]

[1] Department of Plastic, Reconstructive & Hand Surgery, Amsterdam UMC, University of Amsterdam, 1081 HV Amsterdam, The Netherlands; roosmarck@me.com
[2] Burn Center, Red Cross Hospital, 1942 LE Beverwijk, The Netherlands; kgardien@rkz.nl (K.L.M.G.); breed@kpnplanet.nl (R.S.B.)
[3] Department of Plastic, Reconstructive & Hand Surgery, Amsterdam Movement Sciences Research Institute, Amsterdam UMC, Vrije Universiteit Amsterdam, 1081 HV Amsterdam, The Netherlands
[4] Association of Dutch Burn Centers, 1942 LE Beverwijk, The Netherlands; mvlig@burns.nl
[5] Department of Surgery, Leiden University Medical Center, 2333 ZA Leiden, The Netherlands
* Correspondence: e.middelkoop@vumc.nl; Tel.: +31-251275500

Received: 24 November 2018; Accepted: 8 January 2019; Published: 12 January 2019

check for updates

Abstract: Platelet rich plasma (PRP) is blood plasma with a platelet concentration above baseline. When activated, PRP releases growth factors involved in all stages of wound healing, potentially boosting the healing process. To expand our knowledge of the effectiveness of PRP, it is crucial to know the content and composition of PRP products. In this study, growth factor quantification measurements of PRP from burn patients and gender- and age-matched controls were performed. The PRP of burn patients showed levels of growth factors comparable to those of the PRP of healthy volunteers. Considerable intra-individual variation in growth factor content was found. However, a correlation was found between the platelet count of the PRP and most of the growth factors measured.

Keywords: platelets; burns; growth factors; platelet rich plasma; quantification

---

1. Introduction

Platelet rich plasma (PRP) is produced from blood plasma, and results in a platelet concentration above baseline. When PRP is activated, platelets release their growth factors, such as platelet-derived growth factor (PDGF), fibroblast growth factor (FGF), transforming growth factor β (TGF-β), epidermal growth factor (EGF), and vascular endothelial growth factor (VEGF). These growth factors are involved in all stages of wound healing. Improved wound healing qualities have been attributed to PRP, by the multitude of growth factors delivered to a wound [1].

There are numerous types of PRP products and preparation methods. An even larger number of different application areas exist, varying from sports medicine and orthopedics to chronic and acute wounds, as well as aesthetic applications. These are described in an extensive body of literature; however, most studies advocating the use of PRP comprise case reports and patient cohorts. Randomized controlled trials are rare, and systematic reviews repeatedly fail to show strong conclusive evidence of the effects of PRP [1–3]. This could be partly due to the great variability of PRP products, namely, variability in preparation protocols; different composition (with/without leukocytes and fibrin content); variability in platelet baseline count and PRP yield, growth factor content per platelet;

and finally activation and application methods. Furthermore, for all the different applications, the most desirable number of platelets and amount of growth factors that should be used are unknown.

Recently, a new classification system for PRP was proposed by Harrison et al., in an effort to systematize studies done on PRP [4]. This paper also emphasizes the importance of quality control of the platelet preparations. To expand our knowledge of the effectiveness of PRP, it is essential to know the content and composition of the PRP products. Growth factor quantification still seems the best type of quality control of PRP, since platelet count and growth factor quantification do not appear to correlate in a consistent way [5,6]. A recent systematic review of commercial PRP separation systems showed a large heterogeneity in the concentrations of platelets, leukocytes, and growth factors [7]. One of the inclusion criteria of this systematic review was that the studies had to investigate 'healthy volunteers.' This is somewhat curious, because autologous PRP is mostly applied in patients and not healthy volunteers. An extensive search of the literature was carried out; however, we could not find studies describing the quantification of PRP content in actual patients.

In burn patients, the use of PRP has been ascribed potential positive effects on burn wound healing [1,8]. The current study was part of a recent randomized trial, which failed to show significant added value of PRP in acute burns [9]. In addition to the variables in PRP in general described above, a few more can be added for burn injury. Burn injury has a severe impact on the internal physiology of patients [10], and platelet counts show a distinct pattern post-burn injury, with a nadir at day 3, a peak around day 14, followed by a gradual return to normal values [11], thus affecting the baseline platelet count from which the PRP is produced. Since platelets are the core ingredient of PRP, it is crucial to know if and how the quality of the PRP could be affected by the burn injury. In a recent study, it was found that the platelets in burn patients were not overly activated and remained functional and not deprived of growth factors; however, this was tested in platelets in whole blood samples [12]. The current study investigated the quality of PRP, classified as L-PRPIIB-1 according to the new classification system, which implicates leukocyte-rich PRP, activated before application (II), with a mean platelet count between 900–1700 (B), and prepared with a gravitational centrifugation technique (1) [4], from burn patients compared with age and gender matched healthy controls.

2. Results

2.1. Demographics and Hematology

The demographics and hematology results are listed in Table 1. By chance, the patients included were sampled on longitudinal days post-burn injury (Figure 1). The platelet counts follow the known time course post-burn injury as has been described, with only patient 3 still having a lower count than expected. A possible explanation could be that this patient suffered the largest burn [11].

Int. J. Mol. Sci. **2019**, *20*, 288

Table 1. Demographics and hematology results.

	Age	Sex	Post-Burn Day	TBSA * (%)	Platelet Count × 10^3/µL Whole Blood	Platelet Count × 10^3/µL Platelet Rich Plasma (PRP)	Leukocyte Count × 10^3/µL Whole Blood	Leukocyte Count × 10^3/µL PRP	Erythrocyte Count × 10^6/µL Whole Blood	Erythrocyte Count × 10^6/µL PRP
P1	35	F	3	16	212	1141	9.2	29.0	3.0	1.2
P2	67	F	6	9	467	1792	7.5	30.0	3.8	0.5
P3	40	M	10	61	173	1003	8.1	30.0	2.6	1.1
P4	61	F	13	12	524	2500	20.3	94.1	2.6	1.9
P5	72	M	17	5	343	1326	8.10	29.4	4.0	0.5
V1	41	F			282	713	6.3	16.7	4.5	1.5
V2	65	F			311	1248	5.8	24.5	4.4	0.7
V3	42	M			298	1277	7.5	33.2	4.6	0.9
V4	53	F			356	1448	3.8	19.8	4.4	0.7
V5	61	M			284	1678	7.5	48.2	4.7	0.9

* TBSA % = percentage total body surface area percentage burned; P = patient; V = Volunteer.

2.2. Platelet Concentration Ratio

The mean ratio of platelet concentration from whole blood platelet to PRP was 4.44 (SD1.04 range: 2.5 to 5.9) (Figure 1). There was no difference between patients and volunteers, 4.7 vs. 4.2 respectively (p = 0.78 Mann–Whitney Test).

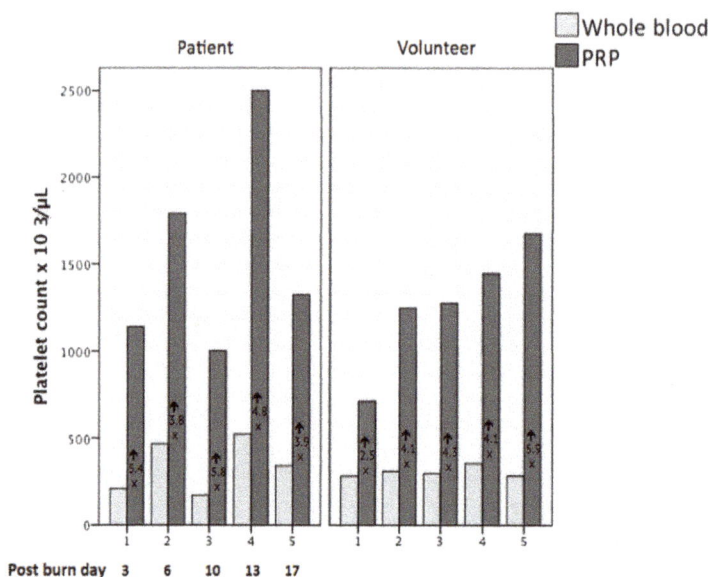

Figure 1. Platelet count in whole blood versus platelet count platelet rich plasma (PRP), in patient group and in volunteer group; the platelet concentration factor is depicted underneath the arrow; under patient group the post- burn day is shown.

2.3. Growth Factor Content

No significant difference was found in mean growth factor content between PRP from burn patients and that from matched healthy controls (Mann–Whitney tests: transforming growth factor β (TGFβ-1) (mean patient 57,542 pg/mL vs. volunteers: 45,389 pg/mL) p = 0.2; TGFβ-2 (mean patients 1292 pg/mL vs. volunteers 934 pg/mL) p = 0.2; TGFβ-3 (mean patients 21 pg/ml vs. volunteers 21 pg/mL) p = 0.9; platelet derived growth factor (PDGF-AA) (mean patients 36,327 pg/mL vs. volunteers 32,113 pg/mL) p = 0.4; PDGF-BB (mean patients 56,031 pg/mL vs. volunteers 44,566 pg/mL) p = 0.5; vascular endothelial growth factor (VEGF) (mean patients 701 pg/mL vs. volunteers 756 pg/mL) p = 0.8; epidermal growth factor (EGF) (mean patients 73 pg/mL vs. volunteers 60 pg/mL) p = 0.7; fibroblast growth factor (FGF-2) (mean patients 224 pg/mL vs. 220 volunteers pg/mL) p = 0.8), nor in growth factor per platelet ratio (data not shown).

There was a noticeable correlation between platelets in PRP and growth factor concentration, when volunteer 5 (which was considered an outlier, because it was more than 2SD outside the mean ratio) was eliminated, except for VEGF and FGF (Figures 2–4 and Supplemental Figures S1–S5) Spearman's rho correlation tests: TGFβ1 R = 0.95, p = 0.008; TGFβ-2 R = 0.9, p = 0.001; TGFβ-3 R = 0.8 p = 0.02; PDGF-AA R = 0.9, p = 0.002; PDGF-BB R = 0.8, p = 0.008; VEGF R = 0.3, p = 0.4; FGF-2 R = 0.1, p = 0.7; EGF R = 0.7, p = 0.03).

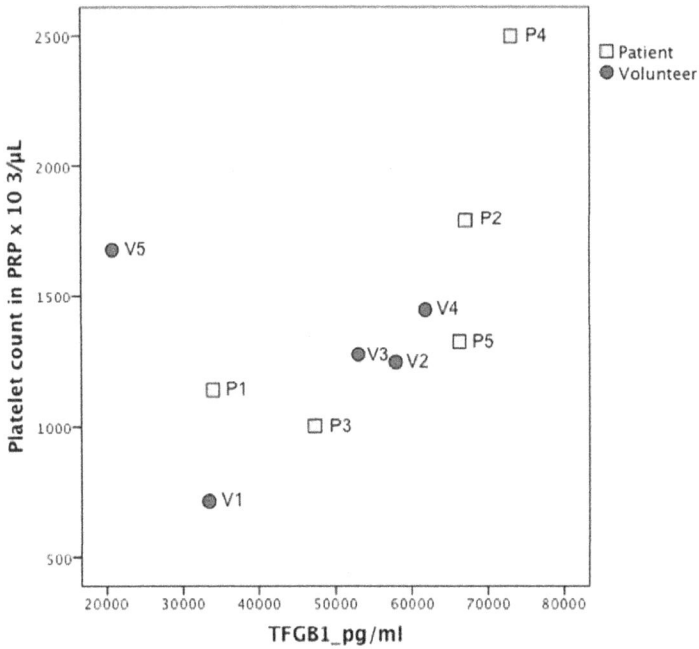

Figure 2. Growth factor quantification per platelet count in platelet rich plasma (PRP) for transforming growth factor β (TGFβ1).

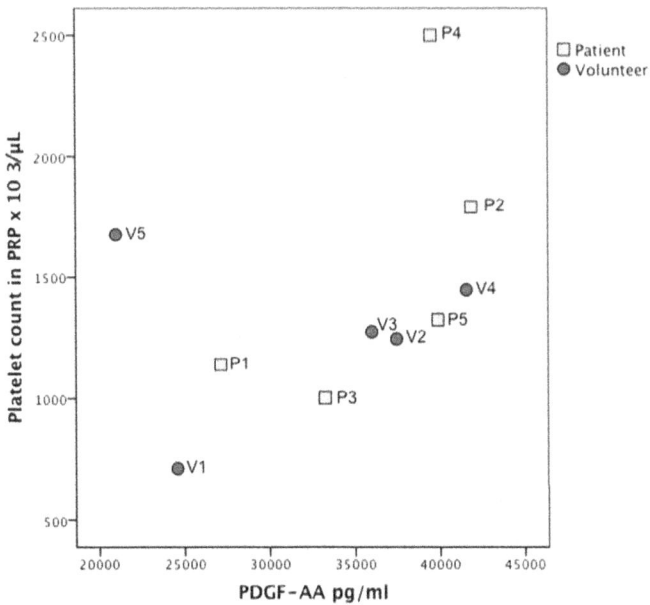

Figure 3. Growth factor quantification per platelet count in platelet rich plasma (PRP) for platelet derived growth factor (PDGF) AA.

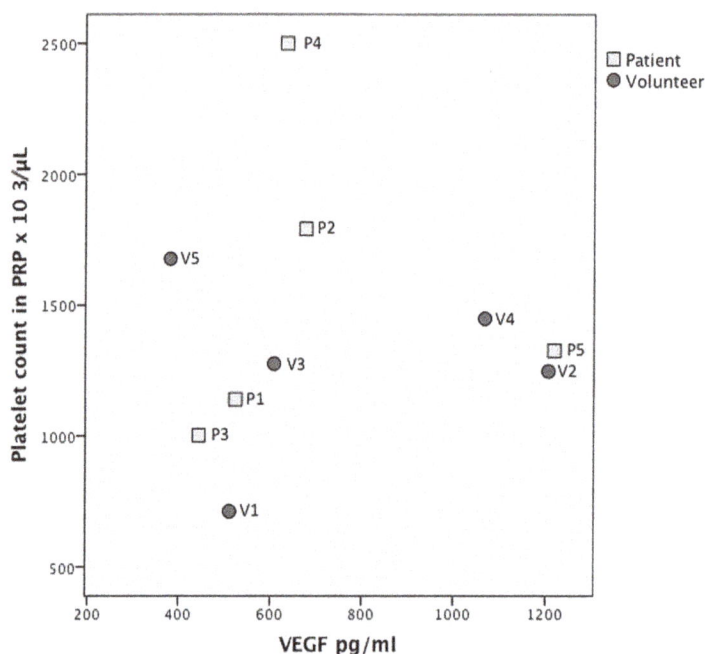

Figure 4. Growth factor quantification per platelet count in platelet rich plasma (PRP) for vascular endothelial growth factor (VEGF).

3. Discussion

In this study it was shown that PRP of burn patients, L-PRPIIB-1, according to the new classification system [4], had comparable levels of growth factors to that of the same type of PRP of healthy volunteers. This is despite the systemic effects that burn injury has on the physiology of burn patients. This is relevant additional information to the main RCT, of which the current study was a part [9], that showed that the addition of PRP to the treatment of burn wounds did not result in improved graft take and epithelialization, nor in better scar quality. Only minor beneficial effects in certain subgroups were seen. From the current study, it can be concluded that the lack of substantial clinical effect of the PRP in acute burns does not seem to be explained by a general lack of available growth factors in the PRP of burn patients.

We did find a considerable variation in growth factor concentrations, which is in accordance with the literature on PRP products [7]. More research is required to determine an optimum platelet and growth factor concentration for burns, as well as for other applications. There is some consensus on the minimum platelet counts required in PRP; it is generally advocated that a minimum platelet count of $0.8–1 \times 10^6/\mu L$ should be obtained, however, there is no compelling evidence for this. Interestingly enough, we found a correlation between the platelet count in PRP and most of the growth factors measured. This has not always been demonstrated in previous studies [5,6]. The platelet count in PRP did not correlate with the outcome in sub-analyses of the main RCT, of which the current study was a part [9]. Nevertheless, platelet count can potentially be used as a quality control parameter for future research, since it is far more feasible to routinely determine the platelet count in PRP than it is to analyze growth factors. We recommend that further research be done to confirm this finding.

A limitation of this study is that only a small cohort of patients was tested, so the results should be considered preliminary. Furthermore, subgroup analyses were not feasible. The effect of gender and age could not be studied; this may influence the growth factor content, as has recently been suggested [6]. Nor could the effect of the percentage total body surface area burned (TBSA %) or timing of the post-burn injury be clarified. It would also have been very interesting if we had been able to correlate the growth factor content with the clinical outcome in the RCT; however, this was not realistic in this small adjunct study.

In conclusion, in this preliminary study, burn patients have a comparable platelet growth factor content in L-PRPIIB-1 to that of matched healthy volunteers. In accordance with the literature, considerable individual variation in growth factor content was found; however, a correlation between growth factor concentration and platelet count in PRP was seen.

4. Materials and Methods

This study was performed as a sub-study (amendment NL28331.094.09) of a randomized controlled trial (ISRCTN14946762) performed in the burn center of Beverwijk, the Netherlands, which compared autologous platelet-rich plasma with standard treatment for burn wounds [9]. All ethical committee and institutional permissions were obtained to recruit five consecutive patients, who were already included in the main RCT, after additional informed consent had been obtained, between December 2011 and March 2012. The PRP was prepared with the Gravitational Platelet Separation System (GPS-III system, Biomet Merck Biomaterials, Darmstadt, Germany). The instructions of the manufacturer were strictly followed. For details of the trial and preparation methods see previous report [9]. From 27 ml blood from five patients, we prepared PRP with an additional GPS-III mini-kit. We matched the patients by gender and age with five healthy volunteers and also prepared PRP with a GPS-III mini-kit.

A small amount of PRP and non-citrated whole blood (WB) was collected in an EDTA (ethylene di-amine tetra-acetic acid) tube, and analyzed for baseline measurements, using the Cell-Dyn Sapphire 2 hematology analyzer (Abbott Diagnostics Division, IL, USA). The platelet, erythrocyte, and leukocyte counts were determined.

The PRP was activated with autologous thrombin according to the manufacturer's protocol (i.e., PRP:thrombin = 10:1) and incubated for one hour at room temperature to mimic clinical application as accurately as possible. Activated PRP was centrifuged ($10,000 \times g$ at 4 °C for 15 min), clots were removed, and supernatants were collected and stored at -80 °C until further analysis. Magnetic bead panel Milliplex MAP kits (EMD Millipore, Billerica, MA, USA) were used to analyze FGF-2, EGF, VEGF, TGFβ-1, TGFβ-2, TGFβ-3, PDGF-AA, and PDGF-BB. Separate kits were used to analyze TGFβ and PDGF. All the kits were used according to the manufacturers' protocol. The Milliplex MAP kits were measured using Bio-Plex 200 (Bio-Rad, Hercules, CA, USA) and the data were analyzed using Bio-Plex manager software.

For statistical analyses, SPSS statistics 21 (IBM) software was used. For the comparison of means, a Mann–Whitney test was used. Correlation was tested with the non-parametric Spearman's rho test. Significance was set at $p \leq 0.05$.

Supplementary Materials: Supplementary materials can be found at http://www.mdpi.com/1422-0067/20/2/288/s1.

Author Contributions: The authors of this paper contributed in the following ways: conceptualization, R.E.M., R.S.B. and E.M.; methodology, R.E.M.; software, R.E.M. and M.V.; validation, R.E.M., K.L.M.G. and M.V.; formal analysis, M.V.; investigation, R.E.M. and K.L.M.G.; resources, R.E.M.; data curating, R.E.M., K.L.M.G. and M.V.; writing—original draft preparation, R.E.M. and E.M.; writing—review and editing, R.E.M., E.M. and R.S.B.; visualization, R.E.M.; supervision, E.M. and R.S.B.; project administration, R.E.M. and K.L.M.G.; funding acquisition, R.E.M. and E.M.

Funding: Biomet (Biomet Europe BV, Dordrecht, the Netherlands) provided the PRP-preparation kits and an unrestricted educational grant, which covered some of the remaining costs of this study. Any remaining costs were covered by a research grant to Association of Dutch Burn Center, from the Dutch Burns Foundation Grant nr.12.02.

Conflicts of Interest: The authors declare no conflict of interest. The funders had no role in the design of the study; in the collection, analyses, or interpretation of data; in the writing of the manuscript, or in the decision to publish the results.

References

1. Marck, R.E.; Middelkoop, E.; Breederveld, R.S. Considerations on the use of platelet-rich plasma, specifically for burn treatment. *J. Burn Care Res. Off. Publ. Am. Burn Assoc.* **2014**, *35*, 219–227. [CrossRef] [PubMed]
2. Grassi, A.; Napoli, F.; Romandini, I.; Samuelsson, K.; Zaffagnini, S.; Candrian, C.; Filardo, G. Is platelet-rich plasma (PRP) effective in the treatment of acute muscle injuries? A systematic review and meta-analysis. *Sports Med.* **2018**, *48*, 971–989. [CrossRef] [PubMed]
3. Martinez-Zapata, M.J.; Marti-Carvajal, A.J.; Sola, I.; Exposito, J.A.; Bolibar, I.; Rodriguez, L.; Garcia, J.; Zaror, C. Autologous platelet-rich plasma for treating chronic wounds. *Cochrane Database Syst. Rev.* **2016**, CD006899. [CrossRef] [PubMed]
4. Harrison, P. The use of platelets in regenerative medicine and proposal for a new classification system: Guidance from the SSC of the ISTH. *J. Thromb. Haemost.* **2018**, *16*, 1895–1900. [CrossRef] [PubMed]
5. Weibrich, G.; Kleis, W.K.; Hafner, G.; Hitzler, W.E. Growth factor levels in platelet-rich plasma and correlations with donor age, sex, and platelet count. *J. Craniomaxillofac. Surg.* **2002**, *30*, 97–102. [CrossRef] [PubMed]
6. Xiong, G.; Lingampalli, N.; Koltsov, J.C.B.; Leung, L.L.; Bhutani, N.; Robinson, W.H.; Chu, C.R. Men and women differ in the biochemical composition of platelet-rich plasma. *Am. J. Sports Med.* **2018**, *46*, 409–419. [CrossRef] [PubMed]
7. Oudelaar, B.W.; Peerbooms, J.C.; Huis In't Veld, R.; Vochteloo, A.J.H. Concentrations of blood components in commercial platelet-rich plasma separation systems: A review of the literature. *Am. J. Sports Med.* **2018**, 363546517746112. [CrossRef] [PubMed]
8. Picard, F.; Hersant, B.; Bosc, R.; Meningaud, J.P. Should we use platelet-rich plasma as an adjunct therapy to treat "acute wounds", "burns" and "laser therapies": A review and a proposal of a quality criteria checklist for further studies. *Wound Repair Regener. Off. Publ. Wound Heal. Soc. Eur. Tissue Repair Soc.* **2015**, *23*, 163–170. [CrossRef] [PubMed]
9. Marck, R.E.; Gardien, K.L.; Stekelenburg, C.M.; Vehmeijer, M.; Baas, D.; Tuinebreijer, W.E.; Breederveld, R.S.; Middelkoop, E. The application of platelet-rich plasma in the treatment of deep dermal burns: A randomized, double-blind, intra-patient controlled study. *Wound Repair Regener. Off. Publ. Wound Heal. Soc. Eur. Tissue Repair Soc.* **2016**, *24*, 712–720. [CrossRef] [PubMed]
10. Evers, L.H.; Bhavsar, D.; Mailander, P. The biology of burn injury. *Exp. Dermatol.* **2010**, *19*, 777–783. [CrossRef] [PubMed]
11. Marck, R.E.; Montagne, H.L.; Tuinebreijer, W.E.; Breederveld, R.S. Time course of thrombocytes in burn patients and its predictive value for outcome. *Burns J. Int. Soc. Burn Inj.* **2013**, *39*, 714–722. [CrossRef] [PubMed]
12. Marck, R.E.; van der Bijl, I.; Korsten, H.; Lorinser, J.; de Korte, D.; Middelkoop, E. Activation, function and content of platelets in burn patients. *Platelets* **2018**, 1–7. [CrossRef] [PubMed]

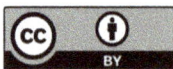

International Journal of
Molecular Sciences

MDPI

Article

Assessment of the Efficacy of Platelet-Rich Plasma in the Treatment of Traumatic Canine Fractures

Sergio López [1], José M. Vilar [1], Joaquín J. Sopena [2,3], Elena Damià [2], Deborah Chicharro [2], José M. Carrillo [2,3,*], Belén Cuervo [2] and Mónica Rubio [2,3]

[1]   Animal Pathology Department, Instituto Universitario de Investigaciones Biomédicas y Universitarias, Universidad de Las Palmas de Gran Canaria, 35416 Trasmontaña S/N, Arucas, Spain; sergiolopezbarbeta@gmail.com (S.L.); jose.vilar@ulpgc.es (J.M.V.)
[2]   Bioregenerative Medicine and Applied Surgery Research Group, Animal Medicine and Surgery Department, Veterinary Faculty, Universidad Cardenal Herrera-CEU, CEU Universities, 46115 Valencia, Spain; jsopena@uchceu.es (J.J.S.); elena.damia@uchceu.es (E.D.); debora.chicharro@uchceu.es (D.C.); belen.cuervo@uchceu.es (B.C.); mrubio@uchceu.es (M.R.)
[3]   García Cugat Foundation CEU-UCH Chair of Medicine and Regenerative Surgery, 08006 Barcelona, Spain
*   Correspondence: jcarrill@uchceu.es; Tel.: +34-96-136-9000 (ext. 66216)

Received: 5 February 2019; Accepted: 27 February 2019; Published: 1 March 2019

check for
updates

Abstract: The role of platelet-rich plasma (PRP) in promoting the healing of bone fractures has not yet been clearly stated. The aim of this prospective clinical study was to evaluate the effectiveness of plasma rich in growth factors (PRGF, a PRP derivate) in the treatment of naturally-occurring bone fractures in dogs. With this objective, sixty-five dogs with radius/ulna or tibia/fibula bone fractures were randomly divided into two groups (PRGF and saline solution (SS) groups) and checked at days 0, 7, 14, 21, 28, 35, 42, 49, 56, 60, 63, 70, 120, and 180. All the fractures were treated with an external skeletal fixation, and pain was controlled with Carprofen. Healing was evaluated by physical examination, limb function, radiography, and by a Likert-type owner satisfaction questionnaire. A faster fracture healing was observed in the PRGF group, with statistically significant differences with respect to the SS group. Swelling at the fracture site was significantly greater at day 14 and 28 in animals injected with PRGF, and more pain on palpation was found in the area at day 28. The injection of PRGF in acute bone fractures accelerates bone healing.

Keywords: PRGF; Carprofen; dog; fracture; bone healing

1. Introduction

Plasma-rich growth factors (PRGF) are currently being used to promote bone healing in reconstructive surgeries [1–3]. In canine models, several experimental studies have published the effect of this platelet rich plasma derivate in osteoarthritis with differing results [4–7]. Platelets are very important in the wound healing process [1]; they rapidly arrive at the wound side and begin the coagulation process. In addition, they release multiple wound-healing growth factors and cytokines within 10 min [1–3]. Platelets are viable for seven days and will continue to release growth factors into the tissue during this time [8].

The use of PRGF is based on the assumption that higher platelet concentrations release significant quantities of growth factors, which aids in bone healing [9–11]. Specifically, growth factors are thought to be a contributing factor in bone regeneration and in increasing vascularization, which are vital features of the bone-healing process [6].

Treatments with PRGF have given excellent clinical results in oral and maxillofacial surgery in humans [9,12], and in bone and cartilage healing in animal studies [7,13,14]. Growth factors have also been used in the treatment of large wounds and skin defects in burn patients [15–17]. However, some controversial results can be found in the cited literature; therefore, the effectiveness of this technique requires further research.

To the authors' knowledge, articles discussing fresh fractures and delayed fracture healing are very scarce [18,19]. In the veterinary field, no publications were found regarding the use of PRGF in fractures.

In this study, the dogs used were clinical patients, but also clinical animal models. In the present study, we hypothesize that treating canine bone fractures with PRGF would accelerate bone healing. Thus, the aim of this clinical trial is to evaluate the use of PRGF in the treatment of naturally occurring bone fractures in dogs.

2. Results

A total of 68 dogs were initially evaluated; however, only 43 met the necessary requirements to be included in the study.

The dogs were randomly assigned to either PGRF or SS groups. Twenty dogs were included in the PRGF group (47%) and 23 in the SS group (53%). The results for each dog belonging to either the PRGF or the SS groups are summarized in their respective tables (Tables 1 and 2).

The mean weight for each group was 16.27 kg for the PRGF group and 13.07 kg for the SS group. Mean age was 40.85 and 57.17 months, respectively, with no statistical differences between groups in these parameters ($p \geq 0.08$).

During the study, all the animals received Carprofen as a rescue analgesia at least one time during the first seven days except for 2 and 4 patients in the PRGF and SS groups, respectively, with no statistical differences between groups ($p \geq 0.05$).

The time (mean $\pm$ SD) for implant removal was 41.3 $\pm$ 11.73 days in the PRGF group and 49 $\pm$ 12.12 days in the SS group. This difference was statistically significant ($p = 0.03$) (Figure 1).

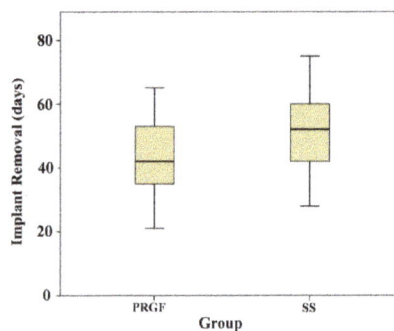

Figure 1. Boxplot corresponding to the days of implant removal for both PRGF and SS groups. Mean time was significantly higher in the SS group.

The time when full weight support was detected was 22.1 $\pm$ 13.64 days and 25.47 $\pm$ 14.9 days in the PRGF and SS groups, respectively; however, this difference was not statistically significant ($p = 0.45$). All animals were sound within six months post-surgery.

Swelling in the fracture site was present in both groups up to day 14 without statistically significant differences between the groups. Between days 14 and 28, swelling was still present in the PRGF group ($p < 0.048$).

The joint movement evaluation showed almost 100% joint mobility without differences between groups in any of the checking periods.

The evaluation of pain on palpation showed statistically significant differences at day 28 between groups, where pain was still present in the PRGF group ($p = 0.041$).

Table 1. Individual data and main results for PRGF group.

Dog #	Breed	Gender	Weight (kg)	Age (months)	Fracture L	Configuration	Weight Support	Time I Removal (days) *	Complications	Analgesia
1	G DANE	M	53	11	U/R	TYPE IIB 2X3	7	35 (39)	NO	Y
2	CROSSBREED	F	4	24	U/R	TYPE IIB 1X2	7	42 (45)	NO	N
3	CROSSBREED	M	17,8	36	U/R	TYPE IIB 2x4	21	28 (32)	NO	Y
4	CROSSBREED	F	8,5	96	U/R	TYPE IIB 2X3	14	56 (60)	GE	Y
5	CROSSBREED	F	4	3	T/F	TYPE IIB 2X3	7	21 (21)	NO	Y
6	CROSSBREED	M	4	36	U/R	TYPE IIB 2X3	28	63 (63)	NO	Y
7	CROSSBREED	M	7	48	T/F	TYPE IIB 2X3	21	35 (40)	PL	Y
8	CROSSBREED	F	6	6	T/F	TYPE IIB	21	28 (30)	NO	Y
9	CROSSBREED	F	2,3	60	U/R	TYPE IIB 2X3	21	42 (42)	PL	Y
10	CROSSBREED	F	22	12	U/R	TYPE IIB 2X3	14	35 (36)	NO	Y
11	CROSSBREED	F	72	20	U/R	TYPE IIB 2X3	60	56 (56)	NO	Y
12	CROSSBREED	M	6,3	48	U/R	TYPE IIB 2X3	60	42 (45)	NO	Y
13	CROSSBREED	M	4	12	U/R	TYPE IIB 2X3	7	56 (56)	NO	Y
14	BELG SHEPH	F	16	96	U/R	TYPE IIB 2X3	21	49 (49)	PL	Y
15	CROSSBREED	M	4,5	24	U/R	TYPE IIB 2X3	21	28 (30)	NO	Y
16	PODENCO	M	22	56	U/R	TYPE IIB 2X3	28	28 (28)	NO	Y
17	CROSSBREED	M	6	70	U/R	TYPE IIB 2X3	21	63 (65)	NO	Y
18	RAT VAL	F	2	24	U/R	TYPE IIB 2X3	21	49 (50)	NO	Y
19	MASTIFF	M	52	36	T/F	TYPE IIB 2X3	28	35 (40)	NO	Y
20	CROSSBREED	M	12	99	U/R	TYPE IIB 2X3	14	35 (35)	NO	N

* The first number references the checking day when stage 4/5 was reached radiographically and the implant was ready for removal; the number in parenthesis refers to the day the implant was removed. RAT VAL: Ratonero Valenciano.

Table 2. Individual data and main results for SS group.

Dog #	Breed	Gender	Weight (kg)	Age (months)	Fracture L	Configuration	Weight Support	Time I Removal (days) *	Complications	Analgesia
1	SIB HUSK	M	27	15	U/R	TYPE IIB	60	63 (69)	PL	Y
2	RAT VAL	F	1,7	6	U/R	TYPE IIB 1X2	21	35 (35)	NO	N
3	CROSSBREED	F	5,5	12	T/F	TYPE IIB1.5X2	7	28 (34)	NO	N
4	CROSSBREED	F	5,5	12	U/R	TYPE IIB1.5X2	7	28 (31)	PL	N
5	AM STAFFORD	M	30	72	U/R	TYPE IIB 2X3	21	35 (36)	NO	Y
6	CROSSBREED	M	4,5	60	U/R	TYPE IIB 2X3	7	56 (58)	NO	Y
7	CROSSBREED	M	20	72	U/R	TYPE IIB 2X3	21	70 (75)	NO	Y
8	GRIFFON	M	15	50	U/R	TYPE IIB 2X3	28	42 (42)	NO	Y
9	GER SHEPH	F	34	70	T/F	TYPE IIB 2X3	21	42 (44)	NO	Y
10	W HIGH W TERR	F	5,6	48	U/R	TYPE IIB 2X3	21	42 (42)	GE	Y
11	CROSSBREED	M	18	48	U/R	TYPE IIB 2X3	21	42 (45)	NO	Y
12	CROSSBREED	F	12	60	T/F	TYPE IIB 2X3	21	42 (45)	NO	Y
13	CROSSBREED	F	3	24	U/R	TYPE IIB 2X3	21	56 (57)	NO	Y
14	MALTESE	F	9	192	T/F	TYPE IIB 2X3	60	56 (60)	NO	Y
15	RAT VAL	F	5	111	T/F	TYPE IIB	21	63 (68)	NO	Y
16	BELG SHEPH	M	34	86	T/F	TYPE IIB	28	63 (65)	NO	N
17	BELG SHEPH	F	9	20	T/F	TYPE IIB 2X3	28	63 (64)	NO	Y
18	YORKSHIRE	F	1,5	35	U/R	TYPE IIB 2X3	21	35 (38)	PL	Y
19	POODLE	F	8	122	U/R	TYPE IIB 2X3	21	49 (50)	NO	Y
20	CROSSBREED	M	25	75	U/R	TYPE IIB 2X3	21	56 (60)	NO	Y
21	DALMATIAN	M	22	46	T/F	TYPE IIB 2X3	21	49 (52)	NO	Y
22	YORKSHIRE	F	1,5	24	U/R	TYPE IIB 2X3	60	56 (60)	NO	Y
23	CROSSBREED	M	4	55	U/R	TYPE IIB 2X3	28	56 (60)	NO	Y

* The first number references the checking day when stage 4/5 was radiographically reached and the implant was ready for removal; the number in parenthesis refers to the day the implant was removed. SIB HUSK: Siberian Husky; RAT VAL: Ratonero Valenciano; AM STAFFORD: American Staffordshire Terrier; GER SHEPH: German Shepherd; W HIGH W TERR: West Highland White Terrier; BELG SHEPH: Belgian Shepherd.

No significant differences were found in the assessment of owner satisfaction at implant removal, with a satisfaction between 4 (24% in PRGF, 25% in SS) and 5 (76% in PRGF, 75% in SS).

Complications were recorded. One dog suffered gastroenteritis, and three dogs had pins become loose in the PRGF group. The same number of complications occurred in SS group (Tables 1 and 2).

3. Discussion

In the present study, the beneficial effect of PRGF in acute ulna/radius and tibia/fibula fracture healing has been proven, achieving a faster healing compared with controls. However, in all cases, a primary and non-complicated healing was present.

To the authors' knowledge, there is no published clinical research discussing the use of PRGF in fractures in a canine model. Experimentally, some studies proved there was faster bone regeneration when PRGF or other autologous platelet concentrates were applied [20,21]. In human medicine, there was only one clinical study evaluating the healing of fresh fractures using PRGF with no positive effect [18]. On the contrary, a clinical case with a delayed union fracture treated with autologous PRGF showed a favorable healing and concluded to be a safe technology for patients [19].

PRGF has also been used by other authors in combination with other therapeutics, showing positive results. Ya-dong Zhang et al. [22] proved that the use of PRGF combined with a degradable bioactive borate glass promotes functional bone repair. On the other hand, other authors [4] found no effect of PRGF on non-grafted implants in dogs; nevertheless, we cannot compare these results with our study because a different process was used to obtain the PRGF: using thrombin (100U/mL) to stimulate growth factor release rather than calcium chloride.

It is known that Carprofen is suitable alone or in combination with other NSAIDs for the control of pain and swelling in dogs [23,24]. Gastrointestinal inflammation and ulceration are among the most common side defects reported in the literature [25]. In our study, there were only two animals with gastroenteritis, and they responded positively to the conventional treatment.

In the present study, it has been observed that the surgical application of PRGF at the fracture site is associated with increased swelling and oedema during the first days, probably due to the activation of angiogenesis and cell activation [26]. The enhancement of the arrival and formation of blood vessels increases heat, pain, and redness of the area. This swelling associated with oedema has been effectively treated with oral Carprofen.

In any case, increased swelling did not affect the animals' gait nor the functional ability of the joint. In this sense, some papers reported the inhibitory effect of interleukins, which may be attributed to PRP [27]. This effect may be related to a reduction of acute pain in the fracture site, even though the activation of angiogenesis may cause an increased perception of discomfort and inflammation [26]. Thus, even if the application of PRGF increases oedema and swelling on the area, the limb's function was minimally affected during the first days.

Good results have been obtained using PRP to accelerate bone fusion [28]. In our case, the group receiving the PRGF injection presented an earlier implant removal, which is in agreement with those who state that chemotactic and mitogenic effect on mesenchymal cells (stem cells) and osteoblasts accelerate bone healing [29,30].

A rapid return to functionality is crucial for quick and correct healing; when the limb bears weight, a transmission of forces takes place that stimulates osteoinduction. Likewise, early activity boosts vascularization and avoids muscle atrophy, which are factors that clearly activate bone healing. Moreover, the Carprofen helped to control pain and acute swelling at the fracture site, facilitating an earlier return to functionality [29]. This shows that swelling control and post-surgical analgesia are fundamental for early functionality of the affected limb and represent an important parameter to be assessed by the pet owners.

Regarding external fixation, all the animals showed limb weight bearing 48 h after surgery. Very few complications arose in relation to the use of external skeletal fixation. One animal presented a secondary infection, which is a usual side effect, and only six animals presented pin loosening. Other studies show a larger number of cases presenting pin loosening as the most frequent complication [31].

The present study has three main limitations. First, the use of dogs with a wide weight range potentially limited results that are more accurate. A narrow weight range could provide more reliable and accurate results, at least for a specific weight range. Second, a biomechanical analysis of gait could provide full objective results regarding limb function. Third, statistical analysis of the variable "swelling at the fracture site" could provide more accurate results if it is considered a continuous variable instead of categorical, avoiding detection, performance, and reporting biases; however, the presence of hematoma or callous formation at the fracture site could potentially hinder precise measurements.

4. Materials and Methods

A multicentric study was designed and formed by four surgeons in four different veterinary clinical centers.

4.1. Animal Model

A total of 68 dogs were evaluated. The follow-up of the animals took place until six months after treatment. The inclusion criteria required the presence of a fresh, single, closed fracture and the absence of significant muscular soft tissue damage or abrasions.

The exclusion criteria for the present study were the following:

- Animals presenting concurrent systemic disease (*Leishmania* spp., *Ehrlichia* spp., etc.).
- Animals with hematological disorders.
- Animals with multiple fractures.
- Animals with internal lesions due to traumatism.
- Animals with open fractures or with significant damage to the surrounding soft-tissue.
- Animals with a significant weight loss or functional disabilities due to the treatment or other non-related causes.
- Animals needing different concurrent fixation methods due to the nature or clinical features of the fracture.

Fractures were classified according to the affected bone. In order to acquire similar healing conditions during the study, only tibia/fibula and radius/ulna fractures were included because of their poor vascularization due to their small surrounding muscular mass. The individual data of each dog for the PGRF and SS groups are summarized in Tables 1 and 2, respectively.

4.2. Fracture Treatment

All fractures were treated with conventional open or closed reduction and external fixation. The external skeletal fixation configuration frame was the most appropriate for each fracture, using type IIa or type IIb [32]. In all cases smooth pins of different diameters, connecting bars, and Meynard clamps were used.

After an initial clinical examination, animals were randomly assigned to one of the following groups depending on the treatment received:

- PRGF group: A single infiltration of PRGF in the fracture site during the surgery.
- SS group: A single infiltration of saline solution in the fracture site during the surgery.

All groups were treated with morphine (0.2 mg IM every 6 h), and Carprofen 4 mg/kg IV (Rimadyl®, Zoetis®, Spain) for 24 h. Cephalexin was administered as a post-surgery antibiotic.

After 24 h, the owners were allowed to give Carprofen (4 mg/kg/day) as a rescue analgesic if their pet presented clear signs of distress or discomfort. This fact should be reported during the clinical follow-up.

4.3. PRGF Preparation

For the present study, the extraction, isolation, activation, and administration model of the PRGF was standardized in all clinics following Anitua´s technique [9]. Briefly, 20 mL of blood were aseptically collected in four 4.5 mL citrate tubes, then centrifuged during 8 min at 460 G. Care has to be taken to avoid the buffy coat. Before the infiltration, the PRGF was activated with 5% of its volume with 10% calcium chloride. This obtained PRP derivate is enriched in platelets 2-fold over peripheral blood and less than 0.2 leucocytes $\times 10^6$/mL.

4.4. Evaluation

The limb function was evaluated on days 0 (pre-surgery), 7, 14, 21, 28, 60, 120, and 180 after the treatment began. This parameter was assessed by the same researcher evaluating animals when standing (1: weight-bearing; 2: no weight-bearing; or 3: no limb support), by observing swelling on the fracture site (0: presence or 1: absence), pain on palpation (0: presence or 1: absence), and joint movement (1: <40%; 2: 40–70%; 3: 70–90%; or 4: >90%).

The same radiologist, unaware of the group of treatment, patient, and surgeon involved, examined all radiographs. Each radiograph was evaluated by a stage score of 1–5 points (1: not visible callus formation; 2: barely visible callus formation; 3: scattered, not homogeneous callus; 4: uniform, mature callus formation; 5: very active, hyperthrophic callus formation). Radiographical examination started for each dog at day 21 and for every two weeks thereafter until the animal reached stage 2; beyond this period, radiographs were taken weekly, coinciding with the checkpoints for the other parameters. When a final score of 4/5 was achieved, implant removal was performed and recorded. The researcher who performed the evaluation of limbs and who read the radiographies were blind to the given treatment (PGRF or SS).

The use of the rescue analgesic and the presence of side effects were registered by the owner. The level of owner satisfaction with the clinical outcome of their pets during the first 28 days and at implant removal was evaluated with the following questionnaire referring to the level of satisfaction measured with a Likert-type scale (Table 3).

Table 3. Likert-type questionnaire of satisfaction for dog owners at time of implant removal.

How do you consider the lameness of (name of the pet) has progressed?				
Excellent	Good	Average	Fair	Poor
5	4	3	2	1
Do you think the treatment given to (name of the pet) has been effective?				
Strongly agree	Agree	Neutral	Disagree	Strongly disagree
How Do You Think (Name of the Pet) has Responded to the Treatment?				
Excellent	Good	Average	Fair	Poor
5	4	3	2	1

4.5. Statistical Analysis

Statistical analysis was performed with the computer program SPSS 18® for Windows® (IBM Co., Chicago, IL, USA). A value of $p < 0.05$ was considered statistically significant. The descriptive study of the population was shown as the mean ± SD. To determine the differences between the groups for non-categorical variables (weight, age, and total doses of Carprofen), a Kruskal–Wallis and Mann–Whitney test was done. To determine the effect of PRGF on implant removal time, a Kaplan–Meier curve and a log-rank test were used. The impact evaluation of total doses of Carprofen, age, weight, and bone fractured, within time to implant removal, a multivariable analysis was made using a Cox regression. Categorical variables (evaluation when walking, evaluation when standing, swelling, pain on palpation, joint movement, use of the recue analgesic, owner satisfaction, and

Int. J. Mol. Sci. **2019**, *20*, 1075

presence of side effects) were assessed using crosstabs with chi square, contingency coefficient, or the Fisher's exact test used when necessary in each variable.

The experimental procedure was approved by the ethics committee of the Research Institute in Biomedical and Health Sciences (ULPGC, Spain). The owners were informed about the aims of the study, and a written consent was required before including their pets in the study.

5. Conclusions

The use of PRGF for bone repair accelerates fracture consolidation and simultaneously promoted healing, achieving clearly shorter implant removal times.

Author Contributions: M.R., E.D., J.J.S., and J.M.C. performed and designed the experiment; S.L. and D.C. wrote the manuscript and participated in performing the experiment; M.R. performed statistical analysis; B.C. and S.L. participated in performing the experiment; and J.M.V. proofread the manuscript and gave approval of the final version.

Acknowledgments: The authors would like to acknowledge the pet owners for their cooperation in this study.

Conflicts of Interest: The authors declare no conflict of interest.

Abbreviations

PRGF	Plasma rich in growth factors
SS	Saline solution
Fracture L	Fracture location
U/R	Ulna/radius
T/F	Tibia/fibula
Time I removal	Time for implant removal
GE	Gastroenteritis
PL	Pin loosening
Y	Yes
N	No

References

1. Anitua, E. The use of plasma-rich growth factors (PRGF) in oral surgery. *Pract. Proc. Aesth. Dent.* **2001**, *13*, 487–493.
2. Anitua, E.A. Enhancement of osseointegration by generating a dynamic implant surface. *J. Oral Implantol.* **2006**, *32*, 72–76. [CrossRef] [PubMed]
3. Taschieri, S.; Rosano, G.; Weinstein, T.; Bortolin, M.; Del Fabbro, M. Treatment of through-and-through bone lesion using autologous growth factors and xenogeneic bone graft: A case report. *Oral Maxillofac. Surg.* **2012**, *16*, 57–64. [CrossRef] [PubMed]
4. Vilar, J.M.; Morales, M.; Santana, A.; Spinella, G.; Rubio, M.; Cuervo, B.; Cugat, R.; Carrillo, J.M. Controlled, blinded force platform analysis of the effect of intraarticular injection of autologous adipose-derived mesenchymal stem cells associated to PRGF-Endoret in osteoarthritic dogs. *BMC Vet. Res.* **2013**, *9*, 131. [CrossRef] [PubMed]
5. Jensen, T.B.; Bechtold, J.E.; Chen, X.; Vestermark, M.; Soballe, K. No effect of autologous growth factors (AGF) around ungrafted loaded implants in dogs. *Int. Orthop.* **2010**, *34*, 925–930. [CrossRef] [PubMed]
6. Li, N.Y.; Chen, L.Q.; Chen, T.; Jin, X.M.; Yuan, R.T. Effect of platelet-rich plasma and latissimus dorsi myofascia with blood vessel on vascularization of tissue engineered bone in dogs. *Hua Xi Kou Qiang Yi Xue Za Zhi* **2007**, *25*, 408–411. [PubMed]
7. Thor, A.L.; Hong, J.; Kjeller, G.; Sennerby, L.; Rasmusson, L. Correlation of platelet growth factor release in jawbone defect repair—A study in the dog mandible. *Clin. Implant Dent. Relat. Res.* **2013**, *15*, 759–768. [CrossRef] [PubMed]
8. Marx, R.E.; Carlson, E.R.; Eichstaedt, R.M.; Schimmele, S.R.; Strauss, J.E.; Georgeff, K.R. Platelet-rich plasma: Growth factor enhancement for bone grafts. *Oral Surg. Oral Med. Oral Pathol. Oral Radiol.* **1998**, *85*, 638–646.

9.   Anitua, E.; Sanchez, M.; Zalduendo, M.M.; de la Fuente, M.; Prado, R.; Orive, G.; Andia, I. Fibroblastic response to treatment with different preparations rich in growth factors. *Cell Prolif.* **2009**, *42*, 162–170. [CrossRef] [PubMed]

10. Marx, R.E.; Garg, A.K. The biology of platelets and the mechanism of platelet-rich plasma. In *Dental and Craniofacial Applications of Platelet-Rich Plasma*; Marx, R.E., Garg, A.K., Eds.; Quintessence Publishing Co.: Chicago, IL, USA, 2005; pp. 3–65.

11. Mishra, A.; Pavelko, T. Treatment of chronic elbow tendinosis with buffered platelet-rich plasma. *Am. J. Sports Med.* **2006**, *34*, 1774–1778. [CrossRef] [PubMed]

12. Anitua, E. Plasma rich in growth factors. Preliminary results of use in the preparation of future sites for implants. *Int. J. Oral Maxillofac. Implants* **1999**, *14*, 529–535. [PubMed]

13. Serra, C.I.; Soler, C.; Carrillo, J.M.; Sopena, J.J.; Redondo, J.I.; Cugat, R. Effect of autologous platelet-rich plasma on the repair of full-thickness articular defects in rabbits. *Knee Surg. Sports Traumatol. Arthrosc.* **2013**, *21*, 1730–1736. [PubMed]

14. Cugat, R.; Alentorn-Geli, E.; Steinbacher, G.; Alvarez-Diaz, P.; Cusco, X.; Seijas, R.; Barastegui, D.; Navarro, J.; Laiz, P.; Garcia-Balletbo, M. Treatment of Knee Osteochondral Lesions Using a Novel Clot of Autologous Plasma Rich in Growth Factors Mixed with Healthy Hyaline Cartilage Chips and Intra-Articular Injection of PRGF. *Case rep. Orthop.* **2017**, *2017*, 8284548. [CrossRef] [PubMed]

15. Nicoletti, G.; Saler, M.; Villani, L.; Rumolo, A.; Tresoldi, M.M.; Faga, A. Platelet Rich Plasma Enhancement of Skin Regeneration in an ex-vivo Human Experimental Model. *Front. Bioeng. Biotechnol.* **2019**, *7*, 2. [CrossRef] [PubMed]

16. Yang, H.S.; Shin, J.; Bhang, S.H.; Shin, J.Y.; Park, J.; Im, G.I.; Kim, C.S.; Kim, B.S. Enhanced skin wound healing by a sustained release of growth factors contained in platelet-rich plasma. *Exp. Mol. Med.* **2011**, *43*, 622–629. [CrossRef] [PubMed]

17. Cieslik-Bielecka, A.; Choukroun, J.; Odin, G.; Dohan Ehrenfest, D.M. L-PRP/L-PRF in esthetic plastic surgery, regenerative medicine of the skin and chronic wounds. *Curr. Pharm. Biotechnol.* **2012**, *13*, 1266–1277. [CrossRef] [PubMed]

18. Zhang, C.Q.; Yuan, T.; Zeng, B.F. Experimental study on effect of platelet-rich plasma in repair of bone defect. *Zhongguo Xiu Fu Chong Jian Wai Ke Za Zhi* 2003, *17*, 355–358. [PubMed]

19. Seijas, R.; Santana-Suarez, R.Y.; Garcia-Balletbo, M.; Cusco, X.; Ares, O.; Cugat, R. Delayed union of the clavicle treated with plasma rich in growth factors. *Acta Orthop. Belgica* 2010, *76*, 689–693.

20. Molina-Minano, F.; Lopez-Jornet, P.; Camacho-Alonso, F.; Vicente-Ortega, V. Plasma rich in growth factors and bone formation: A radiological and histomorphometric study in New Zealand rabbits. *Braz. Oral Res.* **2009**, *23*, 275–280. [CrossRef] [PubMed]

21. Marcazzan, S.; Taschieri, S.; Weinstein, R.L.; Del Fabbro, M. Efficacy of platelet concentrates in bone healing: A systematic review on animal studies—Part B: Large-size animal models. *Platelets* **2018**, *29*, 338–346. [CrossRef] [PubMed]

22. Zhang, Y.D.; Wang, G.; Sun, Y.; Zhang, C.Q. Combination of platelet-rich plasma with degradable bioactive borate glass for segmental bone defect repair. *Acta Orthop. Belgica* **2011**, *77*, 110–115.

23. Karrasch, N.M.; Lerche, P.; Aarnes, T.K.; Gardner, H.L.; London, C.A. The effects of preoperative oral administration of carprofen or tramadol on postoperative analgesia in dogs undergoing cutaneous tumor removal. *Can. Vet. J.* **2015**, *56*, 817–822. [PubMed]

24. Kalchofner Guerrero, K.S.; Schwarz, A.; Wuhrmann, R.; Feldmann, S.; Hartnack, S.; Bettschart-Wolfensberger, R. Comparison of a new metamizole formulation and carprofen for extended post-operative analgesia in dogs undergoing ovariohysterectomy. *Vet. J.* **2015**, *204*, 99–104. [CrossRef] [PubMed]

25. Khan, S.A.; McLean, M.K. Toxicology of frequently encountered nonsteroidal anti-inflammatory drugs in dogs and cats. *Vet. Clin. N. Am. Small Anim. Pract.* **2012**, *42*, 289–306. [CrossRef] [PubMed]

26. Martinez, C.E.; Smith, P.C.; Palma Alvarado, V.A. The influence of platelet-derived products on angiogenesis and tissue repair: A concise update. *Front. Physiol.* **2015**, *6*, 290. [PubMed]

27. Tong, S.; Liu, J.; Zhang, C. Platelet-rich plasma inhibits inflammatory factors and represses rheumatoid fibroblast-like synoviocytes in rheumatoid arthritis. *Clin. Exp. Med.* **2017**, *17*, 441–449. [CrossRef] [PubMed]

28. Kubota, G.; Kamoda, H.; Orita, S.; Inage, K.; Ito, M.; Yamashita, M.; Furuya, T.; Akazawa, T.; Shiga, Y.; Ohtori, S. Efficacy of Platelet-Rich Plasma for Bone Fusion in Transforaminal Lumbar Interbody Fusion. *Asian Spine J.* **2018**, *12*, 112–118. [CrossRef] [PubMed]

29. Holtsinger, R.H.; Parker, R.B.; Beale, B.S.; FRIEDMAN, R.L. The therapeutic efficacy of carprofen (Rimadyl-V™) in 209 clinical cases of canine degenerative joint disease. *Vet. Comp. Orthop. Traumatol.* **1992**, *5*, 140–144.
30. Mehta, S.; Watson, J.T. Platelet rich concentrate: Basic science and current clinical applications. *J. Orthop. Trauma* **2008**, *22*, 432–438. [CrossRef] [PubMed]
31. Gemmill, T.J.; Cave, T.A.; Clements, D.N.; Clarke, S.P.; Bennett, D.; Carmichael, S. Treatment of canine and feline diaphyseal radial and tibial fractures with low-stiffness external skeletal fixation. *J. Small Anim. Pract.* **2004**, *45*, 85–91. [PubMed]
32. Piermattei, D.L.; Flo, G.L.; De Camp, C.E. Fractures: Classification, Diagnoses and Treatment. In *Brinker, Piermattei and Flo's Handbook of Small Animal Orthopaedics and Fracture Repair*; Piermattei, D.L., Flo, G.L., DeCamp, C.E., Eds.; Inter-Médica: Buenos Aires, Argentina, 2006; pp. 25–159.

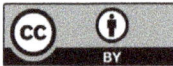

International Journal of
Molecular Sciences

MDPI

Review

Influence of Platelet-Rich and Platelet-Poor Plasma on Endogenous Mechanisms of Skeletal Muscle Repair/Regeneration

Flaminia Chellini, Alessia Tani, Sandra Zecchi-Orlandini and Chiara Sassoli *

Department of Experimental and Clinical Medicine—Section of Anatomy and Histology, University of Florence, Largo Brambilla 3, 50134 Florence, Italy; flaminia.chellini@unifi.it (F.C.); alessia.tani@unifi.it (A.T.); sandra.zecchi@unifi.it (S.Z.-O.)
* Correspondence: chiara.sassoli@unifi.it; Tel.: +39-055-2758-063

Received: 17 January 2019; Accepted: 1 February 2019; Published: 5 February 2019

check for
updates

Abstract: The morpho-functional recovery of injured skeletal muscle still represents an unmet need. None of the therapeutic options so far adopted have proved to be resolutive. A current scientific challenge remains the identification of effective strategies improving the endogenous skeletal muscle regenerative program. Indeed, skeletal muscle tissue possesses an intrinsic remarkable regenerative capacity in response to injury, mainly thanks to the activity of a population of resident muscle progenitors called satellite cells, largely influenced by the dynamic interplay established with different molecular and cellular components of the surrounding niche/microenvironment. Other myogenic non-satellite cells, residing within muscle or recruited via circulation may contribute to post-natal muscle regeneration. Unfortunately, in the case of extended damage the tissue repair may become aberrant, giving rise to a maladaptive fibrotic scar or adipose tissue infiltration, mainly due to dysregulated activity of different muscle interstitial cells. In this context, plasma preparations, including Platelet-Rich Plasma (PRP) and more recently Platelet-Poor Plasma (PPP), have shown advantages and promising therapeutic perspectives. This review focuses on the contribution of these blood-derived products on repair/regeneration of damaged skeletal muscle, paying particular attention to the potential cellular targets and molecular mechanisms through which these products may exert their beneficial effects.

Keywords: fibrosis; myoblasts; myofibroblasts; myogenesis; Platelet-Rich Plasma (PRP); Platelet-Poor Plasma (PPP); satellite cells; skeletal muscle regeneration; stem cell niche; regenerative medicine

1. Introduction

Skeletal muscle can be considered as the largest organ of the human body, accounting for 40–45% of the total body mass, responsible for generating forces that guarantee breathing and movement. In addition, it represents an important metabolic and endocrine organ [1,2]. The incidence of skeletal muscle injuries as a consequence of trauma (e.g., sport injuries), inherited genetic diseases (e.g., muscular dystrophies), pathology (cancer and endocrinological disorders) or systemic conditions such as aging is very high worldwide, thus representing a serious socio-economic concern with relevant Health Care System costs [2,3]. Indeed skeletal muscle damage is the most common cause of severe long-term pain and physical disability, restricting patient daily living activities and imposing lost working days.

It is well known that skeletal muscle tissue possesses an intrinsic remarkable regenerative potential, which, however, becomes compromised in the case of severe and extended damage. In particular, it has been reported that skeletal muscle tissue is able to compensate for up to 20% of muscle mass loss but beyond this threshold the restoration of the native muscle tissue structure and function cannot be achieved [2].

Traditional therapeutic options for the treatment of damaged muscles include RICE (Rest, Ice, Compression and Elevation) treatment, rehabilitation therapies, corticosteroid administration and, in the worst conditions, even reconstructive surgical intervention. The progress of scientific research, that allowed a deeper understanding of the cellular and molecular mechanisms driving skeletal muscle tissue repair/regeneration, together with the advances of regenerative medicine and biotechnology, pushed the development and application of alternative and innovative strategies to promote or improve muscle repair/regeneration, such as cell-based therapy with different kinds of stem cells [4–10], tissue engineering [11,12] and Low Level Laser Therapy (LLLT—more recently termed Photobiomodulation) [13–15].

However, none of the therapeutic options so far adopted has proved to be resolutive and satisfactory; in addition, the most innovative therapeutic strategies, despite the encouraging elicited outcomes, still bear several criticisms hindering their clinical application for regenerative purposes. For more detailed information readers are referred to recent reviews [2,9,10] focusing on this topic, which is beyond the aim of this review.

Based on these considerations, the development of new effective treatments for skeletal muscle injury represents a priority and an urgent need. A current scientific challenge remains the identification of appropriate factors capable of limiting muscle degeneration and/or potentiating the endogenous muscle regenerative program. In this context, plasma preparations, including Platelet-Rich Plasma (PRP) and more recently Platelet-Poor Plasma (PPP), have shown several advantages and promising therapeutic perspectives.

This review, besides giving an updated description of the main cell types driving skeletal muscle repair/regeneration, focuses on the contribution of PRP and PPP on repair/regeneration of damaged skeletal muscle, paying particular attention to the cellular and molecular mechanisms through which these blood-derived products may exert their beneficial effects.

2. Adult Skeletal Muscle Repair and Regeneration: Role of Satellite and Non-Satellite Cells

It has been clearly proven that adult skeletal muscle tissue possesses a remarkable ability to regenerate in response to focal injuries. This is mainly thanks to the activity of a small population of resident mononucleated myogenic precursors, called satellite cells, whose name depends on the unique anatomical location at the periphery of a skeletal myofiber, beneath the surrounding basal lamina in intimate association with the myofiber sarcolemma, and in close proximity to capillaries and neuromuscular junction [16–20]. In healthy skeletal muscles, satellite cells are mitotically quiescent and transcriptionally inactive; in this dormant state they express the paired box transcription factor Pax7, necessary for their survival and function, and the myogenic transcription factor Myf5 (~90% of quiescent satellite cells) but not the myogenic regulatory factors, namely MyoD or myogenin [21,22]. In injured muscles, in response to signals coming from damaged myofibers and infiltrating inflammatory cells (neutrophils and macrophages), satellite cells become activated, giving rise to a progeny of proliferating Pax7, Ki67, Myf5 and MyoD positive adult myoblasts which subsequently, down-regulating Pax7 and expressing myogenin and MRF4/Myf6, differentiate into skeletal myocytes that finally either fuse with each other, forming nascent syncytial contractile myofibers, and fuse with injured myofibers, thus repairing the damage [21]. There is evidence indicating that a small percentage of satellite cells are *true* stem cells, capable of self-renewal, thereby ensuring the replenishment of the basal pool of resident satellite cells that are recruitable in the case of muscle re-injury [16,23,24].

The behavior and the fate of satellite cells are largely influenced by the dynamic interplay established with components of the surrounding microenvironment, which changes under homeostatic conditions (*quiescent state*) and during regeneration (*activated state*) [25]. This microenvironment includes the so called "immediate satellite cell niche" and the microenvironment beyond the immediate niche [16]. The immediate satellite niche represents the microenvironment where the satellite cells reside. It consists of several signaling molecules diffusing between the satellite cell and the myofiber, different extracellular matrix (ECM) components, satellite cell and myofiber surface-associated receptors for mediating cell-to-cell or cell-to-ECM interactions or binding different regulatory factors, and receptors present in the basal lamina to sequester inactive growth factor precursors secreted by either satellite cells and myofibers, serving as a local reservoir to be rapidly activated during muscle injury [16,26,27]. The microenvironment beyond this niche comprises the local milieu and the systemic milieu. The local milieu may be identified by the muscle fascicle wrapped by perimysium, consisting of other myofibers surrounded and connected to each other by endomysium sheath, a heterogeneous population of interstitial cells in the stroma between the myofibers [28–30], blood capillaries together with their secretable factors and associated pericytes and mesoangioblasts [31,32] and motor neuron endings. The main interstitial cells types are represented by fibroblasts, mesenchymal stem/stromal cells (MSCs) including fibro-adipogenic progenitors -FAPs- [33], telocytes (CD34+/vimentin+ stromal cells with a small cell body and distinctive extremely long, thin and moniliform cytoplasmic extensions called telopodes alternating slender segments—podomeres- with dilatations-podoms) [34], Abcg2+ side population (SP) [35], skeletal muscle-derived CD34+/45− (Sk-34) myogenic endothelial progenitors [36], interstitial stem cells positive for stress mediator PW1 expression and negative for Pax7 expression termed PICs [37], integrin β4 interstitial cells.

The systemic milieu includes the entire muscle belly along with bones and surrounding skeletal muscles, the immune cells and circulating growth factors, interleukins/chemokines and hormones.

The dynamic and collaborative interaction between satellite cells and the different cell types of the surrounding microenvironment, becomes crucial for a proper execution of the essential events of repair/regeneration process. Indeed, in contrast to the quiescent conditions, in the activated ones, many cells are found close to satellite cells exerting a supportive role for their functionality. On the other hand, this cell interaction is bidirectional since satellite cells can influence the behavior of interacting cells [20,38].

The cells supporting satellite cell-mediated regeneration in the activated niche may include several cell types.

Pro-inflammatory phagocytic macrophages (M1) and anti-inflammatory pro-regenerative macrophages (M2) have been demonstrated to promote proliferation and differentiation of myogenic precursors respectively, via both paracrine and juxtacrine signaling [39–42]. The ability of macrophages to rescue myoblasts and myotubes from apoptosis has also been demonstrated [43].

Fibroblasts-myofibroblasts and FAPs are the major contributors to the deposition and remodeling of the transitional ECM after a muscle lesion, required to rapidly restore tissue integrity [44]; on the other hand the capability of fibroblasts to promote myoblast proliferation and differentiation and to enhance satellite cell renewal as well as pro-myogenic function of FAPs has been documented [38,45–49].

Telocytes have been supposed to play a "nursing" role in satellite cell-mediated regeneration. By means of their telopodes they connect with each other via homocellular junctions, or with neighboring cells including satellite cells via heterocellular ones, thus forming a three-dimensional network in the interstitium: telocytes might act as a guidance stromal scaffold able to carry signals over long distances, driving satellite cell proliferation, migration and differentiation after their recruitment [34]. In addition, telocytes may modulate satellite cell function in a paracrine manner by the release of extracellular vesicles containing myogenic factors (e.g., Vascular Endothelial Growth Factor, VEGF, or microRNAs) [4,34,50,51].

Capillary endothelial cells secrete different paracrine factors strongly stimulating growth of myogenic progenitors and/or protecting them from apoptosis [19,52,53], whereas *periendothelial cells* including *pericytes* are crucial for the re-entry of satellite cells into quiescence at the end of the regeneration process and myofiber growth [54,55].

In addition, *motor neurons and Schwann cells* secreting neurotrophic factors including Insulin Growth Factor (IGF)-1, Nerve Growth Factor (NGF), Brain-Derived Growth Factor (BDNF) and Ciliary Neurotrophic Factor (CNTF) may contribute to the modulation of satellite cell/myoblast viability, proliferation and fusion [16,20,29,56,57].

Furthermore, in regulating satellite cell quiescence, activation, proliferation and differentiation an essential role is played by ECM factors (both of basal lamina and of interstitial matrix) including specific ligands, soluble factors sequestered within the matrix, as well as by the mechanical properties of ECM itself as extensively discussed in the review by Thomas and co-workers [27].

Many works have demonstrated that, in addition to satellite cells, other cell types residing within muscle or recruited via circulation may contribute to muscle regeneration thanks to their inducible myogenic potential [58]. These so-called myogenic non-satellite cells include: the interstitial Abcg2+SP [35,59–61], skeletal muscle-derived CD34+/45− (Sk-34) cells (likely a subpopulation of SP with more pronounced myogenic potential) [36], PICs [37], mesoangioblasts and pericytes [31,62–64], integrin β4 interstitial cells, CD133+ human skeletal muscle derived and blood- derived stem cells [65–67]. However, if these cells represent an independent source of muscle progenitors undergoing unconventional myogenic differentiation or if they give rise to satellite cells, remains to be elucidated. Moreover, also the molecular mechanisms guiding the lineage switch of these muscle interstitial or circulating cells in the regenerating environment are still unclear [28,29]. Based on all of this evidence, it appears clear that, for an effective restoration of muscle structure and function, collaborative and temporally coordinated juxtacrine and paracrine interactions among many myogenic and non-myogenic cells, are required.

Unfortunately, in case of severe and extended damage, with an intense and persisting inflammatory reaction or in disease settings, the muscle repair may become aberrant, occurring with a maladaptive fibrotic scar or adipose tissue infiltration, or even with heterotopic ossification, mainly as a consequence of dysregulated activity and number of fibroblasts and mesenchymal progenitors [3,33,49,68–70], which hamper the muscle regenerative response. Moreover, a critical event that must be considered for the achievement of a regenerating functional muscle tissue after injury is the re-establishment of neuromuscular junctions for the new myofibers, which is mandatory to prevent muscle wasting [71].

On the basis of these considerations, improving the functionality of satellite and non-satellite myogenic cells either directly or by acting on their microenvironment (e.g., modulating the inflammatory response or MSC functionality thus limiting fibrosis or muscle fatty deposition) as well as nerve regeneration, could represent the final goal of effective therapeutic strategies for efficient muscle regeneration.

3. Plasma Preparations: Platelet-Rich Plasma (PRP) and Platelet-Poor Plasma (PPP)

3.1. Definition and Biological Properties

PRP and PPP can be defined as a plasma fraction with a concentration of platelets respectively above and below baseline levels in whole blood. Unfortunately, so far, no univocal guidelines are available for these plasma preparations and protocols show a high variability among authors, thus leading to plasma fractions differing in terms of concentration of blood cells (platelets and leukocytes) and content and type of cytokines and growth factors. For a detailed and updated overview of the different methods of plasma fraction collection, of the commercially available PRP systems and of PRP classification, the readers are referred to several excellent reviews [72–75]. In any case, the rationale for using plasma fractions, in particular PRP, for regenerative purposes in different areas of medicine [76–81] including musculoskeletal and sport medicine [82–85], relies on the fact that they represent a cost-effective reservoir of numerous biologically active molecules, holding a strong potential for improving tissue healing and regeneration [86–89]. Moreover, the prompt availability from whole blood of patients and thus the autologous source of these blood products, posing no risks of disease transmission or immunogenic reactions [90,91], as well as the ease of administration, represent additional advantages for their clinical use. Furthermore, recent findings demonstrating the safety and favorable outcomes of the application of allogenic PRP to treat musculoskeletal conditions have opened new perspectives for off-the-shelf PRP therapy for all patients for whom the use of autologous PRP would not be recommended [92,93].

3.2. Contribution of PRP to Skeletal Muscle Repair/Regeneration

Some studies have reported positive outcomes after administration of PRP in patients with injured skeletal muscles, without negative side effects. Indeed, patients/athletes with acute muscle strains after PRP intralesional injections combined with a rehabilitation treatment, exhibited an earlier "return to play", faster pain relief without a significant increase of the re-injury risk in short and long term, when compared to patients undergoing a rehabilitation program only [94–98]. Improvement of inflammatory state, reduction of fibrotic scar size and parenchymal recovery was also demonstrated in PRP-treated muscle lesions [94,99–101]. However, despite the encouraging findings, these studies do not reach sufficient statistical significance to support the adoption of PRP therapy for skeletal muscle injury in clinical routine, as recently extensively discussed [83,84,102–104]. Therefore, further human studies, to ascertain and validate the effective therapeutic benefits of PRP for skeletal muscle regenerative purpose, are strongly required.

On the other hand, a large body of experimental evidence supporting the contribution of PRP to the morpho-functional recovery of damaged skeletal muscles comes from studies carried out in animal models. Although these studies cannot be directly validated or extrapolated to human species, they do provide a robust and instructive scientific background to design and perform clinical investigations.

In particular, PRP injections into skeletal muscles of rats or mice subjected to different traumatic injuries (incision, laceration, contusion or lengthening/eccentric contractions) or to cardiotoxin injection or into ischemic muscles, have been demonstrated to contribute to the muscle healing process: (i) by modulating the inflammatory response including the increase in M2 macrophage cell recruitment to the injury site and function [105–108]; (ii) by generating a myogenic response, as evaluated by satellite cell activation, increase of the expression of different myogenic regulatory factors, modulation of the expression of muscle specific microRNAs and activation of myogenic signaling pathways leading to myofiber formation [105,106,109–113]; (iii) by attenuating the impairment of myocytes mitochondrial function determined by muscle damage and improving their endogenous antioxidant defense system [114]; and (iv) by protecting cells from apoptosis [108,111].

In addition, the reduction of type-I collagen deposition and scar formation (fibrosis) [106, 110,112,113,115–118] the enhancement of angiogenesis [106,110,112,116,117] and a faster functional recovery [108,109,113,118,119] have been also observed after PRP application on damaged muscles. Takase and co-workers [120] recently demonstrated also the ability of PRP to prevent fatty degenerative changes of rotator cuff muscles in a rat rotator cuff tear model, when administered into subacromial space.

3.3. Impact of PRP on Satellite Cells and on Myogenic and Non-Myogenic Interstitial Cells

The cellular and molecular mechanisms that could mediate the beneficial pro-regenerative and anti-fibrotic effects of PRP-derived growth factors on muscle tissue healing have been investigated in a growing number of in vitro studies.

Satellite cells may represent a direct target of PRP action. Indeed, the capability of PRP to positively influence the behavior of primary myoblasts—human skeletal myoblasts [116,121], human pre-plated muscle derived-progenitor cells [122], rabbit myogenic progenitor cells [123], rat intrinsic skeletal muscle cells [124]—or satellite cell-derived myoblast line namely murine C2C12 myoblasts [120,121,125,126] and human CD56+ myoblasts [127] by promoting their activation and proliferation [116,120–127] and protecting them from apoptosis [116] has been demonstrated.

Among the different growth factors within PRP, Platelet Derived Growth Factor (PDGF) [122], has been identified as a key factor mediating PRP-induced mitogenic response, whereas the involvement of others—demonstrated to be contained in PRP [86–89]—has been proposed on the basis of previous studies investigating their effects on myoblast cell line or primary muscle stem cells, such as VEGF [4,128], Hepatocyte Growth Factor (HGF) [129] or IGF-1 [130]. The involvement of PDGF and VEGF in mediating the PRP effects may be also presumed on the basis of the recent study of Scully and co-workers [131] showing that platelet releasate is capable to drive C2C12 myoblast proliferation and terminal differentiation, as well as the commitment to differentiation of myofiber-derived stem cells, at least in part via PDGF and VEGF signaling pathways.

However, it must be pointed out that the effects of the combination of different growth factors (such as PRP) may be completely different from the ones elicited by the single growth factors, based on the proved antagonistic or synergistic cross-talk between diverse growth factor-mediated signaling.

In addition, primary cultured skeletal muscle cells treated with PRP have also shown an increased motility/migratory ability associated with an up-regulation of different focal adhesion proteins and F-actin cytoskeleton remodeling [132]; these findings are of particular interest given that migration of satellite cells and of satellite derived-myoblasts is a crucial process in muscle regeneration by which the cells reach the injured site.

In line with these findings, our research group has recently shown that PRP used as single treatment, positively influenced C2C12 myoblast viability and proliferation in the same manner of standard culture media containing animal sera, by promoting the activation of AKT-mediated signaling, as well as the activation of cultured murine satellite cells isolated from single skeletal muscle fibers [133].

In this paper, we also demonstrated that PRP treatment induced C2C12 myoblasts to enter and progress into the myogenic program by stimulating MyoD, myogenin, α-sarcomeric actin expression as standard differentiation culture media containing animal sera did, accordingly to a previous study [127]. The pro-myogenic effect of PRP was also recently demonstrated by the study of McClure and co-workers [126] where C2C12 myoblasts cultured on PRP embedded ECM mimicking scaffold, exhibited a PRP-dose dependent increase in myogenin and myosin heavy chain protein expression, mediated by ERK1/2 signaling activation. In addition, our study reported that PRP promoted also the C2C12 myoblast expression of matrix metalloprotease (MMP)-2 [133] whose function has been reported to be required for satellite cell activation [134–136], for basal lamina degradation and, at the elongation stage of the myogenic differentiation process, for completing the successive myoblast cell migration and fusion [6,27,137,138] thus supporting the pro-myogenic effect of PRP. These latter results concerning differentiation seem to question findings in the literature showing a reduction or even inhibition of myogenic differentiation of myoblasts cultured with PRP [120,121,125]. These contradictory PRP-elicited biological responses may be attributed to different experimental settings and more likely to the heterogeneity of PRP preparation techniques and formulations used, which may contain interplaying pro-myogenic growth factors—such as IGF-1 [130], HGF [129] and β-Fibroblast Growth Factor (FGF) [125,139]—and anti-myogenic ones—such as Transforming Growth Factor (TGF)-β [140]—in different concentrations and proportions. In addition, the different PRP dosages used may account for the discrepancy in the literature on whether PRP hampers or improves differentiation, when considering the dose-dependence of some myogenic cell responses as well as the timing of PRP application [116,121,125,126,132,133].

Another very interesting finding of our recent work [133] is the ability of PRP to satisfactorily support and stimulate in vitro viability, survival and proliferation of MSCs. Taking into consideration the close morpho-functional relationship between satellite and the interstitial stromal cells, in particular the reported supportive juxtacrine and paracrine role of different stromal cell types for satellite cells, our results may suggest that the muscle resident stromal cells could also benefit from the treatment with PRP. In other words, PRP might indirectly promote satellite cell-mediated regeneration by potentiating the nursing role of interstitial MSCs.

PRP may impact indirectly on satellite cells also by favoring the appearance and functionality of pro-regenerative macrophage phenotype (M2) within the healing niche on the basis of recent in vitro studies, evaluating the effects of different PRP preparations on human monocyte-derived cells [141,142] and also being consistent with the findings of in vivo research [106].

On the other hand, PRP could also affect the myogenic potential of the so-called non-satellite myogenic cells. In this line, Li and co-workers [122] have reported that pericytes, isolated from post-mortem human skeletal muscle biopsies, exhibited an enhanced proliferative ability when cultured with PRP as compared to standard culture media while maintaining their in vitro myogenic differentiation capability and in vivo myogenic potential.

Interestingly, we have recently demonstrated the capability of PRP to prevent the transition of fibroblasts into myofibroblasts, the main drivers of tissue scarring [143] via VEGF-A/VEGF-A Receptor-1-mediated inhibition of TGF-β1/Smad3 signaling [144]. These findings, in accordance with other studies [145,146], may contribute to the identification of the cellular and molecular mechanisms responsible for the observed reduction in the fibrotic response achieved after injections of PRP in damaged skeletal muscles [106,110,112,113,115–118]. Such reduction is necessary for the recreation of a more hospitable and conductive microenvironment for muscle progenitor functionality and for axonal growth/regeneration and muscle re-innervation [147] and eventually for a complete tissue morpho-functional recovery. On the other hand, the ability of different PRP-derived factors to positively influence Schwann cell function in vitro and to assist peripheral nerve repair/regeneration in vivo has been documented [148–151], thus allowing us to include Schwann cells in the list of the potential cell targets of PRP in the skeletal muscle tissue during tissue repair/regeneration (Figure 1) and to suggest that promotion of muscle re-innervation may represent an additional benefit exerted by PRP for damaged muscles.

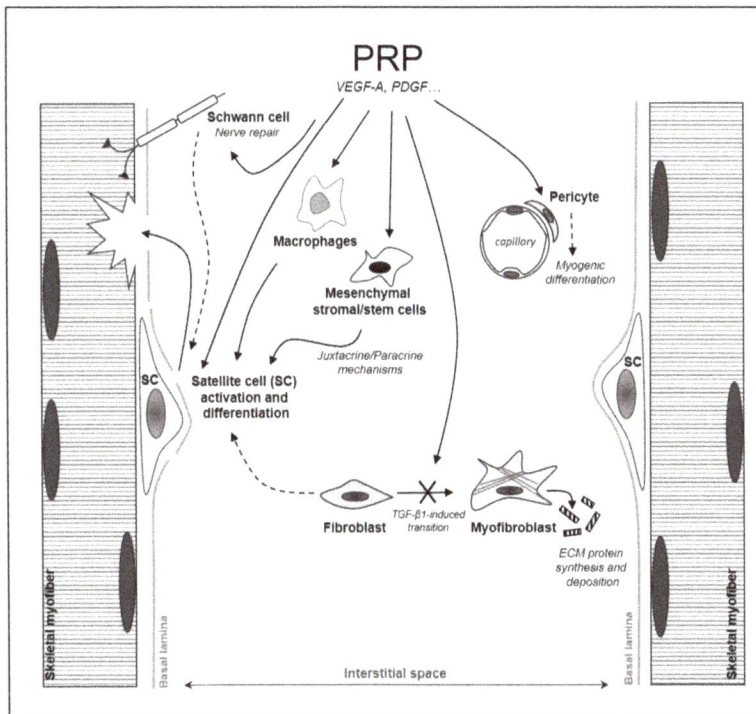

Figure 1. Schematic drawing representing the potential cell targets of PRP during skeletal muscle repair/regeneration, which may mediate its beneficial effects.

3.4. Impact of PPP on Skeletal Myogenesis

PPP, long regarded as the waste product of PRP and used a sham treatment [109], has recently been demonstrated to exert a beneficial effect on myogenesis. In particular, Miroshnychenko and co-workers [121] showed that PPP, differently from PRP, reduced the proliferation rate of human primary skeletal muscle myoblasts but led to a significant induction of differentiation of these cells into the myogenic pathway and myotube formation. The same cell responses were elicited by a modified preparation of PRP, by means of a second spin to remove platelets, suggesting that the beneficial effects of PRP on myogenesis can be mostly due to plasma per se. Indeed, although PPP by its definition contains a very low concentration of platelets and therefore smaller quantities of growth factors, it still represents a reservoir of bioactive molecules (such as PDGF, IGF-1) [87], which may be responsible for the observed pro-myogenic effects on myoblasts. This research is in line with previous studies showing the effectiveness of PPP in evoking biological responses from different cell types involved in the healing process of several tissues, namely fibroblast migration and ECM remodeling [152,153], periodontal ligament stem cell differentiation towards osteoblastic phenotype [154], tenocyte proliferation and collagen production [155], endothelial cell differentiation towards angiogenic cells [156] and macrophage anti-inflammatory activity [157]. Miroshnychenko and co-workers [121] conclude that PPP and platelet deprived-PRP may be more appropriate to promote skeletal muscle regeneration than the traditionally formulated PRP, probably containing a greater quantity of platelet- derived factors detrimental for myoblast differentiation such as TGFβ-1. However, this laboratory evidence does not seem to have received a large consensus from the current literature [103,109].

Therefore, although PPP may hold promise for skeletal muscle injuries, further investigations to assess the exact growth factors contained in this kind of plasma formulation and especially to validate the impact of PPP on myogenic precursors, as well as to disclose its role on skeletal muscle tissue regeneration in vivo are absolutely required. Moreover, to date, no clinical studies evaluating the effect of PPP on skeletal muscle have been conducted.

4. Conclusions and Further Directions

Plasma preparations and especially PRP have been demonstrated to hold a strong therapeutic potential for the healing of injured skeletal muscle tissue due to their ability to potentiate the endogenous mechanisms of tissue repair/regeneration while contributing to limit the aberrant responses such as fibrosis. Nevertheless, despite these encouraging outcomes, evidence from animal studies and even more from human ones, are not still sufficient to attain the effective clinical translation of these blood products for skeletal regenerative purpose. Therefore, further investigations are necessary to validate the regenerative potential of these blood derivates and ultimately drive medical decisions. On the other hand, it must be considered that some human and animal studies have reported limited effectiveness or inefficacy of a PRP therapy for damaged skeletal muscle in terms of tissue regeneration and recovery of functionality, or even an exacerbation of the fibrotic response [158–168]. The main reason for these conflicting results certainly could be due to individual-based variations and muscle lesion type and severity but is most likely due to the great heterogeneity of the injected available products and application timing. Therefore, standardization of PRP preparation techniques as well as of application protocols—considering the cascade of events through which skeletal muscle tissue repair/regeneration progresses—is a priority in order to perform meaningful comparative analyses, to enable reproducibility and reach reliable conclusions. Moreover, a full characterization of plasma preparations is also necessary, evaluating the quantity and the type of the contained bioactive factors, as well as a deep investigation of their effects on the main local cell types involved in the skeletal muscle tissue regeneration. This may lead to novel and optimized plasma formulations for muscle regenerative purposes, based on the selection of factors capable, for instance, of exerting a pro-regenerative and anti-fibrotic action on skeletal muscle tissue.

Int. J. Mol. Sci. **2019**, *20*, 683

Author Contributions: Conceptualization, review of the literature, F.C., A.T., C.S.; writing—original draft preparation, C.S.; preparation of figure, C.S.; writing—review and editing, F.C., A.T., S.Z.-O. and C.S. All the authors have read and approved the submitted version of the review.

Funding: The publication of this review was supported by FFABR-MIUR 2017 (Funding Fund for Basic Research Activities - Ministry of Education, University and Research, Italy) to C.S.

Conflicts of Interest: The authors declare no conflict of interest.

References

1. Giudice, J.; Taylor, J.M. Muscle as a paracrine and endocrine organ. *Curr. Opin. Pharm.* **2017**, *34*, 49–55. [CrossRef] [PubMed]

2. Liu, J.; Saul, D.; Böker, K.O.; Ernst, J.; Lehman, W.; Schilling, A.F. Current Methods for Skeletal Muscle Tissue Repair and Regeneration. *Biomed. Res. Int.* **2018**, *16*, 1984879. [CrossRef] [PubMed]

3. Schaaf, G.; Sage, F.; Stok, M.; Brusse, E.; Pijnappel, W.W.M.; Reuser, A.J.; vd Ploeg, A.T. Ex-vivo Expansion of Muscle-Regenerative Cells for the Treatment of Muscle Disorders. *J. Stem Cell Res.* **2012**, *S11*, 003. [CrossRef]

4. Sassoli, C.; Pini, A.; Chellini, F.; Mazzanti, B.; Nistri, S.; Nosi, D.; Saccardi, R.; Quercioli, F.; Zecchi-Orlandini, S.; Formigli, L. Bone marrow mesenchymal stromal cells stimulate skeletal myoblast proliferation through the paracrine release of VEGF. *PLoS ONE* **2012**, *7*, e37512. [CrossRef] [PubMed]

5. Sassoli, C.; Zecchi-Orlandini, S.; Formigli, L. Trophic actions of bone marrow-derived mesenchymal stromal cells for muscle repair/regeneration. *Cells* **2012**, *1*, 832–850. [CrossRef] [PubMed]

6. Sassoli, C.; Nosi, D.; Tani, A.; Chellini, F.; Mazzanti, B.; Quercioli, F.; Zecchi-Orlandini, S.; Formigli, L. Defining the role of mesenchymal stromal cells on the regulation of matrix metalloproteinases in skeletal muscle cells. *Exp. Cell Res.* **2014**, *323*, 297–313. [CrossRef] [PubMed]

7. Berry, S.E. Concise review: Mesoangioblast and mesenchymal stem cell therapy for muscular dystrophy: Progress, challenges, and future directions. *Stem Cells Transl. Med.* **2015**, *4*, 91–98. [CrossRef] [PubMed]

8. De Albornoz, P.M.; Aicale, R.; Forriol, F.; Maffulli, N. Cell Therapies in Tendon, Ligament, and Musculoskeletal System Repair. *Sports Med. Arthrosc. Rev.* **2018**, *26*, 48–58. [CrossRef]

9. Andia, I.; Maffulli, N. New biotechnologies for musculoskeletal injuries. *Surgeon* **2018**. [CrossRef] [PubMed]

10. Dunn, A.; Talovic, M.; Patel, K.; Patel, A.; Marcinczyk, M.; Garg, K. Biomaterial and stem cell-based strategies for skeletal muscle regeneration. *J. Orthop. Res.* **2019**. [CrossRef]

11. Han, W.M.; Jang, Y.C.; García, A.J. Engineered matrices for skeletal muscle satellite cell engraftment and function. *Matrix Biol.* **2017**, *60–61*, 96–109. [CrossRef] [PubMed]

12. Kwee, B.J.; Mooney, D.J. Biomaterials for skeletal muscle tissue engineering. *Curr. Opin. Biotechnol.* **2017**, *47*, 16–22. [CrossRef] [PubMed]

13. Alves, A.N.; Fernandes, K.P.; Deana, A.M.; Bussadori, S.K.; Mesquita-Ferrari, R.A. Effects of low-level laser therapy on skeletal muscle repair: A systematic review. *Am. J. Phys. Med. Rehabil.* **2014**, *93*, 1073–1085. [CrossRef] [PubMed]

14. Sassoli, C.; Chellini, F.; Squecco, R.; Tani, A.; Idrizaj, E.; Nosi, D.; Giannelli, M.; Zecchi-Orlandini, S. Low intensity 635 nm diode laser irradiation inhibits fibroblast-myofibroblast transition reducing TRPC1 channel expression/activity: New perspectives for tissue fibrosis treatment. *Lasers Surg. Med.* **2016**, *48*, 318–332. [CrossRef] [PubMed]

15. De Oliveira, H.A.; Antonio, E.L.; Silva, F.A.; de Carvalho, P.T.C.; Feliciano, R.; Yoshizaki, A.; Vieira, S.S.; de Melo, B.L.; Leal-Junior, E.C.P.; Labat, R.; et al. Protective effects of photobiomodulation against resistance exercise-induced muscle damage and inflammation in rats. *J. Sports Sci.* **2018**, *36*, 2349–2357. [CrossRef] [PubMed]

16. Yin, H.; Price, F.; Rudnicki, M.A. Satellite cells and the muscle stem cell niche. *Physiol. Rev.* **2013**, *93*, 23–67. [CrossRef] [PubMed]

17. Scicchitano, B.M.; Sica, G.; Musarò, A. Stem Cells and Tissue Niche: Two Faces of the Same Coin of Muscle Regeneration. *Eur. J. Transl. Myol.* **2016**, *26*, 6125. [CrossRef] [PubMed]

18. Le Grand, F.; Rudnicki, M.A. Skeletal muscle satellite cells and adult myogenesis. *Curr. Opin. Cell Biol.* **2007**, *19*, 628–633. [CrossRef] [PubMed]

19. Mounier, R.; Chrétien, F.; Chazaud, B. Blood vessels and the satellite cell niche. *Curr. Top. Dev. Biol.* **2011**, *96*, 121–138. [CrossRef] [PubMed]

20. Dinulovic, I.; Furrer, R.; Handschin, C. Plasticity of the Muscle Stem Cell Microenvironment. *Adv. Exp. Med. Biol.* **2017**, *1041*, 141–169. [CrossRef]

21. Dumont, N.A.; Wang, Y.X.; Rudnicki, M.A. Intrinsic and extrinsic mechanisms regulating satellite cell function. *Development* **2015**, *142*, 1572–1581. [CrossRef] [PubMed]

22. Von Maltzahn, J.; Jones, A.E.; Parks, R.J.; Rudnicki, M.A. Pax7 is critical for the normal function of satellite cells in adult skeletal muscle. *Proc. Natl. Acad. Sci. USA* **2013**, *110*, 16474–16479. [CrossRef] [PubMed]

23. Tierney, M.T.; Sacco, A. Satellite Cell Heterogeneity in Skeletal Muscle Homeostasis. *Trends Cell Biol.* **2016**, *26*, 434–444. [CrossRef] [PubMed]

24. Kuang, S.; Kuroda, K.; Le Grand, F.; Rudnicki, M.A. Asymmetric self-renewal and commitment of satellite stem cells in muscle. *Cell* **2007**, *129*, 999–1010. [CrossRef] [PubMed]

25. Bentzinger, C.F.; Wang, Y.X.; Dumont, N.A.; Rudnicki, M.A. Cellular dynamics in the muscle satellite cell niche. *EMBO Rep.* **2013**, *14*, 1062–1072. [CrossRef] [PubMed]

26. Urciuolo, A.; Quarta, M.; Morbidoni, V.; Gattazzo, F.; Molon, S.; Grumati, P.; Montemurro, F.; Tedesco, F.S.; Blaauw, B.; Cossu, G.; et al. Collagen VI regulates satellite cell self-renewal and muscle regeneration. *Nat. Commun.* **2013**, *4*, 1964. [CrossRef] [PubMed]

27. Thomas, K.; Engler, A.J.; Meyer, G.A. Extracellular matrix regulation in the muscle satellite cell niche. *Connect. Tissue Res.* **2015**, *56*, 1–8. [CrossRef]

28. Malecova, B.; Puri, P.L. "Mix of Mics"-Phenotypic and Biological Heterogeneity of "Multipotent" Muscle Interstitial Cells (MICs). *J. Stem Cell Res.* **2012**, pii:004. [CrossRef]

29. Ceafalan, L.C.; Popescu, B.O.; Hinescu, M.E. Cellular players in skeletal muscle regeneration. *Biomed. Res. Int.* **2014**, *2014*, 957014. [CrossRef]

30. Čamernik, K.; Barlič, A.; Drobnič, M.; Marc, J.; Jeras, M.; Zupan, J. Mesenchymal Stem Cells in the Musculoskeletal System: From Animal Models to Human Tissue Regeneration? *Stem Cell Rev.* **2018**, *14*, 346–369. [CrossRef]

31. Tonlorenzi, R.; Rossi, G.; Messina, G. Isolation and Characterization of Vessel-Associated Stem/Progenitor Cells from Skeletal Muscle. *Methods Mol. Biol.* **2017**, *1556*, 149–177. [CrossRef]

32. Vezzani, B.; Pierantozzi, E.; Sorrentino, V. Not All Pericytes Are Born Equal: Pericytes from Human Adult Tissues Present Different Differentiation Properties. *Stem Cells Dev.* **2016**, *25*, 1549–1558. [CrossRef] [PubMed]

33. Judson, R.N.; Low, M.; Eisner, C.; Rossi, F.M. Isolation, Culture, and Differentiation of Fibro/Adipogenic Progenitors (FAPs) from Skeletal Muscle. *Methods Mol. Biol.* **2017**, *1668*, 93–103. [CrossRef]

34. Marini, M.; Rosa, I.; Ibba-Manneschi, L.; Manetti, M. Telocytes in skeletal, cardiac and smooth muscle interstitium: Morphological and functional aspects. *Histol. Histopathol.* **2018**, *33*, 1151–1165. [CrossRef] [PubMed]

35. Doyle, M.J.; Zhou, S.; Tanaka, K.K.; Pisconti, A.; Farina, N.H.; Sorrentino, B.P.; Olwin, B.B. Abcg2 labels multiple cell types in skeletal muscle and participates in muscle regeneration. *J. Cell Biol.* **2011**, *195*, 147–163. [CrossRef] [PubMed]

36. Tamaki, T.; Akatsuka, A.; Okada, Y.; Matsuzaki, Y.; Okano, H.; Kimura, M. Growth and differentiation potential of main- and side-population cells derived from murine skeletal muscle. *Exp. Cell Res.* **2003**, *291*, 83–90. [CrossRef]

37. Mitchell, K.J.; Pannérec, A.; Cadot, B.; Parlakian, A.; Besson, V.; Gomes, E.R.; Marazzi, G.; Sassoon, D.A. Identification and characterization of a non-satellite cell muscle resident progenitor during postnatal development. *Nat. Cell. Biol.* **2010**, *12*, 257–266. [CrossRef] [PubMed]

38. Farup, J.; Madaro, L.; Puri, P.L.; Mikkelsen, U.R. Interactions between muscle stem cells, mesenchymal-derived cells and immune cells in muscle homeostasis, regeneration and disease. *Cell Death Dis.* **2015**, *6*, e1830. [CrossRef] [PubMed]

39. Tidball, J.G.; Villalta, S.A. Regulatory interactions between muscle and the immune system during muscle regeneration. *Am. J. Physiol. Regul. Integr. Comp. Physiol.* **2010**, *298*, R1173–R1187. [CrossRef] [PubMed]

40. Bencze, M.; Negroni, E.; Vallese, D.; Yacoub-Youssef, H.; Chaouch, S.; Wolff, A.; Aamiri, A.; Di Santo, J.P.; Chazaud, B.; Butler-Browne, G.; et al. Proinflammatory macrophages enhance the regenerative capacity of human myoblasts by modifying their kinetics of proliferation and differentiation. *Mol. Ther.* **2012**, *20*, 2168–2179. [CrossRef] [PubMed]

41. Ceafalan, L.C.; Fertig, T.E.; Popescu, A.C.; Popescu, B.O.; Hinescu, M.E.; Gherghiceanu, M. Skeletal muscle regeneration involves macrophage-myoblast bonding. *Cell Adhes. Migr.* **2018**, *12*, 228–235. [CrossRef] [PubMed]

42. Wang, X.; Zhao, W.; Ransohoff, R.M.; Zhou, L. Infiltrating macrophages are broadly activated at the early stage to support acute skeletal muscleinjury repair. *J. Neuroimmunol.* **2018**, *317*, 55–66. [CrossRef] [PubMed]

43. Sonnet, C.; Lafuste, P.; Arnold, L.; Brigitte, M.; Poron, F.; Authier, F.J.; Chrétien, F.; Gherardi, R.K.; Chazaud, B. Human macrophages rescue myoblasts and myotubes from apoptosis through a set of adhesion molecular systems. *J. Cell Sci.* **2006**, *119*, 2497–2507. [CrossRef] [PubMed]

44. Serrano, A.L.; Mann, C.J.; Vidal, B.; Ardite, E.; Perdiguero, E.; Muñoz-Cánoves, P. Cellular and molecular mechanisms regulating fibrosis in skeletal muscle repair and disease. *Curr. Top. Dev. Biol.* **2011**, *96*, 167–201. [CrossRef] [PubMed]

45. Joe, A.W.; Yi, L.; Natarajan, A.; Le Grand, F.; So, L.; Wang, J.; Rudnicki, M.A.; Rossi, F.M. Muscle injury activates resident fibro/adipogenic progenitors that facilitate myogenesis. *Nat. Cell Biol.* **2010**, *12*, 153–163. [CrossRef] [PubMed]

46. Murphy, M.M.; Lawson, J.A.; Mathew, S.J.; Hutcheson, D.A.; Kardon, G. Satellite cells, connective tissue fibroblasts and their interactions are crucial for muscle regeneration. *Development* **2011**, *138*, 3625–3637. [CrossRef] [PubMed]

47. Heredia, J.E.; Mukundan, L.; Chen, F.M.; Mueller, A.A.; Deo, R.C.; Locksley, R.M.; Rando, T.A.; Chawla, A. Type 2 innate signals stimulate fibro/adipogenic progenitors to facilitate muscle regeneration. *Cell* **2013**, *153*, 376–388. [CrossRef] [PubMed]

48. Mackey, A.L.; Magnan, M.; Chazaud, B.; Kjaer, M. Human skeletal muscle fibroblasts stimulate in vitro myogenesis and in vivo muscle regeneration. *J. Physiol.* **2017**, *595*, 5115–5127. [CrossRef] [PubMed]

49. Malecova, B.; Gatto, S.; Etxaniz, U.; Passafaro, M.; Cortez, A.; Nicoletti, C.; Giordani, L.; Torcinaro, A.; De Bardi, M.; Bicciato, S.; et al. Dynamics of cellular states of fibro-adipogenic progenitors during myogenesis and muscular dystrophy. *Nat. Commun.* **2018**, *9*, 3670. [CrossRef] [PubMed]

50. Cretoiu, S.M.; Popescu, L.M. Telocytes revisited. *Biomol. Concepts* **2014**, *5*, 353–369. [CrossRef] [PubMed]

51. Nakamura, Y.; Miyaki, S.; Ishitobi, H.; Matsuyama, S.; Nakasa, T.; Kamei, N.; Akimoto, T.; Higashi, Y.; Ochi, M. Mesenchymal-stem-cell-derived exosomes accelerate skeletal muscle regeneration. *FEBS Lett.* **2015**, *589*, 1257–1265. [CrossRef] [PubMed]

52. Christov, C.; Chrétien, F.; Abou-Khalil, R.; Bassez, G.; Vallet, G.; Authier, F.J.; Bassaglia, Y.; Shinin, V.; Tajbakhsh, S.; Chazaud, B.; et al. Muscle satellite cells and endothelial cells: Close neighbors and privileged partners. *Mol. Biol. Cell* **2007**, *18*, 1397–1409. [CrossRef] [PubMed]

53. Verma, M.; Asakura, Y.; Murakonda, B.S.R.; Pengo, T.; Latroche, C.; Chazaud, B.; McLoon, L.K.; Asakura, A. Muscle Satellite Cell Cross-Talk with a Vascular Niche Maintains Quiescence via VEGF and Notch Signaling. *Cell Stem Cell* **2018**, *23*, 530–543.e9. [CrossRef] [PubMed]

54. Abou-Khalil, R.; Mounier, R.; Chazaud, B. Regulation of myogenic stem cell behavior by vessel cells: The "menage a trois" of satellite cells, periendothelial cells and endothelial cells. *Cell Cycle* **2010**, *9*, 892–896. [CrossRef] [PubMed]

55. Kostallari, E.; Baba-Amer, Y.; Alonso-Martin, S.; Ngoh, P.; Relaix, F.; Lafuste, P.; Gherardi, R.K. Pericytes in the myovascular niche promote post-natal myofiber growth and satellite cell quiescence. *Development* **2015**, *142*, 1242–1253. [CrossRef] [PubMed]

56. Menetrey, J.; Kasemkijwattana, C.; Day, C.S.; Bosch, P.; Vogt, M.; Fu, F.H.; Moreland, M.S.; Huard, J. Growth factors improve muscle healing in vivo. *J. Bone Jt. Surg. Br.* **2000**, *82*, 131–137. [CrossRef]

57. De Perini, A.; Dimauro, I.; Duranti, G.; Fantini, C.; Mercatelli, N.; Ceci, R.; Di Luigi, L.; Sabatini, S.; Caporossi, D. The p75NTR-mediated effect of nerve growth factor in L6C5 myogenic cells. *BMC Res. Notes* **2017**, *10*, 686. [CrossRef] [PubMed]

58. Judson, R.N.; Zhang, R.H.; Rossi, F.M. Tissue-resident mesenchymal stem/progenitor cells in skeletal muscle: Collaborators or saboteurs? *FEBS J.* **2013**, *280*, 4100–4108. [CrossRef] [PubMed]

59. Asakura, A.; Seale, P.; Girgis-Gabardo, A.; Rudnicki, M.A. Myogenic specification of side population cells in skeletal muscle. *J. Cell Biol.* **2002**, *159*, 123–134. [CrossRef] [PubMed]

60. Uezumi, A.; Ojima, K.; Fukada, S.; Ikemoto, M.; Masuda, S.; Miyagoe-Suzuki, Y.; Takeda, S. Functional heterogeneity of side population cells in skeletal muscle. *Biochem. Biophys. Res. Commun.* **2006**, *341*, 864–873. [CrossRef]

61. Tanaka, K.K.; Hall, J.K.; Troy, A.A.; Cornelison, D.D.; Majka, S.M.; Olwin, B.B. Syndecan-4-expressing muscle progenitor cells in the SP engraft as satellite cells during muscle regeneration. *Cell Stem Cell* **2009**, *4*, 217–225. [CrossRef] [PubMed]

62. Dellavalle, A.; Maroli, G.; Covarello, D.; Azzoni, E.; Innocenzi, A.; Perani, L.; Antonini, S.; Sambasivan, R.; Brunelli, S.; Tajbakhsh, S.; et al. Pericytes resident in postnatal skeletal muscle differentiate into muscle fibres and generate satellite cells. *Nat. Commun.* **2011**, *2*, 499. [CrossRef] [PubMed]

63. Díaz-Manera, J.; Gallardo, E.; de Luna, N.; Navas, M.; Soria, L.; Garibaldi, M.; Rojas-García, R.; Tonlorenzi, R.; Cossu, G.; Illa, I. The increase of pericyte population in human neuromuscular disorders supports their role in muscle regeneration in vivo. *J. Pathol.* **2012**, *228*, 544–553. [CrossRef] [PubMed]

64. Birbrair, A.; Zhang, T.; Wang, Z.M.; Messi, M.L.; Enikolopov, G.N.; Mintz, A.; Delbono, O. Skeletal muscle pericyte subtypes differ in their differentiation potential. *Stem Cell Res.* **2013**, *10*, 67–84. [CrossRef] [PubMed]

65. Benchaouir, R.; Meregalli, M.; Farini, A.; D'Antona, G.; Belicchi, M.; Goyenvalle, A.; Battistelli, M.; Bresolin, N.; Bottinelli, R.; Garcia, L.; et al. Restoration of human dystrophin following transplantation of exon-skipping-engineered DMD patient stem cells into dystrophic mice. *Cell Stem Cell* **2007**, *1*, 646–657. [CrossRef] [PubMed]

66. Negroni, E.; Riederer, I.; Chaouch, S.; Belicchi, M.; Razini, P.; Di Santo, J.; Torrente, Y.; Butler-Browne, G.S.; Mouly, V. In vivo myogenic potential of human CD133+ muscle-derived stem cells: A quantitative study. *Mol. Ther.* **2009**, *17*, 1771–1778. [CrossRef] [PubMed]

67. Meng, J.; Chun, S.; Asfahani, R.; Lochmüller, H.; Muntoni, F.; Morgan, J. Human skeletal muscle-derived CD133(+) cells form functional satellite cells after intramuscular transplantation in immunodeficient host mice. *Mol. Ther.* **2014**, *22*, 1008–1017. [CrossRef]

68. Dulauroy, S.; Di Carlo, S.E.; Langa, F.; Eberl, G.; Peduto, L. Lineage tracing and genetic ablation of ADAM12(+) perivascular cells identify a major source of profibrotic cells during acute tissue injury. *Nat. Med.* **2012**, *18*, 1262–1270. [CrossRef]

69. Uezumi, A.; Ikemoto-Uezumi, M.; Tsuchida, K. Roles of non myogenic mesenchymal progenitors in pathogenesis and regeneration of skeletal muscle. *Front. Physiol.* **2014**, *5*, 68. [CrossRef]

70. Lemos, D.R.; Babaeijandaghi, F.; Low, M.; Chang, C.K.; Lee, S.T.; Fiore, D.; Zhang, R.H.; Natarajan, A.; Nedospasov, S.A.; Rossi, F.M. Nilotinib reduces muscle fibrosis in chronic muscle injury by promoting TNF-mediated apoptosis of fibro/adipogenic progenitors. *Nat. Med.* **2015**, *21*, 786–794. [CrossRef]

71. Rudolf, R.; Deschenes, M.R.; Sandri, M. Neuromuscular junction degeneration in muscle wasting. *Curr. Opin. Clin. Nutr. Metab. Care* **2016**, *19*, 177–181. [CrossRef] [PubMed]

72. DeLong, J.M.; Russell, R.P.; Mazzocca, A.D. Platelet-rich plasma: The PAW classification system. *Arthroscopy* **2012**, *28*, 998–1009. [CrossRef] [PubMed]

73. De Pascale, M.R.; Sommese, L.; Casamassimi, A.; Napoli, C. Platelet derivatives in regenerative medicine: An update. *Transfus. Med. Rev.* **2015**, *29*, 52–61. [CrossRef] [PubMed]

74. Mautner, K.; Malanga, G.A.; Smith, J.; Shiple, B.; Ibrahim, V.; Sampson, S.; Bowen, J.E. A call for a standard classification system for future biologic research: The rationale for new PRP nomenclature. *PM R* **2015**, *7*, S53–S59. [CrossRef] [PubMed]

75. Le, A.D.K.; Enweze, L.; DeBaun, M.R.; Dragoo, J.L. Platelet-Rich Plasma. *Clin. Sports Med.* **2019**, *38*, 17–44. [CrossRef] [PubMed]

76. Cervelli, V.; Gentile, P.; Scioli, M.G.; Grimaldi, M.; Casciani, C.U.; Spagnoli, L.G.; Orlandi, A. Application of platelet-rich plasma in plastic surgery: Clinical and in vitro evaluation. *Tissue Eng. Part C Methods* **2009**, *15*, 625–634. [CrossRef] [PubMed]

77. Agrawal, A.A. Evolution, current status and advances in application of platelet concentrate in periodontics and implantology. *World J. Clin. Cases* **2017**, *5*, 159–171. [CrossRef]

78. Giannaccare, G.; Versura, P.; Buzzi, M.; Primavera, L.; Pellegrini, M.; Campos, E.C. Blood derived eye drops for the treatment of cornea and ocular surface diseases. *Transfus. Apher. Sci.* **2017**, *56*, 595–604. [CrossRef]

79. Tandulwadkar, S.R.; Naralkar, M.V.; Surana, A.D.; Selvakarthick, M.; Kharat, A.H. Autologous intrauterine platelet-rich plasma instillation for suboptimal endometrium in frozen embryo transfer cycles: A pilot study. *J. Hum. Reprod. Sci.* **2017**, *10*, 208–212. [CrossRef]

80. Santos, S.C.N.D.S.; Sigurjonsson, O.E.; Custodio, C.A.; Mano, J.F.C.D.L. Blood plasma derivatives for tissue engineering and regenerative medicine therapies. *Tissue Eng. Part B Rev.* **2018**, *24*, 454–462. [CrossRef]

81. Chicharro-Alcántara, D.; Rubio-Zaragoza, M.; Damiá-Giménez, E.; Carrillo-Poveda, J.M.; Cuervo-Serrato, B.; Peláez-Gorrea, P.; Sopena-Juncosa, J.J. Platelet rich plasma: New insights for cutaneous wound healing management. *J. Funct. Biomater.* **2018**, *9*, 10. [CrossRef] [PubMed]

82. Nguyen, R.T.; Borg-Stein, J.; McInnis, K. Applications of platelet-rich plasma in musculoskeletal and sports medicine: An evidence-based approach. *PM R* **2011**, *3*, 226–250. [CrossRef] [PubMed]

83. Andia, I.; Abate, M. Platelet-rich plasma in the treatment of skeletal muscle injuries. *Expert. Opin. Biol.* **2015**, *15*, 987–999. [CrossRef] [PubMed]

84. Andia, I.; Abate, M. Platelet-rich plasma: Combinational treatment modalities for musculoskeletal conditions. *Front. Med.* **2018**, *12*, 139–152. [CrossRef] [PubMed]

85. Andia, I.; Martin, J.I.; Maffulli, N. Advances with platelet rich plasma therapies for tendon regeneration. *Expert Opin. Biol.* **2018**, *18*, 389–398. [CrossRef] [PubMed]

86. Amable, P.R.; Carias, R.B.; Teixeira, M.V.; da Cruz Pacheco, I.; Corrêa do Amaral, R.J.; Granjeiro, J.M.; Borojevic, R. Platelet-rich plasma preparation for regenerative medicine: Optimization and quantification of cytokines and growth factors. *Stem Cell Res.* **2013**, *4*, 67. [CrossRef] [PubMed]

87. Martínez, C.E.; Smith, P.C.; Palma Alvarado, V.A. The influence of platelet-derived products on angiogenesis and tissue repair: A concise update. *Front. Physiol.* **2015**, *6*, 290. [CrossRef] [PubMed]

88. Pochini, A.C.; Antonioli, E.; Bucci, D.Z.; Sardinha, L.R.; Andreoli, C.V.; Ferretti, M.; Ejnisman, B.; Goldberg, A.C.; Cohen, M. Analysis of cytokine profile and growth factors in platelet-rich plasma obtained by open systems and commercial columns. *Einstein* **2016**, *14*, 391–397. [CrossRef] [PubMed]

89. Qiao, J.; An, N.; Ouyang, X. Quantification of growth factors in different platelet concentrates. *Platelets* **2017**, *28*, 774–778. [CrossRef]

90. San Sebastian, K.M.; Lobato, I.; Hernández, I.; Burgos-Alonso, N.; Gomez-Fernandez, M.C.; López, J.L.; Rodríguez, B.; March, A.G.; Grandes, G.; Andia, I. Efficacy and safety of autologous platelet rich plasma for the treatment of vascular ulcers in primary care: Phase III study. *BMC Fam. Pract.* **2014**, *15*, 211. [CrossRef]

91. Suthar, M.; Gupta, S.; Bukhari, S.; Ponemone, V. Treatment of chronic non-healing ulcers using autologous platelet rich plasma: A case series. *J. Biomed. Sci.* **2017**, *24*, 16. [CrossRef] [PubMed]

92. Bottegoni, C.; Farinelli, L.; Aquili, A.; Chiurazzi, E.; Gigante, A. Homologous platelet-rich plasma for the treatment of knee involvement in primary Sjögren's syndrome. *J. Biol. Regul. Homeost. Agents* **2016**, *30*, 63–67. [PubMed]

93. Anitua, E.; Prado, R.; Orive, G. Allogeneic Platelet-Rich Plasma: At the Dawn of an Off-the-Shelf Therapy? *Trends Biotechnol.* **2017**, *35*, 91–93. [CrossRef] [PubMed]

94. Bubnov, R.; Yevseenko, V.; Semeniv, I. Ultrasound guided injections of platelets rich plasma for muscle injury in professional athletes. Comparative study. *Med. Ultrason.* **2013**, *15*, 101–105. [CrossRef] [PubMed]

95. Wetzel, R.J.; Patel, R.M.; Terry, M.A. Platelet-rich plasma as an effective treatment for proximal hamstring injuries. *Orthopedics* **2013**, *36*, e64–e70. [CrossRef] [PubMed]

96. A Hamid, M.S.; Mohamed Ali, M.R.; Yusof, A.; George, J.; Lee, L.P. Platelet-rich plasma injections for the treatment of hamstring injuries: A randomized controlled trial. *Am. J. Sports Med.* **2014**, *42*, 2410–2418. [CrossRef] [PubMed]

97. Rossi, L.A.; Molina Rómoli, A.R.; Bertona Altieri, B.A.; Burgos Flor, J.A.; Scordo, W.E.; Elizondo, C.M. Does platelet-rich plasma decrease time to return to sports in acute muscle tear? A randomized controlled trial. *Knee Surg. Sports Traumatol. Arthrosc.* **2017**, *25*, 3319–3325. [CrossRef]

98. Borrione, P.; Fossati, C.; Pereira, M.T.; Giannini, S.; Davico, M.; Minganti, C.; Pigozzi, F. The use of platelet-rich plasma (PRP) in the treatment of gastrocnemius strains: A retrospective observational study. *Platelets* **2018**, *29*, 596–601. [CrossRef]

99. Bernuzzi, G.; Petraglia, F.; Pedrini, M.F.; De Filippo, M.; Pogliacomi, F.; Verdano, M.A.; Costantino, C. Use of platelet-rich plasma in the care of sports injuries: Our experience with ultrasound-guided injection. *Blood Transfus.* **2014**, *12*, s229–s234. [CrossRef]

100. Zanon, G.; Combi, F.; Combi, A.; Perticarini, L.; Sammarchi, L.; Benazzo, F. Platelet-rich plasma in the treatment of acute hamstring injuries in professional football players. *Joints* **2016**, *4*, 17–23. [CrossRef]

101. Punduk, Z.; Oral, O.; Ozkayin, N.; Rahman, K.; Varol, R. Single dose of intra-muscular platelet rich plasma reverses the increase in plasma iron levels in exercise-induced muscle damage: A pilot study. *J. Sport Health Sci.* **2016**, *5*, 109–114. [CrossRef] [PubMed]

Int. J. Mol. Sci. **2019**, *20*, 683

102. Sheth, U.; Dwyer, T.; Smith, I.; Wasserstein, D.; Theodoropoulos, J.; Takhar, S.; Chahal, J. Does Platelet-Rich Plasma Lead to Earlier Return to Sport When Compared With Conservative Treatment in Acute Muscle Injuries? A Systematic Review and Meta-analysis. *Arthroscopy* **2018**, *34*, 281–288.e1. [CrossRef] [PubMed]

103. Scully, D.; Naseem, K.M.; Matsakas, A. Platelet biology in regenerative medicine of skeletal muscle. *Acta Physiol. (Oxf.)* **2018**, *223*, e13071. [CrossRef] [PubMed]

104. Grassi, A.; Napoli, F.; Romandini, I.; Samuelsson, K.; Zaffagnini, S.; Candrian, C.; Filardo, G. Is Platelet-Rich Plasma (PRP) Effective in the Treatment of Acute Muscle Injuries? A Systematic Review and Meta-Analysis. *Sports Med.* **2018**, *48*, 971–989. [CrossRef] [PubMed]

105. Borrione, P.; Grasso, L.; Chierto, E.; Geuna, S.; Racca, S.; Abbadessa, G.; Ronchi, G.; Faiola, F.; Di Gianfrancesco, A.; Pigozzi, F. Experimental model for the study of the effects of platelet-rich plasma on the early phases of muscle healing. *Blood Transfus.* **2014**, *12*, s221–s228. [CrossRef] [PubMed]

106. Li, H.; Hicks, J.J.; Wang, L.; Oyster, N.; Philippon, M.J.; Hurwitz, S.; Hogan, M.V.; Huard, J. Customized platelet-rich plasma with transforming growth factor β1 neutralization antibody to reduce fibrosis in skeletal muscle. *Biomaterials* **2016**, *87*, 147–156. [CrossRef] [PubMed]

107. Garcia, T.A.; Camargo, R.C.T.; Koike, T.E.; Ozaki, G.A.T.; Castoldi, R.C.; Camargo Filho, J.C.S. Histological analysis of the association of low level laser therapy and platelet-rich plasma in regeneration of muscle injury in rats. *Braz. J. Phys.* **2017**, *21*, 425–433. [CrossRef] [PubMed]

108. Tsai, W.C.; Yu, T.Y.; Chang, G.J.; Lin, L.P.; Lin, M.S.; Pang, J.S. Platelet-Rich Plasma Releasate Promotes Regeneration and Decreases Inflammation and Apoptosis of Injured Skeletal Muscle. *Am. J. Sports Med.* **2018**, *46*, 1980–1986. [CrossRef] [PubMed]

109. Hammond, J.W.; Hinton, R.Y.; Curl, L.A.; Muriel, J.M.; Lovering, R.M. Use of autologous platelet-rich plasma to treat muscle strain injuries. *Am. J. Sports Med.* **2009**, *37*, 1135–1142. [CrossRef] [PubMed]

110. Gigante, A.; Del Torto, M.; Manzotti, S.; Cianforlini, M.; Busilacchi, A.; Davidson, P.A.; Greco, F.; Mattioli-Belmonte, M. Platelet rich fibrin matrix effects on skeletal muscle lesions: An experimental study. *J. Biol. Regul. Homeost. Agents* **2012**, *26*, 475–484. [PubMed]

111. Dimauro, I.; Grasso, L.; Fittipaldi, S.; Fantini, C.; Mercatelli, N.; Racca, S.; Geuna, S.; Di Gianfrancesco, A.; Caporossi, D.; Pigozzi, F.; et al. Platelet-rich plasma and skeletal muscle healing: A molecular analysis of the early phases of the regeneration process in an experimental animal model. *PLoS ONE* **2014**, *9*, e102993. [CrossRef] [PubMed]

112. Cianforlini, M.; Mattioli-Belmonte, M.; Manzotti, S.; Chiurazzi, E.; Piani, M.; Orlando, F.; Provinciali, M.; Gigante, A. Effect of platelet rich plasma concentration on skeletal muscle regeneration: An experimental study. *J. Biol. Regul. Homeost. Agents* **2015**, *29*, 47–55. [PubMed]

113. Contreras-Muñoz, P.; Torrella, J.R.; Serres, X.; Rizo-Roca, D.; De la Varga, M.; Viscor, G.; Martínez-Ibáñez, V.; Peiró, J.L.; Järvinen, T.A.H.; Rodas, G.; et al. Postinjury Exercise and Platelet-Rich Plasma Therapies Improve Skeletal Muscle Healing in Rats But Are Not Synergistic When Combined. *Am. J. Sports Med.* **2017**, *45*, 2131–2141. [CrossRef] [PubMed]

114. Martins, R.P.; Hartmann, D.D.; de Moraes, J.P.; Soares, F.A.; Puntel, G.O. Platelet-rich plasma reduces the oxidative damage determined by a skeletal muscle contusion in rats. *Platelets* **2016**, *27*, 784–790. [CrossRef] [PubMed]

115. Cunha, R.C.; Francisco, J.C.; Cardoso, M.A.; Matos, L.F.; Lino, D.; Simeoni, R.B.; Pereira, G.; Irioda, A.C.; Simeoni, P.R.; Guarita-Souza, L.C.; et al. Effect of platelet-rich plasma therapy associated with exercise training in musculoskeletal healing in rats. *Transpl. Proc.* **2014**, *46*, 1879–1881. [CrossRef] [PubMed]

116. Anitua, E.; Pelacho, B.; Prado, R.; Aguirre, J.J.; Sánchez, M.; Padilla, S.; Aranguren, X.L.; Abizanda, G.; Collantes, M.; Hernandez, M.; et al. Infiltration of plasma rich in growth factors enhances in vivo angiogenesis and improves reperfusion and tissue remodeling after severe hind limb ischemia. *J. Control. Release* **2015**, *202*, 31–39. [CrossRef] [PubMed]

117. Terada, S.; Ota, S.; Kobayashi, M.; Kobayashi, T.; Mifune, Y.; Takayama, K.; Witt, M.; Vadalà, G.; Oyster, N.; Otsuka, T.; et al. Use of an antifibrotic agent improves the effect of platelet-rich plasma on muscle healing after injury. *J. Bone Jt. Surg. Am.* **2013**, *95*, 980–988. [CrossRef] [PubMed]

118. Denapoli, P.M.; Stilhano, R.S.; Ingham, S.J.; Han, S.W.; Abdalla, R.J. Platelet-Rich Plasma in a Murine Model: Leukocytes, Growth Factors, Flt-1, and Muscle Healing. *Am. J. Sports Med.* **2016**, *44*, 1962–1971. [CrossRef]

119. Pinheiro, C.L.; Peixinho, C.C.; Esposito, C.C.; Manso, J.E.; Machado, J.C. Ultrasound biomicroscopy and claudication test for in vivo follow-up of muscle repair enhancement based on platelet-rich plasma therapy in a rat model of gastrocnemius laceration. *Acta Cir. Bras.* **2016**, *31*, 103–110. [CrossRef] [PubMed]

120. Takase, F.; Inui, A.; Mifune, Y.; Sakata, R.; Muto, T.; Harada, Y.; Ueda, Y.; Kokubu, T.; Kurosaka, M. Effect of platelet-rich plasma on degeneration change of rotator cuff muscles: In vitro and in vivo evaluations. *J. Orthop. Res.* **2017**, *35*, 1806–1815. [CrossRef] [PubMed]

121. Miroshnychenko, O.; Chang, W.T.; Dragoo, J.L. The Use of Platelet-Rich and Platelet-Poor Plasma to Enhance Differentiation of Skeletal Myoblasts: Implications for the Use of Autologous Blood Products for Muscle Regeneration. *Am. J. Sports Med.* **2017**, *45*, 945–953. [CrossRef] [PubMed]

122. Li, H.; Usas, A.; Poddar, M.; Chen, C.W.; Thompson, S.; Ahani, B.; Cummins, J.; Lavasani, M.; Huard, J. Platelet-rich plasma promotes the proliferation of human muscle derived progenitor cells and maintains their stemness. *PLoS ONE* **2013**, *8*, e64923. [CrossRef] [PubMed]

123. Im, W.; Ban, J.J.; Lim, J.; Lee, M.; Chung, J.Y.; Bhattacharya, R.; Kim, S.H. Adipose-derived stem cells extract has a proliferative effect on myogenic progenitors. *In Vitro Cell. Dev. Biol. Anim.* **2014**, *50*, 740–766. [CrossRef] [PubMed]

124. Tsai, W.C.; Yu, T.Y.; Lin, L.P.; Lin, M.S.; Wu, Y.C.; Liao, C.H.; Pang, J.S. Platelet rich plasma releasate promotes proliferation of skeletal muscle cells in association with upregulation of PCNA, cyclins and cyclin dependent kinases. *Platelets* **2017**, *28*, 491–497. [CrossRef] [PubMed]

125. McClure, M.J.; Garg, K.; Simpson, D.G.; Ryan, J.J.; Sell, S.A.; Bowlin, G.L.; Ericksen, J.J. The influence of platelet-rich plasma on myogenic differentiation. *J. Tissue Eng. Regen. Med.* **2016**, *10*, E239–E249. [CrossRef] [PubMed]

126. McClure, M.J.; Clark, N.M.; Schwartz, Z.; Boyan, B.D. Platelet-rich plasma and alignment enhance myogenin via ERK mitogen activated protein kinase signaling. *Biomed. Mater.* **2018**, *13*, 055009. [CrossRef] [PubMed]

127. Kelc, R.; Trapecar, M.; Gradisnik, L.; Rupnik, M.S.; Vogrin, M. Platelet-rich plasma, especially when combined with a TGF-β inhibitor promotes proliferation, viability and myogenic differentiation of myoblasts in vitro. *PLoS ONE* **2015**, *10*, e0117302. [CrossRef]

128. Deasy, B.M.; Feduska, J.M.; Payne, T.R.; Li, Y.; Ambrosio, F.; Huard, J. Effect of VEGF on the regenerative capacity of muscle stem cells in dystrophic skeletal muscle. *Mol. Ther.* **2009**, *17*, 1788–1798. [CrossRef]

129. Walker, N.; Kahamba, T.; Woudberg, N.; Goetsch, K.; Niesler, C. Dose-dependent modulation of myogenesis by HGF: Implications for c-Met expression and downstream signalling pathways. *Growth Factors* **2015**, *33*, 229–241. [CrossRef]

130. Duan, C.; Ren, H.; Gao, S. Insulin-like growth factors (IGFs), IGF receptors, and IGF-binding proteins: Roles in skeletal muscle growth and differentiation. *Gen. Comp. Endocrinol.* **2010**, *167*, 344–351. [CrossRef]

131. Scully, D.; Sfyri, P.; Verpoorten, S.; Papadopoulos, P.; Muñoz-Turrillas, M.C.; Mitchell, R.; Aburima, A.; Patel, K.; Gutiérrez, L.; Naseem, K.M.; et al. Platelet releasate promotes skeletal myogenesis by increasing muscle stem cell commitment to differentiation and accelerates muscle regeneration following acute injury. *Acta Physiol. (Oxf.)* **2018**, *19*, e13207. [CrossRef] [PubMed]

132. Tsai, W.C.; Yu, T.Y.; Lin, L.P.; Lin, M.S.; Tsai, T.T.; Pang, J.S. Platelet rich plasma promotes skeletal muscle cell migration in association with up-regulation of FAK, paxillin, and F-Actin formation. *J. Orthop. Res.* **2017**, *35*, 2506–2512. [CrossRef] [PubMed]

133. Sassoli, C.; Vallone, L.; Tani, A.; Chellini, F.; Nosi, D.; Zecchi-Orlandini, S. Combined use of bone marrow-derived mesenchymal stromal cells (BM-MSCs) and platelet rich plasma (PRP) stimulates proliferation and differentiation of myoblasts in vitro: New therapeutic perspectives for skeletal muscle repair/regeneration. *Cell Tissue Res.* **2018**, *372*, 549–570. [CrossRef] [PubMed]

134. Yamada, M.; Sankoda, Y.; Tatsumi, R.; Mizunoya, W.; Ikeuchi, Y.; Sunagawa, K.; Allen, R.E. Matrix metalloproteinase-2 mediates stretch-induced activation of skeletal muscle satellite cells in a nitric oxide-dependent manner. *Int. J. Biochem. Cell Biol.* **2008**, *40*, 2183–2191. [CrossRef] [PubMed]

135. Pallafacchina, G.; François, S.; Regnault, B.; Czarny, B.; Dive, V.; Cumano, A.; Montarras, D.; Buckingham, M. An adult tissue-specific stem cell in its niche: A gene profiling analysis of in vivo quiescent and activated muscle satellite cells. *Stem Cell Res.* **2010**, *4*, 77–91. [CrossRef] [PubMed]

136. Bellayr, I.; Holden, K.; Mu, X.; Pan, H.; Li, Y. Matrix metalloproteinase inhibition negatively affects muscle stem cell behavior. *Int. J. Clin. Exp. Pathol.* **2013**, *6*, 124–141. [PubMed]

137. Chen, X.; Li, Y. Role of matrix metalloproteinases in skeletal muscle: Migration, differentiation, regeneration and fibrosis. *Cell Adhes. Migr.* **2009**, *3*, 337–341. [CrossRef]

138. Miyazaki, D.; Nakamura, A.; Fukushima, K.; Yoshida, K.; Takeda, S.; Ikeda, S. Matrix metalloproteinase-2 ablation in dystrophin-deficient mdx muscles reduces angiogenesis resulting in impaired growth of regenerated muscle fibers. *Hum. Mol. Genet.* **2011**, *20*, 1787–1799. [CrossRef] [PubMed]

139. Cassano, M.; Dellavalle, A.; Tedesco, F.S.; Quattrocelli, M.; Crippa, S.; Ronzoni, F.; Salvade, A.; Berardi, E.; Torrente, Y.; Cossu, G.; et al. Alpha sarcoglycan is required for FGF-dependent myogenic progenitor cell proliferation in vitro and in vivo. *Development* **2011**, *138*, 4523–4533. [CrossRef]

140. Sartori, R.; Gregorevic, P.; Sandri, M. TGFβ and BMP signaling in skeletal muscle: Potential significance for muscle-related disease. *Trends Endocrinol. Metab.* **2014**, *25*, 464–471. [CrossRef] [PubMed]

141. Escobar, G.; Escobar, A.; Ascui, G.; Tempio, F.I.; Ortiz, M.C.; Pérez, C.A.; López, M.N. Pure platelet-rich plasma and supernatant of calcium-activated P-PRP induce different phenotypes of human macrophages. *Regen. Med.* **2018**, *13*, 427–441. [CrossRef] [PubMed]

142. Papait, A.; Cancedda, R.; Mastrogiacomo, M.; Poggi, A. Allogeneic platelet-rich plasma affects monocyte differentiation to dendritic cells causing an anti-inflammatory microenvironment, putatively fostering wound healing. *J. Tissue Eng. Regen. Med.* **2018**, *12*, 30–43. [CrossRef] [PubMed]

143. Pakshir, P.; Hinz, B. The big five in fibrosis: Macrophages, myofibroblasts, matrix, mechanics, and miscommunication. *Matrix Biol.* **2018**, *68–69*, 81–93. [CrossRef] [PubMed]

144. Chellini, F.; Tani, A.; Vallone, L.; Nosi, D.; Pavan, P.; Bambi, F.; Zecchi Orlandini, S.; Sassoli, C. Platelet-Rich Plasma Prevents In Vitro Transforming Growth Factor-β1-Induced Fibroblast to Myofibroblast Transition: Involvement of Vascular Endothelial Growth Factor (VEGF)-A/VEGF Receptor-1-Mediated Signaling. *Cells* **2018**, *7*, 142. [CrossRef] [PubMed]

145. Anitua, E.; Troya, M.; Orive, G. Plasma rich in growth factors promote gingival tissue regeneration by stimulating fibroblast proliferation and migration and by blocking transforming growth factor-β1-induced myodifferentiation. *J. Periodontol.* **2012**, *83*, 1028–1037. [CrossRef] [PubMed]

146. Anitua, E.; de la Fuente, M.; Muruzabal, F.; Riestra, A.; Merayo-Lloves, J.; Orive, G. Plasma rich in growth factors (PRGF) eye drops stimulates scarless regeneration compared to autologous serum in the ocular surface stromal fibroblasts. *Exp. Eye Res.* **2015**, *135*, 118–126. [CrossRef] [PubMed]

147. Wang, M.L.; Rivlin, M.; Graham, J.G.; Beredjiklian, P.K. Peripheral nerve injury, scarring, and recovery. *Connect. Tissue Res.* **2018**, *6*, 1–7. [CrossRef] [PubMed]

148. Giannessi, E.; Coli, A.; Stornelli, M.R.; Miragliotta, V.; Pirone, A.; Lenzi, C.; Burchielli, S.; Vozzi, G.; De Maria, C.; Giorgetti, M. An autologously generated platelet-rich plasma suturable membrane may enhance peripheral nerve regeneration after neurorraphy in an acute injury model of sciatic nerve neurotmesis. *J. Reconstr. Microsurg.* **2014**, *30*, 617–626. [CrossRef]

149. Zheng, C.; Zhu, Q.; Liu, X.; Huang, X.; He, C.; Jiang, L.; Quan, D.; Zhou, X.; Zhu, Z. Effect of platelet-rich plasma (PRP) concentration on proliferation, neurotrophic function and migration of Schwann cells in vitro. *J. Tissue Eng. Regen. Med.* **2016**, *10*, 428–436. [CrossRef]

150. Sánchez, M.; Garate, A.; Delgado, D.; Padilla, S. Platelet-rich plasma, an adjuvant biological therapy to assist peripheral nerve repair. *Neural Regen. Res.* **2017**, *12*, 47–52. [CrossRef]

151. Teymur, H.; Tiftikcioglu, Y.O.; Cavusoglu, T.; Tiftikcioglu, B.I.; Erbas, O.; Yigitturk, G.; Uyanikgil, Y. Effect of platelet-rich plasma on reconstruction with nerve autografts. *Kaohsiung J. Med. Sci.* **2017**, *33*, 69–77. [CrossRef] [PubMed]

152. Cáceres, M.; Martínez, C.; Martínez, J.; Smith, P.C. Effects of platelet-rich and -poor plasma on the reparative response of gingival fibroblasts. *Clin. Oral Implant. Res.* **2012**, *23*, 1104–1111. [CrossRef] [PubMed]

153. Creeper, F.; Ivanovski, S. Effect of autologous and allogenic platelet-rich plasma on human gingival fibroblast function. *Oral Dis.* **2012**, *18*, 494–500. [CrossRef] [PubMed]

154. Martínez, C.E.; González, S.A.; Palma, V.; Smith, P.C. Platelet-Poor and Platelet-Rich Plasma Stimulate Bone Lineage Differentiation in Periodontal Ligament Stem Cells. *J. Periodontol.* **2016**, *87*, e18–e26. [CrossRef] [PubMed]

155. de Mos, M.; van der Windt, A.E.; Jahr, H.; van Schie, H.T.; Weinans, H.; Verhaar, J.A.; van Osch, G.J. Can platelet-rich plasma enhance tendon repair? A cell culture study. *Am. J. Sports Med.* **2008**, *36*, 1171–1178. [CrossRef] [PubMed]

Int. J. Mol. Sci. **2019**, *20*, 683

156. Shahidi, M.; Vatanmakanian, M.; Arami, M.K.; Sadeghi Shirazi, F.; Esmaeili, N.; Hydarporian, S.; Jafari, S. A comparative study between platelet-rich plasma and platelet-poor plasma effects on angiogenesis. *Med. Mol. Morphol.* **2018**, *51*, 21–31. [CrossRef] [PubMed]

157. Renn, T.Y.; Kao, Y.H.; Wang, C.C.; Burnouf, T. Anti-inflammatory effects of platelet biomaterials in a macrophage cellular model. *Vox Sang.* **2015**, *109*, 138–147. [CrossRef] [PubMed]

158. Rettig, A.C.; Meyer, S.; Bhadra, A.K. Platelet-Rich Plasma in Addition to Rehabilitation for Acute Hamstring Injuries in NFL Players: Clinical Effects and Time to Return to Play. *Orthop. J. Sports Med.* **2013**, *1*, 2325967113494354. [CrossRef] [PubMed]

159. Delos, D.; Leineweber, M.J.; Chaudhury, S.; Alzoobaee, S.; Gao, Y.; Rodeo, S.A. The effect of platelet-rich plasma on muscle contusion healing in a rat model. *Am. J. Sports Med.* **2014**, *42*, 2067–2074. [CrossRef] [PubMed]

160. Hamid, M.S.; Yusof, A.; Mohamed Ali, M.R. Platelet-rich plasma (PRP) for acute muscle injury: A systematic review. *PLoS ONE* **2014**, *9*, e90538. [CrossRef]

161. Hamilton, B.; Tol, J.L.; Almusa, E.; Boukarroum, S.; Eirale, C.; Farooq, A.; Whiteley, R.; Chalabi, H. Platelet-rich plasma does not enhance return to play in hamstring injuries: A randomised controlled trial. *Br. J. Sports Med.* **2015**, *49*, 943–950. [CrossRef] [PubMed]

162. Reurink, G.; Goudswaard, G.J.; Moen, M.H.; Weir, A.; Verhaar, J.A.; Bierma-Zeinstra, S.M.; Maas, M.; Tol, J.L. Dutch HIT-study Investigators. Rationale, secondary outcome scores and 1-year follow-up of a randomised trial of platelet-rich plasma injections in acute hamstring muscle injury: The Dutch Hamstring Injection Therapy study. *Br. J. Sports Med.* **2015**, *49*, 1206–1212. [CrossRef] [PubMed]

163. Kelc, R.; Vogrin, M. Concerns about fibrosis development after scaffolded PRP therapy of muscle injuries: Commentary on an article by Sanchez et al.: Muscle repair: Platelet-rich plasma derivates as a bridge from spontaneity to intervention. *Injury* **2015**, *46*, 428. [CrossRef] [PubMed]

164. Martinez-Zapata, M.J.; Orozco, L.; Balius, R.; Soler, R.; Bosch, A.; Rodas, G.; Til, L.; Peirau, X.; Urrútia, G.; Gich, I.; et al. PRP-RICE group. Efficacy of autologous platelet-rich plasma for the treatment of muscle rupture with haematoma: A multicentre, randomised, double-blind, placebo-controlled clinical trial. *Blood Transfus.* **2016**, *14*, 245–254. [CrossRef] [PubMed]

165. Guillodo, Y.; Madouas, G.; Simon, T.; Le Dauphin, H.; Saraux, A. Platelet-rich plasma (PRP) treatment of sports-related severe acute hamstring injuries. *Muscles Ligaments Tendons J.* **2016**, *5*, 284–288. [CrossRef] [PubMed]

166. Navani, A.; Li, G.; Chrystal, J. Platelet rich plasma in musculoskeletal pathology: A necessary rescue or a lost cause? *Pain Physician* **2017**, *20*, E345–E356. [PubMed]

167. Tonogai, I.; Hayashi, F.; Iwame, T.; Takasago, T.; Matsuura, T.; Sairyo, K. Platelet-rich plasma does not reduce skeletal muscle fibrosis after distraction osteogenesis. *J. Exp. Orthop.* **2018**, *5*, 26. [CrossRef]

168. Manduca, M.L.; Straub, S.J. Effectiveness of PRP Injection in Reducing Recovery Time of Acute Hamstring Injury: A Critically Appraised Topic. *J. Sport Rehabil.* **2018**, *27*, 480–484. [CrossRef]

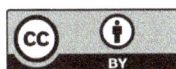

MDPI

St. Alban-Anlage 66

4052 Basel

Switzerland

Tel. +41 61 683 77 34

Fax +41 61 302 89 18

www.mdpi.com

International Journal of Molecular Sciences Editorial Office

E-mail: ijms@mdpi.com

www.mdpi.com/journal/ijms

www.ingramcontent.com/pod-product-compliance
Lightning Source LLC
Chambersburg PA
CBHW051858210326
41597CB00033B/5939